ABC of
Rheumatology

Fourth edition

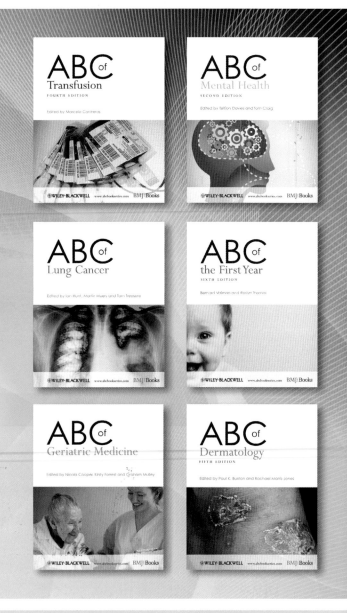

ABC of
Rheumatology

Fourth edition

EDITED BY

Ade Adebajo

Associate Director of Teaching
University of Sheffield Medical School
Honorary Senior Lecturer and Consultant Rheumatologist/
Director of Undergraduate Medical Education
Academic Rheumatology Group
Faculty of Medicine, University of Sheffield and Barnsley Hospital
South Yorkshire, UK

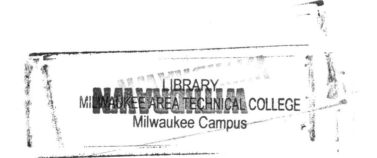

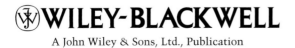

WILEY-BLACKWELL
A John Wiley & Sons, Ltd., Publication

BMJ|Books

BMJ Books is an imprint of BMJ Publishing Group Limited, used under licence by Blackwell Publishing which was acquired by John Wiley & Sons in February 2007. Blackwell's publishing programme has been merged with Wiley's global Scientific, Technical and Medical business to form Wiley-Blackwell.

Registered office: John Wiley & Sons Ltd, The Atrium, Southern Gate, Chichester, West Sussex, PO19 8SQ, UK

Editorial offices: 9600 Garsington Road, Oxford, OX4 2DQ, UK
The Atrium, Southern Gate, Chichester, West Sussex, PO19 8SQ, UK
111 River Street, Hoboken, NJ 07030-5774, USA

For details of our global editorial offices, for customer services and for information about how to apply for permission to reuse the copyright material in this book please see our website at www.wiley.com/wiley-blackwell

Library of Congress Cataloging-in-Publication Data

ABC of rheumatology. – 4th ed. / [edited by] Adewale Adebajo.
    p. ; cm.
  Includes bibliographical references and index.
  ISBN 978-1-4051-7068-0
1. Rheumatology.   2. Joints–Diseases.   I. Adebajo, Adewale.
  [DNLM: 1. Rheumatic Diseases. WE 544 A134 2008]
  RC927.A23 2008
  616.7′23–dc22
                                  2008009429

A catalogue record for this book is available from the British Library.

Set in 9.25 on 12 pt Minion by SNP Best-set Typesetter Ltd., Hong Kong
Printed and bound in Malaysia by KHL Printing Co Sdn Bhd

1   2010

Contents

Contributors

Ade Adebajo
Associate Director of Teaching
University of Sheffield Medical School
Honorary Senior Lecturer and Consultant Rheumatologist/
Director of Undergraduate Medical Education
Academic Rheumatology Group
Faculty of Medicine, University of Sheffield and Barnsley Hospital
South Yorkshire, UK

Mohammed Akil
Consultant Rheumatologist
Royal Hallamshire Hospital
Sheffield, UK

Cynthia Aranow
Associate Investigator
Feinstein Institute for Medical Research
Manhassett, NY, USA

Howard A Bird
Professor
Chapel Allerton Hospital
Leeds, UK

Carol M Black
Professor and Centre Director
Centre for Rheumatology
Royal Free Hospital
London, UK

Rachelle Buchbinder
Professor/Consultant Rheumatologist
Monash Department of Clinical Epidemiology
Cabrini Hospital School of Public Health and Preventative Medicine
Monash University
Melbourne, Australia

Anita Campbell
General Practitioner
Richmond Medical Centre
Sheffield, UK

Edwin S L Chan
Assistant Professor of Medicine
Department of Medicine
New York University School of Medicine
New York, NY, USA

Bruce N Cronstein
Paul R Esserman Professor of Medicine
Director, Clinical and Translational Science Institute
New York University School of Medicine
New York, NY, USA

Janet Cushnaghan
Research Fellow MRC ERC
Southampton General Hospital
Southampton, UK

Paul Davis
Professor of Medicine
University of Alberta
Edmonton, AB, Canada

Chris Deighton
Consultant Rheumatologist
Derbyshire Royal Infirmary
Derby, UK

Christopher P Denton
Professor of Experimental Rheumatology
Centre for Rheumatology
Royal Free Hospital
London, UK

D John Dickson
Community Specialist in Primary Care Rheumatology
Redcar & Cleveland Primary Care Trust
Redcar, UK

Rajiv K Dixit
Associate Clinical Professor of Medicine
University of California
San Francisco, CA, USA
Director
Northern California Arthritis Center
Walnut Creek, CA, USA

Michael Doherty
Professor of Rheumatology
University of Nottingham
Department of Academic Rheumatology
Nottingham City Hospital
Nottingham, UK

Adrian Dunbar
General Practitioner with Special Interest in Musculoskeletal
Medicine and Chronic Pain Management
Skipton, UK

Richard Eastell
Professor
Division of Clinical Sciences
Northern General Hospital
Sheffield, UK

Helen Foster
Professor of Paediatric Rheumatology
Newcastle University
Newcastle upon Tyne, UK

Caroline Gordon
Professor of Rheumatology
Division of Immunity and Infection
The Medical School
University of Birmingham
Birmingham, UK

Kamran Hameed
Associate Professor
Consultant Rheumatologist
Agakhan University Hospital
Karachi, Pakistan

Andrew J Hamer
Consultant Orthopaedic Surgeon
Northern General Hospital
Sheffield, UK

Elaine M Hay
Professor and Honorary Consultant in Community Rheumatology
Staffordshire Rheumatology Centre
The Haywood
Stoke-on-Trent, UK

Philip S Helliwell
Senior Lecturer in Rheumatology
Academic Unit of Musculoskeletal Disease
University of Leeds
Leeds, UK

Jackie Hill
Arthritis Research Campaign Senior Lecturer in Rheumatology Nursing
& Co-Director Academic and Clinical Unit for Musculoskeletal Nursing
(ACUMeN) University of Leeds
Chapel Allerton Hospital
Leeds, UK

Robert Inman
Toronto Hospital Western Division
Toronto, ON, Canada

David A Isenberg
Professor of Rheumatology
University College Hospital
London, UK

Jeffrey N Katz
Case Western Reserve University
Cleveland, OH, USA

Andrew Keat
Arthritis Centre
Northwick Park Hospital
Harrow, UK

Virginia Byers Kraus
Associate Professor Medicine
Duke University Medical Center
Durham, NC, USA

Margaret J Larché
McMaster University
Hamilton, ON, Canada

Peter J Maddison
Consultant Rheumatologist
North West Wales NHS Trust
Professor of Musculoskeletal Medicine
School of Medical Sciences
Bangor University
Bangor, UK

Eric L Matteson
Mayo Clinic
Rochester, MN, USA

Eugene McCloskey
Reader in Adult Bone Disease
Academic Unit of Bone Metabolism and WHO Collaborating Centre for Metabolic Bone Diseases
University of Sheffield
Sheffield, UK

Caroline Mitchell
Senior Clinical Lecturer General Practitioner
Academic Unit of Primary Medical Care
University of Sheffield
Sheffield, UK

Jacqueline Oliver
Research Associate
Arthritis Research Campaign
Chesterfield, UK

Nicola Peel
Northern General Hospital
Sheffield, UK

Rosalind Ramsey-Goldman
Solovy Arthritis Research Society Research Professor of Medicine
Northwestern University Feinberg School of Medicine
Chicago, IL, USA

Sarah Ryan
Nurse Consultant in Rheumatology
Haywood Hospital
Stoke-on-Trent Community Health Service
Stoke-on-Trent, UK

David G I Scott
Consultant Rheumatologist
Norfolk and Norwich University Hospital NHS Trust
Honorary Professor
University of East Anglia
Norwich, UK

Michael Shipley
University College London Hospitals
The Middlesex Hospital
London, UK

Alan Silman
Medical Director
Arthritis Research Campaign
Chesterfield, UK

Taunton R Southwood
Professor of Paediatric Rheumatology
University of Birmingham, Birmingham
Birmingham Children's Hospital
NHS Foundation Trust
Birmingham, UK

Cathy Speed
Honorary Consultant
Rheumatology and Sports Medicine
Cambridge University Hospital
Cambridge, UK

Ilona S Szer
Director, Pediatric Rheumatology
Rady Children's Hospital and Health Center
San Diego, CA, USA

Mohammed Tikly
Professor of Rheumatology
Chris Hani Baragwanath Hospital
University of the Witwatersrand
Johannesburg, South Africa

Lori Tucker
Division of Pediatric Rheumatology
British Columbia's Children's Hospital
Vancouver, BC, Canada

Martin Underwood
Professor of Primary Care Research
Warwick Medical School
University of Warwick
Coventry, UK

Louise Warburton
Shawbirch Medical Practice
Shawbirch
Telford, UK

Richard A Watts
Consultant Rheumatologist
Clinical Senior Lecturer University of East Anglia, Norwich
Ipswich Hospital NHS Trust
Ipswich, UK

Mark Wilkinson
Clinical Senior Lecturer, Orthopaedics
Academic Unit of Bone Metabolism
University of Sheffield
Northern General Hospital
Sheffield, UK

Anthony G Wilson
Professor of Rheumatology
University of Sheffield
Sheffield, UK

Elspeth Wise
General Practitioner
Belmont Surgery
Durham, UK

James Woodburn
Professor of Rehabilitation
Glasgow Caledonian University
Glasgow, UK

Preface

The fourth edition of the ABC of Rheumatology marks a change in Editor. I would like to thank my predecessor Mike Snaith for his sterling work in producing such excellent previous editions of this book which has led to its worldwide recognition and appeal. The fact that the book is now in its fourth edition is testimony to the great foundation that he laid.

I have kept the tradition as well as enriched the strengths of previous editions to ensure that this book continues to provide a good and up to date foundational knowledge of Rheumatology and Musculoskeletal Medicine for a wide spectrum of those interested in this field. This ranges from family doctors, medical students, nurse specialists, allied health professionals to doctors in training and others besides.

I would like to thank all those who have contributed to this current edition including my colleagues, not only in Sheffield but also across the United Kingdom and indeed other parts of the world. I am particularly pleased to have so many authors from North America where this book is increasingly being used.

Finally, I wish to thank the publishers for their dedication and professionalism.

Ade Adebajo

List of Abbreviations

ACE	angiotensin-converting enzyme		ICP	integrated-care pathway
AHPS	allied health professionals		IL-1	interleukin-1 etc.
ANA	antinuclear antibody		IPJ	interphalangeal joint
ANCA	anti-neutrophil cytoplasmic antibodies		JDM	juvenile dermatomyositis
APLA	antiphospholipid antibody		JIA	juvenile idiopathic arthritis
APLS	antiphospholipid antibody syndrome		JCA	juvenile chronic arthritis
arc	The Arthritis Research Campaign		JRA	juvenile rheumatoid arthritis
ARMA	Arthritis and Muskuloskeletal Alliance		KD	Kawasaki disease
AS	ankylosing spondylitis		LBP	low back pain
BMD	bone mineral density		MCPJ	metacarpophalangeal joint
BMI	body mass index		MCTD	mixed connective tissue disease
BSR	British Society for Rheumatology		MDT	multidisciplinary team
CATS	clinical assessment and treatment services		MMP-3	matrix metalloproteinase-3
CHB	congenital heart block		MPO	myloperoxidase
CMCJ	carpometacarpal joint		MRI	magnetic resonance imaging
CRP	C-reactive protein		NICE	National Institute for Health and Clinical Excellence
CTGF	connective tissue growth factor		NOGG	National Osteoporosis Guideline Group
CWP	chronic widespread pain		NSAID	non-steroidal anti-inflammatory drug
DIPJ	distal interphalangeal joint		OA	osteoarthritis
DMARDs	disease-modifying antirheumatic drugs		PAH	pulmonary arterial hypertension
DMS	dermatomyositis		PIPJ	proximal interphalangeal joint
DRUJ	distal radio-ulnar joint		PMR	polymyalgia rheumatica
DXA	dual X-ray absorptiometry		PsA	psoriatic arthritis
ELISA	enzyme-linked immunosorbent assay		RA	rheumatoid arthritis
ERA	enthesitis-related arthritis		ReA	reactive arthritis
ESP	extended-scope physiotherapist		RVSP	right ventricular systolic pressure
ESR	erythrocyte sedimentation rate		SAA	serum amyloid A
ESWT	extracorporeal shock wave therapy		SCLE	subacute cutaneous lupus erythematosus
GCA	giant cell arteritis		SLE	systemic lupus erythematosus
GI	gastrointestinal		SpA	spondyloarthritides
GP	general practitioner		SRC	scleroderma renal crisis
GPsSI	GP with special interest		SSc	systemic sclerosis
GU	genito-urinary		ST	spinal stenosis
HRCT	high-resolution computed tomography		TGF	transforming growth factor
HSP	Henoch–Schönlein purpura		TNF	tumour necrosis factor
IBD	inflammatory bowel disease			

CHAPTER 1

Community Rheumatology: Delivering Care Across Boundaries

Elaine M Hay[1], Jackie Hill[2] and Ade Adebajo[3]

[1]Staffordshire Rheumatology Centre, Stoke-on-Trent, UK
[2]University of Leeds, Leeds, UK
[3]University of Sheffield, Sheffield, UK

OVERVIEW

- The importance of a multidisciplinary care pathway in the management of musculoskeletal patients is now well recognized globally.

- The need to provide a whole-community approach to the management of these patients is also being increasingly recognized globally.

- The shared-care monitoring of rheumatology patients on disease-modifying drugs between primary and secondary care is an example of a successful model using this approach.

- A community-wide approach encompassing the involvement and education of both patient and primary care physician will lead to earlier diagnosis, speedier and more appropriate secondary care referrals, quicker treatment and ultimately improved clinical outcomes.

- A community-wide approach will ensure that psychosocial factors are not overlooked and that "red flags" for regional pain syndromes are not missed.

- This approach will also ensure that evidence-based primary care treatments for musculoskeletal problems are developed and implemented.

The ever-increasing demand upon the acute hospitals to deliver emergency medicine, together with technological (but time-consuming and expensive) advances means that in the UK and elsewhere follow-up of many chronic conditions has been squeezed out of the acute setting and, by default, delegated to primary care. Unfortunately this shift in activity has not always been mirrored by an appropriate shift in resources and skills. This chapter discusses new ways of working to try to ensure that patients with musculoskeletal conditions receive timely, appropriate treatments within the limitations imposed by restricted resources.

Shared care—how to make it work

With hospital services running at full (or over) capacity, one way

ABC of Rheumatology, 4th edn. Edited by Ade Adebajo.
©2010 Blackwell Publishing Ltd. 9781405170680.

forwards is to develop models of shared care appropriate to local need, responsive to local demands and in the patients' best interests. Simply transferring the workload from rheumatologists to general practitioners (GPs) will not work—primary care is also bursting at the seams. One way of transferring rheumatological expertise to the community, without increasing the burden on the primary care team, is to develop the roles of health professionals such as nurses, physiotherapists and occupational therapists. Such practitioners, working in an extended role, operate at a high level of clinical practice and cross traditional professional boundaries. Their expertise includes assessment (of the disease and psychosocial factors), follow-up and management of patients with musculoskeletal conditions and inflammatory arthritis. Their roles and responsibilities have recently been defined (Carr, 2001).

What is the role of the specialist nurse?

Specialist nurses are highly skilled and provide holistic care for patients and their significant others by addressing their physical, psychological and social needs. They can play a pivotal role in the management of people with musculoskeletal conditions, acting as effective communicators between the patient, their GP and hospital consultant. Like GPs, they tend to stay in post for many years and become a "constant presence" in the patient's illness journey, thus ensuring the continuity of care that those with a chronic disease value so highly. The role of the specialist nurse is essentially to provide care management, education and support for patients and their families, and to act as an educator and resource for other health professionals. The role includes those activities shown in Box 1.1. Some nurse specialists also undertake advanced practices such as intra-articular injections (Meadows and Sheehan, 2005). This can be particularly useful to GPs, who may be inexperienced in this procedure. After specialist training these nurses can also prescribe drug therapy (Carr, 2001). Of all these activities, patient education remains one of the priorities of the specialist nurse (Department of Health, 2006).

Why educate patients?

Patient education enables people with complex chronic diseases to care for themselves, bringing benefits for everyone. Supporting patients to self care has been shown to reduce their GP visits by 40–69% (Schillinger *et al.*, 2003). Patient education is not a treatment in itself but a treatment enhancer, magnifying the effects of standard treatments by persuading patients to adhere to them more closely, or to adopt actions that are believed to be beneficial. To do this, patients must be active collaborators in their care and believe in their ability to perform a specific task or achieve a certain objective. This is known as "self-efficacy". For changes to occur patients must acquire knowledge and skills, and so patient education involves the multidisciplinary team and the patient and their partner/carers in both primary and secondary care. Every consultation is an opportunity to educate and provide information. In order to care for themselves, patients will need to know about the topics shown in Box 1.2.

Patients should be given both verbal and written explanations. The Arthritis Research Campaign (arc), Arthritis Care, and the National Rheumatoid Arthritis Society are good reliable sources of the latter.

Skill enhancement can be gained from attendance at an Expert Patients Programme, and giving the patient the address of local and national community support networks offers great benefits.

It is important to remember that simply because information has been provided does not mean that it has been understood or acted upon. One quick and easy method to ensure assimilation is the "teach me back" method (Schillinger *et al.*, 2003), which involves the patient being asked to "teach me" or "show me" as if the professional does not understand the problem. This quickly identifies any misunderstandings and allows purposeful correction.

Who should be referred to secondary care?

Waiting times for new rheumatology appointments vary widely and depend on local resources but also, to some extent, on how clinicians triage referrals from GPs. To make the system work effectively, care pathways need to be developed in which the patient is a partner, and which take psychosocial as well as biomechanical factors into consideration. The outcome, in terms of whether the patient is given an appropriate priority with an appropriate heath-care professional, depends largely upon the information contained within the referral letter. Standardized referral forms may help but have the disadvantages that they are time-consuming to complete and rather impersonal. Helpful information to include in a referral letter is shown in Box 1.3.

It has been estimated that 15–30% of all GP consultations are for musculoskeletal conditions. Most of these are for osteoarthritis in the over 50s age group and back pain in the under 50s. One challenge for the GP is how to spot the small number of patients with early inflammatory arthritis among this caseload who will benefit from early referral to hospital and prompt treatment with DMARDs. There are no specific clinical, radiological or immunological markers for rheumatoid arthritis (RA). Normal blood test results and X-rays do not exclude RA, but equally a positive rheumatoid factor does not clinch the diagnosis. Most rheumatology departments encourage an "inclusive approach" to referral and encourage GPs to maintain a high index of suspicion and not delay patients with possible inflammatory arthritis. Ideally, patients suspected of having inflammatory problems will be fast-tracked to secondary care. Box 1.4 highlights certain features thought to be indicative of early RA.

Box 1.1 **Role of the specialist nurse**

- Supervise treatment safety—e.g. monitoring disease-modifying antirheumatic drugs (DMARDS)
- Review treatment effectiveness
- Coordinate the multidisciplinary team
- Provide a communication channel between the patient and the team
- Act as the patient's advocate
- Promote continuity of care
- Identify and address psychosocial patients' issues
- Man telephone advice lines
- Facilitate education for patients, carers and health professionals

---

Box 1.3 **Important information to include in a rheumatology referral letter**

- Length of history
- Pattern of joint involvement
- Presence of joint swelling
- Presence of early morning stiffness
- Previous treatments and response
- Level of distress/disability
- Results of investigations
- Other relevant medical or psychosocial factors

Box 1.2 **Knowledge necessary for self care**

- Disease aetiology and progress
- Drugs and how to take them; what the side effects are and what to do if they occur
- How to exercise
- How to protect joints and acquire appropriate devices and home changes
- How to control pain
- Coping strategies

Box 1.4 **Symptoms and signs suggestive of early inflammatory arthritis**

- Symmetrical soft-tissue swelling (synovitis) of wrists and/or metacarpophalangeal joints and/or proximal interphalangeal joints
- Joint stiffness a significant problem—especially in the early mornings for >30 minutes
- Soft-tissue swelling of any joints
- Good response to a trial of non-steroidal anti-inflammatory drugs

Primary care management of musculoskeletal problems

Clearly, the majority of patients presenting to GPs will not have inflammatory arthritis. Indeed, often a precise pathological diagnosis based on symptoms and signs and results of investigations will not be possible, and may not be the most appropriate approach to management. This "medical model" of care often fails to address other important influences on pain perception, such as emotional and behavioural factors, and may encourage chronicity by using terms such as "arthritis", "wear and tear" or "degeneration", which emphasise the unchanging nature of the condition. Doctors are trained to diagnose "disease", whereas the patient's concern is what to do about their musculoskeletal pain, not just what to call it.

An alternative approach, which may be more useful in primary care, limits the diagnostic process to identifying potentially serious pathology—the so-called "red flag" disorders—and other specific diseases or disorders. This system was initially developed for back pain, and has been effective in changing the primary care management of this condition. It is equally applicable to other widespread or regional pain disorders, however (Box 1.5) (reviewed in Carr, 2001). Patients with "red flags" and certain other patients with specific diagnoses, including inflammatory arthropathies and connective-tissue disorders, should be considered for referral to secondary care for further investigation and management.

Having excluded and dealt with the small proportion of patients with potential serious pathology and specific diagnoses, the next step is to decide how best to manage the remainder. Two areas need to be addressed: how to deal with the presenting pain and distress (discussed below), and how to prevent future disability. Guidelines for the management of low back pain highlight the importance of identifying factors that predict chronicity. It is important to give positive messages about likely recovery and lack of long-term

harm, taking particular account of psychosocial barriers to recovery ("yellow flags"). These principles have been described elsewhere (Department of Health, 2007) and are summarized in Box 1.6.

Evidence-based primary care treatments for musculoskeletal problems

The shift in emphasis towards self-management of musculoskeletal problems means that the primary health-care team is of central importance. There is a growing evidence base supporting the effectiveness of a number of simple primary care interventions for musculoskeletal problems (reviewed in Schillinger et al., 2003). Direct access physiotherapy reduces wait times and costs for treatment and is one way to facilitate the use of exercise and self-management regimes. These have been demonstrated to be beneficial for patients with a variety of regional and widespread musculoskeletal conditions, including osteoarthritis, back pain, fibromyalgia and shoulder problems. Prescribed exercise need not be the province of the physiotherapist alone. Often, wait times to see a physiotherapist are excessively long, and many self-limiting musculoskeletal conditions can be managed with sensible exercise regimes undertaken outside the hospital setting. This has the advantage of promoting self-help and "demedicalizing" common musculoskeletal problems. arc publishes a wide range of patient information leaflets and booklets, which are useful adjuncts to advice and education provided by health-care professionals (Box 1.7).

Local steroid injections are effective for reducing pain from soft-tissue problems such as tennis elbow and shoulder problems in the short term but do not improve long-term outcome. They should be reserved for patients in whom pain is restricting rehabilitation

---

Box 1.5 **"Red flags" for regional pain syndromes**

History of significant trauma
- Fracture
- Major soft-tissue injury

Localized joint swelling and/or redness
- Septic arthritis
- Inflammatory arthritis
- Haemarthrosis

Unremitting night pain
- Malignancy
- Inflammation/infection

Bone tenderness
- Fracture
- Malignancy
- Infection

Systemic disturbance

Significant co-morbidity

Box 1.6 **Psychosocial factors that predict chronicity**

- Belief that pain is due to progressive pathology
- Belief that pain represents harm or injury
- Belief that avoiding activity will speed up recovery
- Tendency to social isolation
- Tendency to anxiety/depression
- Expectation that passive treatments rather than self-help programmes will be of benefit

---

Box 1.7 **arc publications**

Arthritis Research Campaign (arc) leaflets, booklets and other publications are available from:

Dept RD
arc Trading Ltd
Brunel Drive
Northern Road Industrial Estate
Newark
Notts. NG24 2DE
www.arc.org.uk

with the measures discussed above. Although the risks from local steroid injections are minimal, certain precautions need to be adhered to (Box 1.8).

Non-steroidal anti-inflammatory drugs may be beneficial for the short-term treatment of osteoarthritis but have a worrying side-effect profile in the patient group most likely to be prescribed them (elderly females). Simple analgesics are the preferred option where possible.

Global issues

The issues discussed in this chapter have global application, as the burden of illness from musculoskeletal conditions is high in both the developed world and developing countries alike, particularly with an ever-increasing elderly population worldwide. In developing countries, it is essential to involve local community leaders and community health workers in the management of patients with these conditions. Awareness of the importance of musculoskeletal conditions, in terms of morbidity but also mortality, needs to be raised among all health-care workers, governments and members of the public. With increasing travel and migration, knowledge of the global spectrum of musculoskeletal conditions is important. There also needs to be an increasing emphasis on prevention through encouraging healthy lifestyles and joint protection and by tackling modifiable risk factors such as falls prevention. Whether in primary or secondary care, or whether in a developing or developed country, what is key is not where musculoskeletal care takes place, but that it is appropriately given.

Conclusion

Over the last 10 years there has been a shift in thinking about how best to care for patients with rheumatological disorders (Box 1.9). For those with inflammatory arthritis the emphasis is on prompt referral to secondary care so that treatment with potentially disease-modifying agents can be instituted early, before irreversible joint damage has occurred. For patients with non-inflammatory conditions, such as osteoarthritis and regional or widespread musculoskeletal pain, optimal management depends on developing an efficient triage system that can identify those with "red flags" who will benefit from referral to secondary care for further investigation and management. The first-line management for the remainder should be by health-care professionals in primary care, using the strategies outlined above.

References

Carr A. *Defining the Extended Clinical Role for Allied Health Professionals in Rheumatology. arc Conference Proceedings No. 12.* Arthritis Research Campaign, Chesterfield, 2001.

Department of Health. Self care for people with long term conditions. Department of Health Long Term Conditions Team, 2006; available online at http://www.dh.gov.uk/en/Healthcare/Longtermconditions/DH_087281

Linton SJ. A review of psychological factors in back and neck pain. *Spine* 2000; **25**: 1148–1156.

Meadows A, Sheehan NJ. Prescribing and injecting: the expanding role of the rheumatology nurse. *Musculoskeletal Care* 2005; **3**: 176–178.

O'Dell JR. Combinations of conventional disease-modifying antirheumatic drugs. *Rheumatic Disease Clinics of North America* 2001; **27**: 415–426.

Schillinger D, Piette J, Grumbach K *et al.* Closing the loop: physician communication with diabetic patients who have low health literacy. *Archives of Internal Medicine* 2003; **163**: 83–90.

Smidt N, Assendelft WJJ, Windt van der DAWM *et al.* Corticosteroid injections for lateral epicondylitis: a systematic review. *Pain* 2002; **96**: 23–40.

Further reading

Dziedzic K, Jordan J, Sim J *et al.* Treatment options for regional musculoskeletal pain: what is the evidence? In: Breivik H & Shipley M, eds. *Pain: Best Practice and Research Compendium.* Elsevier, Toronto, 2007: 183–197.

Doherty M, Dougados M, eds. Osteoarthritis: current treatment strategies. *Best Practice and Research. Clinical Rheumatology* 2001; **15**: 517–656.

Main CJ, Williams A. ABC of psychological medicine: musculoskeletal pain. *BMJ* 2002; **325**: 534–537.

White C, Cooper RG. *In Practice: Prescribing and Monitoring of Disease-Modifying Anti-Rheumatic Drugs (DMARDs) for Inflammatory Arthritis.* Arthritis Research Campaign, Chesterfield, 2005.

CHAPTER 2

Pain in the Wrist and Hand

Michael Shipley[1] and Elspeth Wise[2]

[1]University College London Hospitals, London, UK
[2]Belmont Surgery, Durham, UK

OVERVIEW

- Nodal osteoarthritis affecting the distal interphalangeal joints is very common and generally painful only for a few months.
- If a patient presents with swollen and painful joints in the hand, consider inflammatory arthritis as a diagnosis.
- The hand and wrist are common sites for overuse and injury. Remember to ask about precipitating factors, especially work/occupation and hobbies.
- Carpal tunnel syndrome is a common peripheral nerve entrapment syndrome and has a classical presentation.
- Raynaud's syndrome generally requires symptomatic treatment only, but consider secondary causes if seen in older people.

Hand or wrist pain and resultant impaired function are often the cause of great anxiety for patients. Hands, as prehensile organs, give us a great deal of information about the world in which we live. They are capable of performing incredibly fine and delicate movements and are essential for work, sport, hobbies and social interaction.

Functional anatomy

The wrist is a complex structure comprising three groups of joints: the radiocarpal joints, which allow flexion, extension, abduction, adduction and circumduction; the inferior radio-ulnar joint, which allows pronation and supination; and the intercarpal joints (Figure 2.1).

The eight carpal bones, in two rows of four, form a bony gutter and are the base of the carpal tunnel. The flexor retinaculum, a strong fascial band, forms the palmar side of the tunnel. Running through the carpal tunnel are the deep and superficial flexor tendons, the tendons of flexor pollicis longus, flexor carpi radialis and the median nerve. The ulnar nerve lies superficial to the flexor retinaculum but deep to the transverse carpal ligament in Guyon's canal. The extensor tendons are held in position on the extensor surface of the wrist by the extensor retinaculum. Fibrous septa

divide the extensor compartment into six. All of the flexor tendons are encased in a common synovial tendon, which extends from a position just proximal to the wrist to the middle of the palm. Flexor pollicis longus and flexor carpi ulnaris have their own individual sheaths, as do each of the six extensor compartments.

The hand bones are the metacarpals, proximal phalanges, middle phalanges, distal phalanges and sesamoid bones. A sesamoid bone lies at the base of the thumb in the tendons of flexor pollicis brevis. The first metacarpal bone of the thumb is the shortest and most mobile of the metacarpals and lies in a different plane to the others. This is important to allow opposition, i.e. pincer action to grasp objects. The carpometacarpal and trapezoscaphoid joints are prone to osteoarthritis.

Individual tendon sheaths for the deep and superficial flexor tendons start at the level of the distal transverse crease of the palm and end at the bases of the distal phalanxes. The sheath for flexor pollicis longus continues from the carpal tunnel to the distal phalanx. During flexion, five fibrous bands, or pulleys, hold the flexor sheaths in position.

The second to fifth metacarpophalangeal joints flex to about 90°. Active extension is rarely more than 30°. Passive extension varies from 60° to more than 100° in people with hypermobility. The proximal and distal interphalangeal joints are hinge joints. The lumbrical and interossei muscles produce complex movements that involve extension of the interphalangeal joints and flexion at the metacarpophalangeal joints and are essential to fine hand functions, such as writing.

There are many possible causes of pain in the wrist and hand (Table 2.1).

Tendon problems

Flexor tenosynovitis

Unaccustomed or repetitive use of the finger and inflammatory arthritis cause flexor tenosynovitis (Figure 2.2), inflammation of the synovial sheath of the finger flexor tendons, which leads to volar swelling and tenderness just proximal and distal to the wrist. The flexor tendon sheaths in the palm or finger may also be affected. The hand feels stiff, painful and swollen, particularly in the morning. Rest helps. Injection is sometimes needed. Local anaesthetic helps introduce the needle alongside the tendon in the palm just proximal to the metacarpophalangeal joint.

ABC of Rheumatology, 4th edn. Edited by Ade Adebajo.
©2010 Blackwell Publishing Ltd. 9781405170680.

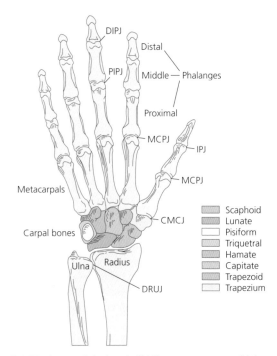

Figure 2.1 The bones of the hand. CMCJ = carpometacarpal joint; DIPJ = distal interphalangeal joint; DRUJ = distal radio-ulnar joint; IPJ = interphalangeal joint; MCPJ = metacarpophalangeal joint; PIPJ = proximal interphalangeal joint

Table 2.1 Causes of pain in the wrist and hand

At all ages	In older patients
• Trauma	• Nodal osteoarthritis
	○ Distal interphalangeal joints (Heberden's nodes)
	○ First carpometacarpal joints
	○ Proximal interphalangeal joints (Bouchard's nodes)
• Flexor tenosynovitis	• Scaphoid fracture
○ Carpal tunnel syndrome	
• Flexor tendonosis	• Pseudogout
○ Trigger finger or thumb	
• De Quervain's tenosynovitis	• Gout
	○ Acute
	○ Chronic tophaceous
• Extensor tenosynovitis	• Dupuytren's contracture
• Ganglion	• Diabetic stiff hand
• Mallet finger	• Septic arthritis
• Cubital tunnel syndrome	
• Inflammatory arthritis	
• Raynaud's syndrome	
• Writer's cramp	
• Chronic upper limb pain	
• Reflex sympathetic dystrophy	
• Scaphoid fracture	
• Osteonecrosis	

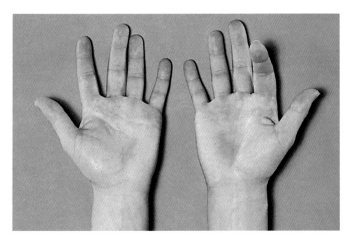

Figure 2.2 Flexor tenosynovitis

Carpal tunnel syndrome

Carpal tunnel syndrome is a peripheral nerve entrapment syndrome of the median nerve, often caused by flexor tenosynovitis. It can occur in the third trimester of pregnancy. Repetitive use of the hand increases the risk of developing carpal tunnel syndrome but its status as a work injury is controversial (Yagev *et al.*, 2001). A ganglion, or very rarely amyloidosis or myxoedema, causes carpal tunnel syndrome. Pain, tingling and numbness in a median nerve distribution (thumb, index finger, middle and radial side of ring finger) are typically present on waking or can wake the patient. The fingers feel swollen and intense aching is felt in the forearm. The symptoms may appear when the patient holds a newspaper or the steering wheel of a car. Permanent numbness and wasting of the thenar eminence (flexor pollicis and opponens pollicis) cause clumsiness. The patient's history often indicates the diagnosis (Pal *et al.*, 2001), or using a scored questionnaire may help (Kamath and Stothard, 2004).

Tests and investigations—Tinel's sign (tapping the median nerve in the carpal tunnel) or Phalen's test (holding the wrist in forced dorsiflexion) may provoke symptoms. Weakness of abduction of the thumb distal phalanx with the thumb adducted towards the fifth digit is typical. The carpal tunnel and median nerve are seen on ultrasonic images, although US and MRI are not usually needed.

Management and injection technique—A splint worn on the wrist at night relieves or reduces the symptoms of carpal tunnel syndrome. This is diagnostic and may be curative. A corticosteroid injection into the carpal tunnel (Figure 2.3) may also be considered, as this often helps rapidly, although recurrence is common. The needle is inserted at the distal wrist skin crease, just to the ulnar side of the palmaris longus tendon, or about 0.5 cm to the ulnar side of flexor carpi radialis at an angle of 45° towards the middle finger. The local anaesthetic is injected superficially. If a small test injection of corticosteroid causes finger pain, the needle is in the nerve and needs to be repositioned. An injection of a locally acting

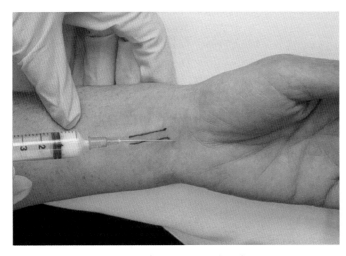

Figure 2.3 Injection technique for carpal tunnel syndrome

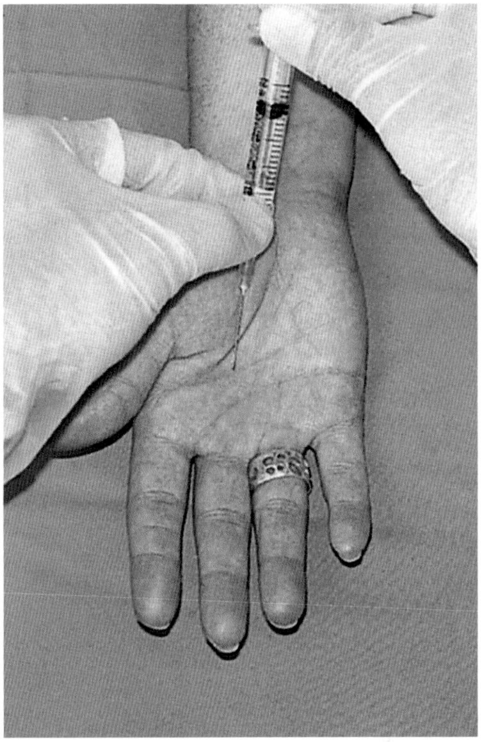

steroid preparation, e.g. hydrocortisone acetate, often precipitates the symptoms, but it is effective and non-toxic (O'Gradaigh and Merry, 2000; Wong *et al.*, 2001).

Recurrent daytime symptoms, unrelieved by splints, warrant nerve-conduction studies. Slowing of median nerve conduction at the wrist suggests demyelination due to local compression. The action potential is reduced or absent due to nerve-fibre loss if the lesion is severe or prolonged. Needle electromyography is unpleasant but detects denervation.

Decompression surgery should be considered for: recurrent symptoms not eased by splints or injection; significant nerve damage; muscle wasting; and/or permanent numbness (Trumble *et al.*, 2001). Pins and needles often worsen briefly post-operatively while the nerve recovers. Recovery of sensation or strength, or both, may be limited or non-existent if the lesion is severe and longstanding.

Finger flexor tendonosis and trigger finger

Gripping and hard manual work cause palpable thickening and nodularity of the finger flexor tendon; tendon sheath synovitis may also be present. The affected fingers are stiff in the morning, when the patient also has pain in the palm and along the dorsum of the finger(s). The pain is reproduced by passive extension of the finger. This is common in rheumatoid arthritis and in dactylitis caused by seronegative arthritis. Nodular flexor tenosynovitis is more common and less responsive to treatment in patients with diabetes than in other patients (Stahl *et al.*, 1997).

Trigger finger is caused by a nodule catching at the pulley that overlies the metacarpophalangeal joint in the palm. The patient wakens with the finger flexed and has to force it straight with a painful or painless click. Triggering also occurs after gripping. The nodule and the "catch" in movement are felt in the palm.

Management and injection technique—A low-pressure injection of local anaesthetic followed by a locally acting steroid preparation alongside the tendon nodule in the palm helps (Rankin and

Figure 2.4 Injection technique for flexor tenosynovitis and trigger finger

Rankin, 1998) (Figure 2.4). If symptoms are persistent or recurrent, surgical release is needed.

Overuse and local injury (after opening a tight jar) are the most common causes of thumb flexor tenosynovitis and trigger thumb. Either the interphalangeal joint cannot be flexed or it sticks in flexion and snaps straight. The sesamoid bone in the flexor pollicis brevis tendon is tender on the volar surface of the thumb's metacarpophalangeal joint. Corticosteroid injection next to the sesamoid bone at the site of maximal tenderness helps.

De Quervain's tenosynovitis

De Quervain's stenosing tenosynovitis affects the tendon sheath of abductor pollicis longus and extensor pollicis brevis at the radial styloid. It causes pain at or just proximal or distal to the styloid, in contrast with first carpometacarpal osteoarthritis, which causes pain at the base of the thumb. Tenderness, swelling and Finkelstein's test—pushing the thumb into the palm while holding the wrist in ulnar deviation—increases the pain. Crepitus or a tendon nodule may cause triggering.

Management and injection technique—Rest is essential, with avoidance of thumb extension and pinching, but immobilization splints are inconvenient. Therapeutic ultrasound or local anti-inflammatory gels help; injection of local anaesthetic, then a locally acting steroid preparation alongside the tendon under low pressure at the point of maximum tenderness rapidly relieves the pain (Figure 2.5). A second injection may be needed. Surgery is rarely necessary, unless stenosis or nodule formation develops.

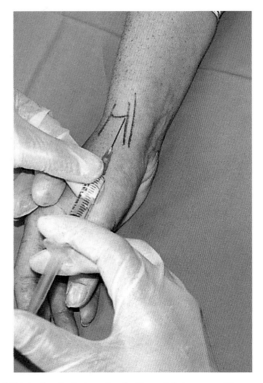

Figure 2.5 Injection technique for de Quervain's tenosynovitis

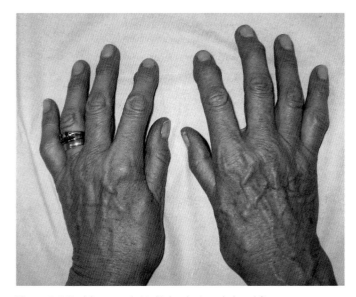

Figure 2.6 Nodal osteoarthritis (Heberden's nodes) and first carpometacarpal osteoarthritis

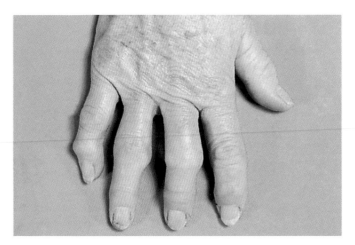

Figure 2.7 Nodal osteoarthritis with Bouchard's nodes

Extensor tenosynovitis

Inflammation of the common extensor (fourth) compartment causes well-defined swelling that extends from the back of the hand to just proximal to the wrist. The extensor retinaculum causes a typical "hourglass" shape proximal and distal to the wrist. This contrasts with wrist synovitis, which causes diffuse swelling distal to the radius and ulna. Repetitive wrist and finger movements, especially with the wrist in dorsiflexion, are the cause, and this is one of the several causes of forearm and wrist pain seen in keyboard workers. It is also common in rheumatoid arthritis. Rest helps extensor tenosynovitis, but often a corticosteroid injection into the tendon sheath is needed. Workplace reviews and wrist supports for those who use a keyboard and mouse help prevent recurrences.

Mallet finger

This is a flexion deformity affecting the distal interphalangeal joint of the finger and is due to either distal extensor tendon rupture or avulsion with a bony fragment after traumatic forced flexion of the extended fingertip. The resultant weakness is often painless and presents with an inability to actively extend the fingertip. Treatment is usually by splinting the distal interphalangeal joint in extension or, rarely, surgery.

Osteoarthritis

Nodal osteoarthritis

Nodal osteoarthritis most commonly involves the distal interphalangeal joints and is familial. The joint swells and becomes inflamed and painful, but the pain subsides over a few weeks or

months and leaves bony swellings (Heberden's nodes). Most patients manage with local anti-inflammatory gels or no treatment once they know the prognosis is good. The appearance sometimes causes distress. Occasionally, the joint becomes unstable and limits pinch gripping. Surgical fusion of the index distal interphalangeal joints or thumb interphalangeal joint in slight flexion improves grip, although this is rarely necessary. Involvement of the proximal interphalangeal joints (Bouchard's nodes) is less common and may be mistaken for early rheumatoid arthritis (Figure 2.6). Stiffness of the proximal joints impairs hand function significantly.

First carpometacarpal osteoarthritis

Pain at the base of the thumb in the early phase of first carpometacarpal osteoarthritis (Figure 2.7) is disabling, but with time the joint stiffens and adducts, and pain and disability decrease. The hand becomes "squared". Management is usually conservative, but

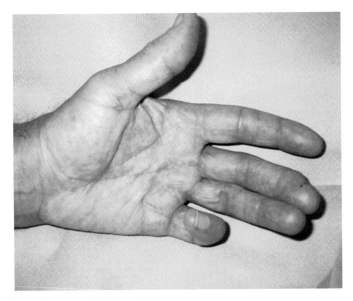

Figure 2.8 Dupuytren's contracture

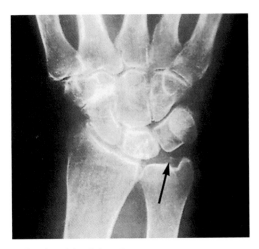

Figure 2.9 Chondrocalcinosis in wrist

a corticosteroid injection helps severe pain associated with local inflammation. Surgical replacement is rarely warranted, although the outcome is good. Some find a splint helpful.

Dupuytren's contracture

Dupuytren's contracture (Figure 2.8) is a relatively common and painless condition that is associated with palpable fibrosis of the palmar aponeurosis, usually in the palm but occasionally at the base of a digit. It is more common in white people, men, heavy drinkers, smokers and patients with diabetes mellitus. The cause is unknown, but repeated trauma may be important. Fibroblast proliferation starts in the superficial fascia and invades the dermis. An early sign is skin pitting or puckering. The contraction eventually causes flexion of the digit(s), most often the ring finger, but disability is often minimal. Disabling and progressive flexion is more common in the familial form. Nodular fibromatosis also affects the sole of the foot, the knuckle pads (Garrod's pads) and the penis (Peyronie's disease), and these conditions may coexist. Specialist hand clinics use magnetic resonance imaging to assess the lesion. The role of local corticosteroid injections and radiotherapy in early disease is unclear (Ketchum and Donahue, 2000; Seegenschmiedt et al., 2001). Surgical excision is helpful but recurrence is common. No controlled studies exist.

Cubital tunnel syndrome

Ulnar nerve compression at the elbow can be caused by direct pressure from leaning on the elbow, stretching the nerve with the elbow in prolonged flexion at night, or holding a telephone. It causes pins and needles in an ulnar distribution (little finger and the ulnar side of the ring finger). Prolonged entrapment causes hypothenar wasting and weakness of the hand's intrinsic muscles. The nerve is tender and sensitive at the elbow, where Tinel's sign is positive. Nerve conduction studies are normal in around 50% of cases. Avoidance of direct pressure and prolonged elbow flexion help.

Surgical anterior transposition of the nerve is occasionally needed. In some cases the ulnar nerve is compressed in Guyon's canal at the wrist.

Systemic disorders causing hand pain

Inflammatory arthritis

The hands are often affected early in rheumatoid arthritis, with symmetrical swelling of the metacarpophalangeal joints, proximal interphalangeal joints and wrists. The feet and other joints are usually also affected. Psoriatic and other forms of seronegative arthritis are less common, are more likely to be asymmetrical, and may be associated with marked skin and tendon changes that produce a "sausage" finger. The distal interphalangeal joints and adjacent nails may also be affected in psoriasis. Morning pain and stiffness are typical. Intra-articular steroids are often useful adjuncts to systemic medication.

Acute pseudogout and chondrocalcinosis of the wrist

Sudden wrist inflammation in an older patient may be due to calcium pyrophosphate arthritis (pseudogout). Marked swelling and inflammation are observed—the joint feels hot, and infection may need to be excluded. Chondrocalcinosis (Figure 2.9), although often asymptomatic, is usually seen in the triangular ligament of the wrist on X-ray radiography. The joint aspirate is turbid and contains weakly positively birefringent crystals under polarized light. Steroid injection or a short course of a non-steroidal anti-inflammatory drug or colchine usually helps; regular use of non-steroidal anti-inflammatory drugs or colchine can be used to manage frequent attacks.

Acute gout and chronic tophaceous gout

Acute urate gout rarely affects the hands. Tophaceous deposits in individuals in renal failure or who have been on long-term diuretic treatment are initially painless, chalky subcutaneous deposits. The tophi can ulcerate and a few such patients also develop acute gout in the hand and elsewhere.

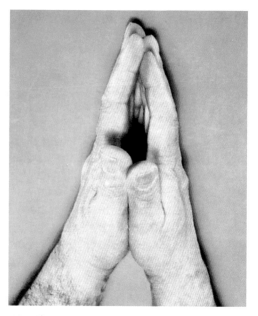

Figure 2.10 Positive prayer sign: diabetic stiff hands (also nodal osteoarthritis and flexor tenosynovitis)

Diabetic stiff hand (cheiroarthropathy—limited joint mobility syndrome)

Stiff hands are seen in 5–10% of patients with type I diabetes. This is more common in those with poor diabetic control and is associated with limited shoulder mobility, diabetic nephropathy and retinopathy. Patients develop waxy, tight skin and a so-called positive prayer sign—inability to hold the fingers and palms together (Figure 2.10). However, limited joint mobility in diabetes is multifactorial, and may also be due to flexor tenosynovitis, Dupuytren's contracture or nodal osteoarthritis. Good diabetic control is essential. Injection for symptomatic flexor tenosynovitis helps. No specific treatment exists for the skin changes.

Raynaud's phenomenon

This disorder, which results from severe vasospasm in response to a temperature change, causes marked and typically sharply demarcated pallor of one or more digits. As circulation recovers, the digit becomes blue (cyanotic) and then bright red because of rebound hyperaemia—the triphasic response. Raynaud's is commoner in females than males. In young women the condition is often a harmless nuisance, requiring warm gloves and sometimes vasodilators. Its onset for the first time in older people warrants investigation. Raynaud's may also be part of a systemic autoimmune disorder (rheumatoid arthritis, systemic lupus erythematosus, or systemic sclerosis), and it occasionally leads to necrosis. Autoimmune-associated Raynaud's can be extremely severe and requires specialist referral. Vibration white finger is a compensational industrial disease in people who use vibrating tools. Roughly two in three patients with primary Raynaud's phenomenon have spontaneous resolution of their symptoms (Spencer-Green, 1998).

> **Box 2.1 Characteristics of chronic upper limb pain syndrome**
>
> - Often starts as carpal tunnel syndrome, flexor tenosynovitis or tennis elbow
> - Spreads to affect the upper arm more diffusely
> - Physical signs may be minimal
> - Often associated with:
>   - use of keyboards
>   - sudden changes in work practices
>   - disharmony at work
>   - anxiety and sleeplessness
> - Neurophysiological and psychosocial mechanisms involved
> - Best dealt with non-judgementally

Other disorders

Ganglion

A ganglion is a cystic swelling in continuity with a joint or tendon sheath through a fault in the capsule. It is filled with clear, viscous fluid rich in hyaluronan. Ganglia are common on the dorsal wrist, are often painless and resolve spontaneously (50% at 6 years; see http://www.medicine.ox.ac.uk/bandolier/booth/miscellaneous/wristgang.html). Often, only reassurance of the patient is required. Wrist splints relieve the pain. Aspiration and injection are rarely effective, and surgical excision is best if the ganglion is persistent and painful.

Chronic (work-related) upper limb pain

The main symptom of chronic upper limb pain is pain (Box 2.1). A local cause (carpal tunnel syndrome, flexor or extensor tenosynovitis, or tennis elbow) may be the initial trigger. The patient develops widespread pain that is often disproportionate to the findings but causes great distress. A prior change in work pattern may exist, and often disharmony is found at the workplace. The cause is unclear, but neurophysiological and psychosocial factors are probably involved. The phenomenon of central "wind up" of pain seen in many chronic pain syndromes probably plays a role. It is easy for the doctor to find the problem exasperating and difficult to understand, but it is best managed non-judgementally. Early reductions in work activities and pain-control measures are important, but it is best not to ask the person to take too much time off. Advice to the employer to review work practices reduces the risk of litigation. Referral to a specialist pain clinic should be considered.

Osteonecrosis (rare)

Kienböck's disease is the late result of a dorsiflexion injury often seen in manual labourers. Fragmentation and collapse of the lunate causes shortening of the carpus and secondary osteoarthritis. Osteonecrosis takes up to 18 months to appear on X-ray radiography.

Scaphoid bone fracture

Pain in the anatomical snuffbox after a fall onto an outstretched hand requires an immediate X-ray examination, although a fracture is not always visible. Any severe wrist injury should be managed as a potential scaphoid fracture with a plaster, and a further X-ray radiograph should be taken 3 weeks later. Unrecognized scaphoid fracture leads to pain associated with failed union, osteonecrosis and secondary osteoarthritis.

Writer's cramp

Writer's cramp is the most common type of focal dystonia and occurs during complex hand activities—writing or playing a musical instrument. Clumsiness and painful tightness in the hand and forearm occur during writing or playing, and abnormal tension and strange posturing develop. Focal dystonias are often inappropriately described as "psychological." Local botulinum toxin injection produces temporary relief. Retraining and learning new techniques help some patients, but the outlook is poor and may lead to the end of musical careers.

Septic arthritis

Septic arthritis of the hand or wrist is rare. It is an important differential diagnosis of acute pseudogout. If septic arthritis is suspected, it should be treated as a medical emergency and referred to Accident and Emergency or a specialist unit for investigation and appropriate intravenous antibiotic treatment. The patient is usually febrile and unwell. It is essential not to start antibiotics before all the necessary samples have been taken for culture. Non-steroidal anti-inflammatory drugs and analgesics can be given for pain, which is often severe.

Local corticosteroid injection technique

During local corticosteroid injections (Box 2.2), an injection of local anaesthetic (or topical anaesthetic) is followed by 0.2–1 ml of a suitable steroid preparation, such as hydrocortisone acetate 25 mg/ml or depot methylprednisolone 40 mg/ml. Methylprednisolone is about five times as powerful as hydrocortisone on a mg per mg basis. It is best first to introduce the needle

> ### Box 2.2 **Local corticosteroid injection technique**
>
> - Hand and arm well supported
> - Equipment readily to hand
> - Clean skin thoroughly
> - Use small-bore needle
> - Inject small volume of local anaesthetic
> - Inject corticosteroid through same needle
> - Always inject under low pressure

with local anaesthetic and then to inject the steroid under low pressure. Patients should be warned that the pain might increase for a day or two after injection. Superficial injections or, very rarely, leakage of the corticosteroid along the needle track, cause local skin depigmentation and atrophy of subcutaneous fat; this is more likely with depot injections of steroid. Consent from the patient should always be obtained.

References

Kamath V, Stothard J. Erratum to: A clinical questionnaire for the diagnosis of carpal tunnel syndrome. *Journal of Hand Surgery (Edinburgh, Scotland)* 2004; **29**: 95.

Ketchum LD, Donahue TK. The injection of nodules of Dupuytren's disease with triamcinolone acetonide. *Journal of Hand Surgery* 2000; **25**: 1157–1162.

O'Gradaigh D, Merry P. Corticosteroid injection for the treatment of carpal tunnel syndrome. *Annals of the Rheumatic Diseases* 2000; **59**: 918–919.

Pal B, O'Gradaigh D, Merry P. Diagnosis of carpal tunnel syndrome. *Rheumatology* 2001; **40**: 595–597.

Rankin ME, Rankin EA. Injection therapy for management of stenosing tenosynovitis (de Quervain's disease) of the wrist. *Journal of the National Medical Association* 1998; **90**: 474–476.

Seegenschmiedt MH, Olschewski T, Guntrum F. Radiotherapy optimization in early-stage Dupuytren's contracture; results of a randomized study. *International Journal of Radiation Oncology, Biology, Physics* 2001; **49**: 785–798.

Spencer-Green G. Outcomes in primary Raynaud's phenomenon: a meta-analysis of the frequency, rates and predictors of transition to secondary diseases. *Archives of Internal Medicine* 1998; **158**; 595–600.

Stahl S, Kanter Y, Karnelli E. Outcome of trigger finger treatment in diabetes. *Journal of Rheumatology* 1997; **24**: 931–936.

Trumble TE, Gilbert M, McCallister WV. Endoscopic versus open surgical treatment of carpal tunnel syndrome. *Neurosurgery Clinics of North America* 2001; **12**: 255–266.

Wong SM, Hui ACF, O'Gradaigh D, Merry P. Corticosteroid injection for the treatment of carpal tunnel syndrome. *Annals of the Rheumatic Diseases* 2001; **60**: 897.

Yagev Y, Carel RS, Yagev R. Assessment of work-related risk factors for carpal tunnel syndrome. *Israel Medical Association Journal* 2001; **3**: 569–571.

Further reading

Bland JDP. Carpal tunnel syndrome. *British Medical Journal* 2007; **335**: 343–346.

Zhang W, Doherty M, Leeb BF *et al.* EULAR evidence based recommendations for the management of hand osteoarthritis: report of a Task Force of the EULAR Standing Committee for International Clinical Studies Including Therapeutics (ESCISIT). *Annals of the Rheumatic Diseases* 2007; **66**: 377–388.

CHAPTER 3

Pain in the Neck, Shoulder and Arm

Rachelle Buchbinder[1] and Caroline Mitchell[2]

[1]Cabrini Hospital and Monash University, Melbourne, Australia
[2]University of Sheffield, Sheffield, UK

OVERVIEW

- Neck, shoulder and lateral elbow pain are common musculoskeletal problems for which patients seek care in general practice.

- Non-specific neck pain is often acute and self-limiting, attributed to a mechanical basis, but persistence or recurrence is common. For most patients with acute neck pain and no "red flags", further investigation is not necessary.

- Neck pain usually responds to analgesia and advice about simple mobilization and exercises. High-quality evidence for the effectiveness of many treatment modalities is limited and often contradictory.

- Most shoulder complaints are due to rotator cuff disease, which is more prevalent with increasing age. Adhesive capsulitis, or "frozen shoulder", is a self-limiting condition, occurring most commonly in middle age. It can be distinguished from rotator cuff disease by the presence of global restriction of shoulder movements. It is also more common in people with diabetes.

- For most patients with shoulder pain the diagnosis can also usually be made clinically. Treatment aims to control pain and restore movement and function of the shoulder.

- Lateral epicondylitis is thought to be an overload injury at the origin of the common extensors at the lateral epicondyle. Patients present with pain and tenderness over the lateral epicondyle and pain with resisted movements. Prognosis is generally favourable, with 80% recovery within a year. Management is directed towards controlling pain, avoiding aggravating activities and maintaining movement.

The neck and shoulder are two of the most common sources of musculoskeletal pain. Neck pain has a self-reported point prevalence of between 10 and 20%. The majority of neck pain is acute and self-limiting and can be attributed to a mechanical or postural basis. However moderate or severe symptoms may persist in up to 30% of patients.

Shoulder pain has a self-reported point prevalence of between 14 and 26% in the general population. The incidence of shoulder pain increases with age, as does its functional impact. About one-quarter of all new episodes presenting for care resolve fully within 1 month, and nearly half have resolved within 3 months of onset. However, persistence or recurrence of shoulder symptoms within a year of initial presentation is common (in up to 50% of people).

Anatomy and function of the neck and shoulder joint

The neck moves almost constantly during waking hours through flexion, extension and rotation at the intervertebral and facet joints of the seven cervical vertebrae, through the actions of the surrounding muscles.

The shoulder is a series of articulations, including the scapulothoracic articulation, where the scapula slides on the ribcage (Figure 3.1). Soft tissue structures—capsules, ligaments, muscles, tendons, bursae and neurovascular elements—complete the framework and allow remarkable mobility to be achieved. The glenohumeral joint is extremely mobile and relies on the rotator cuff for stability. Instability, caused by laxity (congenital or acquired) or lack of muscular control because of pain, is a common feature of shoulder complaints.

The elbow is a compound synovial joint composed of a complex of two closely related articulations between the humerus and both the ulna and radius. It is supported by the ligaments and muscles.

Clinical evaluation

Neck and arm pain have a wide differential diagnosis. It is sometimes hard to distinguish between pain arising from the neck or the shoulder (Figure 3.2). Pain proximal to the shoulder, in the shoulder girdle or over the scapula indicates referred pain from the neck.

It is important to assess the patient's concerns, expectations, functional disability and any psychosocial and occupational issues. Details of hand dominance, any injury, hobbies, sporting activities and treatments for this or any other similar previous musculoskeletal problems should be noted. Significant past and current medical history—prescribed drugs and adverse reactions—should also be explored. The history should elicit the presence of any clinical features that indicate potentially serious pathology.

Determine the mode of onset and duration of the pain, nature, site, radiation, temporal characteristics, exacerbating and relieving

ABC of Rheumatology, 4th edn. Edited by Ade Adebajo.
©2010 Blackwell Publishing Ltd. 9781405170680.

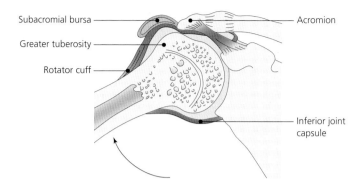

Figure 3.1 The shoulder "complex" of joints. This includes the scapulothoracic articulation, where the scapula slides on the ribcage. Adapted from Speed *et al.*, 2000

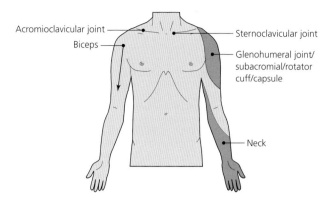

Figure 3.3 Features of cervical-nerve-root lesions

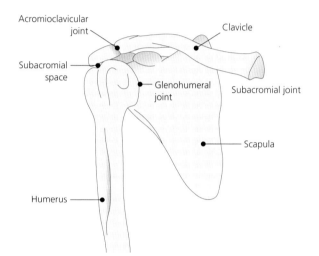

Figure 3.2 Sites and radiation of pain in the shoulder, arm and neck. Adapted from Speed *et al.*, 2000

Box 3.1 **Differential diagnosis of neck pain**

Structural
- Mechanical or non-specific
- Prolapsed intervertebral disc
- Cervical myelopathy

Neoplasm
- Primary or secondary

Inflammatory
- Rheumatoid arthritis
- Polymyalgia rheumatica and giant cell or temporal arteritis
- Spondyloarthropathies

Infection
- Discitis
- Osteomyelitis
- Paraspinal abscess

Metabolic
- Paget's disease

Myofascial
- Myofascial syndromes, fibromyalgia

features, and associated symptoms. Disturbed sleep is common with both neck and shoulder pain. Nevertheless, nocturnal pain should raise suspicion of nerve root pain, bony pathology or underlying malignancy, particularly if there is a history of cancer and/or systemic symptoms.

Radiation of pain distally from the upper arm or elbow suggests referred pain from the neck or peripheral neurological lesions (Figure 3.2). Neurological symptoms should be sought and their distribution ascertained (Figure 3.3).

Other notable symptoms include stiffness, clicking, clunking or locking. Joint swelling around the shoulder or elbow can occur in relation to arthropathy, infection or trauma. Systemic symptoms, such as fevers, night sweats, weight loss, generalized joint pains, new "lumps" (lympadenopathy, mass lesions) and new respiratory symptoms, should be specifically sought.

A structured examination aims to define the source of the pain and the degree of functional deficit and coexisting pathologies.

It includes careful inspection, palpation, movement, special tests, neurological assessment and further investigations, as appropriate.

Neck pain

Pain in the neck usually arises because of poorly defined mechanical influences, although it can occur because of pathology within the spine or be referred from elsewhere. A list of differential diagnoses of neck pain is shown in Box 3.1. When considering the diagnosis it is important to look for "red flags" or clinical features that indicate that there might be a serious underlying cause of the complaint (Table 3.1). Restricted cervical movements and local tenderness help to confirm the local origin of neck pain. Risk

Table 3.1 "Red flags" or clinical features indicative of potentially serious pathology in the neck and/or shoulder

"Red flags"	Potential pathology
History of cancer, symptoms and signs of cancer, unexplained deformity, mass or swelling	Malignancy
Fever, systemically unwell, redness and swelling	Infection
Trauma, epileptic fit, electric shock, loss of rotation and normal shape	Unreduced shoulder dislocation
Recent trauma, acute disabling pain and significant weakness, positive "drop arm" sign	Acute rotator cuff tear
Diffuse poorly localized pain and/or abnormal sensation, unexplained wasting, loss of power or altered reflexes	Neurological lesion, cervical radiculopathy, myelopathy
Referred pain: neck pain, myocardial ischaemia, referred diaphragmatic pain, apical lung cancer, metastases	Pain arising from elsewhere
Bilateral shoulder pain with or without neck pain, early morning stiffness	Polymyalgia rheumatica, rheumatoid arthritis, giant cell arteritis
Rapid swelling after trauma	Haemarthrosis of the shoulder

Table 3.2 Arm dermatomes

Nerve root	Weakness	Reflex change
C5	Shoulder abduction	Biceps
C6	Wrist extension, supination, elbow flexion	Radial
C7	Elbow extension, wrist flexion	Triceps
C8	Finger flexors	NA
T1	Finger abductors	NA

NA = not applicable

factors include manual jobs, heavy workloads, increasing age and depression, while chronicity is weakly predicted by the presence of concomitant low back pain, older age and previous episodes of neck pain.

Simple mechanical neck pain describes a common, usually self-limiting, clinical presentation of pain with or without restricted movement, but without neurological or "red flag" features. Onset may be acute (acute torticollis, or "wry neck") or gradual, and, like low back pain, tends to be recurrent. It usually responds to conservative treatment, although patients should be instructed to return for further assessment if symptoms persist or change in quality. Neck pain may be accompanied by myofascial or diffuse regional pain often involving the shoulder girdle, reproduced by palpation of trigger points ("knots" within muscle).

Radicular pain, due to compression of a nerve root from herniation of a cervical disc, or due to non-compressive causes such as local infection or tumour, refers to neck pain that radiates into the shoulder girdle and/or arm with paraesthesia or numbness in a root distribution. Subjective weakness is less common. Examination may not reveal the nerve root level because of the extensive overlap of dermatomes (Table 3.2). Motor involvement and/or objective sensory loss warrant urgent referral for specialist assessment. In general, 40–80% of people with compressive cervical radiculopathy have complete resolution of their symptoms over time with conservative treatment.

Cervical myelopathy (compression of the spinal cord), which may arise due to midline disc herniation, is suggested by a history of difficulty walking, lower limb symptoms or bladder and bowel dysfunction. Motor signs of myelopathy below the level of spinal cord involvement may include weakness with increased reflexes and tone (upper motor neurone signs), decreased pinprick sensation and loss of position and/or vibration sense. These symptoms warrant urgent referral for specialist assessment.

Whiplash injury, an abrupt flexion/extension movement of the cervical spine as a result of sudden acceleration–deceleration, may occur in road traffic or sporting injuries, and is characterized by quite localized or diffuse neck and arm pain with muscle spasm, and limited neck movements. Symptoms may be persistent, although 50% of patients recover within 3 months and 80% within 12 months. Risk factors for chronicity after whiplash include the severity of the initial symptoms and psychological disturbance.

Neck pain is common in inflammatory arthritis, and atlanto-axial and sub-axial subluxation may develop, particularly in rheumatoid arthritis. Immobility due to osteophytic linking of vertebrae may be seen in ankylosing spondylitis.

Investigation of neck pain

For most patients with acute neck pain and no "red flags", further investigation (radiographs, blood tests) is not necessary. Due to the high prevalence of asymptomatic degenerative changes in the cervical spine, plain radiographs are rarely diagnostic, and pain severity correlates poorly with radiographic abnormalities. Magnetic resonance imaging (MRI) is highly sensitive in detecting disc and cord abnormalities if these are suspected, whereas computed tomography is better for evaluation of bone.

Treatment of neck pain

Patients should be informed of the generally favourable prognosis of neck pain and the fact that serious underlying conditions are very unlikely. Pertinent psychosocial and occupational issues may need to be explored.

Neck pain usually responds to simple analgesia and advice about simple mobilization and exercises. High-quality evidence for the effectiveness of many treatment modalities is limited and often contradictory.

Advice to stay active—Encourage patients to persist with their normal activities. There is no evidence that collars reduce pain or improve function, nor is there evidence about special pillows. In general patients are advised to sleep on their side with a single pillow supporting the neck. Early mobilization and return to normal activity may reduce pain in people with acute whiplash injury more than immobilization or rest with a collar.

Drug therapy—There is limited evidence about the relative benefits of paracetamol, opioid analgesics, non-steroidal anti-inflammatory drugs (NSAIDs) and antidepressants. Potential benefits versus risks of NSAIDs should be considered, particularly in high-risk patients (consider potential drug interactions, the elderly, coexisting asthma, past history of peptic ulcer, renal impairment). All patients on regular analgesia should be reviewed regularly for both efficacy and adverse effects. If there is significant nocturnal pain, a tricyclic antidepressant (e.g. amitriptyline 10 to 50 mg orally, at night) may be helpful.

Exercises—Gentle neck exercises may be a useful and effective treatment for acute neck pain. The best type and mix of exercise has not been defined, but includes stretching, strengthening and proprioceptive retraining exercises (usually prescribed by a physiotherapist). Exercises for cervical radiculopathy are unproven. Exercise therapy is contraindicated in the presence of myelopathy.

Mobilization or manipulative techniques—Mobilization or manipulative techniques for both acute and chronic pain (typically performed by physiotherapists, chiropractors or osteopaths), either alone or in combination with other physical interventions, may have a modest effect, although this is unproven.

Multidisciplinary biopsychosocial rehabilitation—The principle underlying multidisciplinary rehabilitation is to simultaneously address all components (physical, psychological and social) of the patient's pain experience. Cognitive behavioural therapy has been shown to decrease time off work and other behavioural manifestations of pain but not to change the degree of pain.

Other non-operative treatments—The efficacy of most passive non-manipulative therapies (e.g. heat, massage, transcutaneous electrical nerve stimulation, pulsed electromagnetic field treatment) is not supported by evidence. Acupuncture might provide short-term pain relief in people with chronic neck pain, but evidence is limited. There is also limited evidence about the effectiveness of massage for neck pain. There is limited evidence that myofascial trigger-point injections using local anaesthetic into tender points are beneficial in reducing chronic neck pain. There is inconclusive evidence about the effectiveness of traction for neck pain with or without cervical radiculopathy, and it should not be used before imaging to exclude spinal cord compression or a large disc protrusion. A short course of oral glucocorticoids prescribed by a specialist, and after appropriate investigation, may be of benefit for cervical radiculopathy but is unproven. Facet joint injections, medial branch blocks and percutaneous radiofrequency denervation are performed under the premise that pain arises from the facet joint; however, the evidence to support these procedures is very limited. Botulinum A intramuscular injections have been shown to be ineffective for neck pain with or without radiculopathy.

Surgery—Surgery is not indicated for patients with neck pain in the absence of neurological symptoms of radiculopathy or myelopathy. Surgery for cervical radiculopathy is indicated for progressive motor weakness, and it may be also be a reasonable option for those who have failed 6–12 weeks of conservative treatment. In both instances, there should be evidence of nerve root compression at the appropriate level to fit the presentation. Anterior cervical discectomy with or without and fusion is the most commonly used procedure. Surgery may also be indicated in people with myelopathy to prevent neurological progression.

Shoulder pain

The differential diagnosis of shoulder pain is summarized in Box 3.2. Pain may also arise in the scapulothoracic region, and a list of differential diagnoses is shown in Box 3.3. "Red flags" or clinical

---

Box 3.2 **Differential diagnosis of shoulder pain**

Pain arising from the shoulder
- Rotator cuff disease or associated with the rotator cuff
  - Tendinitis, partial- and full-thickness tears
  - Calcific tendonitis
  - Complete rotator cuff tear
  - Rupture of the origin of the long head of biceps
  - Subacromial bursitis
- Adhesive capsulitis ("frozen shoulder")
- Glenohumeral joint
  - Osteoarthritis
  - Rheumatoid arthritis
  - Polymyalgia rheumatica
  - Septic arthritis
  - Instability and dislocation
  - Traumatic labral tears
  - Acromioclavicular and sternoclavicular disorders
  - Malignancy—myeloma, bony metastases

Pain arising from elsewhere
- Referred pain from the neck
- Myocardial ischaemia, referred diaphragmatic pain
- Lesions of axillary, suprascapular, long thoracic, radial, musculocutaneous nerves, brachial plexus, referred pain
- Malignancy—apical lung cancer

Regional or diffuse pain
- Myofascial pain syndromes, fibromyalgia

Box 3.3 **Differential diagnosis of scapulothoracic pain**

- Local muscle injury
- Myofascial pain syndrome
- Subscapular bursitis
- Snapping scapula
- Suprascapular nerve palsy
- Referred pain from cervical or thoracic spine
- Bone injury—e.g. fracture or metastatic deposit in scapula

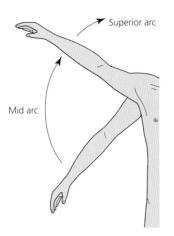

Figure 3.4 Subacromial impingement of the rotator cuff can occur with abduction of the arm. Adapted from Speed *et al.*, 2000

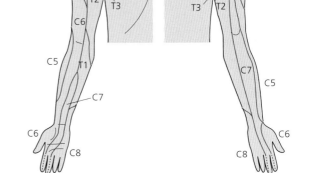

Figure 3.5 Mid or superior painful arcs of abduction represent subacromial impingement or acromioclavicular pathology, respectively

features suggestive of serious underlying pathology in people who present with shoulder pain are shown in Table 3.1.

Rotator cuff disease

Most shoulder complaints (60–70%) are due to rotator cuff disease, a broad term that includes a wide array of diagnostic labels. Some labels derive from clinical features (e.g. painful arc syndrome); some from assumed pathophysiology (e.g. impingement syndrome—impingement upon the cuff tendons between the acromion and head of the humerus (Figure 3.4) and some from the imaging appearance (e.g. calcific tendinitis, rotator cuff tendinitis or tendinopathy, subacromial bursitis and partial- or full-thickness tears).

Based upon MRI scans, asymptomatic cuff tears are common. The incidence increases with age (over half those over 60 years of age have tears), suggesting that it may be part of the normal ageing process combined with repetitive microtrauma. A significant number of asymptomatic tears will become symptomatic over time, and longstanding tears can result in glenohumeral arthritis. Rotator cuff disorders commonly occur in young people engaged in sport involving overhead activities, but are most common in middle and older age. Occupational associations include repetitive movements, working with vibrating tools, working in awkward postures and performing similar work for a prolonged period.

The patient typically complains of pain felt in the shoulder and/or lateral aspect of the upper arm that is worse with overhead activities and at night, particularly when lying on the affected side.

Characteristic features of the examination include pain in the mid-range of active abduction (Figure 3.5) and on resisted shoulder abduction with or without external rotation, and evidence of impingement (production of pain at the anterior shoulder if the arm is flexed forwards to 90°, adducted and internally rotated, elicited by asking the patient to place their hand on the contralateral shoulder and push up against resistance). In contrast to adhesive capsulitis, which causes global restriction of both active and passive movements, passive range of motion is often normal in rotator cuff disease, although certain movements may be restricted by pain. It is therefore important to assess both active (patient moves the shoulder) and passive (the examiner moves the shoulder) movements to distinguish apparent from true restriction of shoulder motion.

Painful weakness and atrophy suggest significant tears. Winging or asymmetry of the scapula may indicate a degree of shoulder instability. The "drop arm" test suggests a complete or large rotator cuff tear.

Calcific tendinitis usually affects women aged 30–50 years and is associated with the formation and resorption of calcific deposits within the cuff. The patient typically presents with acute onset of severe pain, occasionally with a fever and severe limitation of shoulder movements due to pain. In the more chronic stages, pain and catching are reported, and signs of impingement may be noted.

Diagnosis—The diagnosis of rotator cuff disease can usually be made clinically. Blood tests and plain radiographs are not necessary in the absence of "red flags" unless there is a failure to respond to treatment. Plain radiographs may exclude other causes of shoulder pain, such as significant glenohumeral osteoarthritis. If calcific tendinitis is suspected, there may be fluffy calcific deposits, situated just proximal to the rotator cuff insertion (Figure 3.6), and the erythrocyte sedimentation rate and white cell count may also be raised. The diagnostic utility of shoulder ultrasound and MRI in primary care is unknown. Due to the high prevalence of asymptomatic abnormalities in the rotator cuff, these investigations have little to add to the largely conservative management of rotator cuff disease in primary care. Ultrasound and MRI can detect full-thickness rotator cuff tears but have less accuracy for detecting partial-thickness tears.

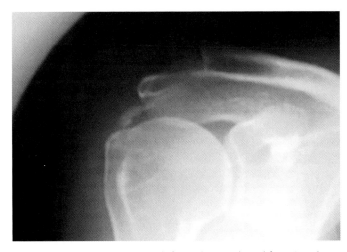

Figure 3.6 Plain X-ray showing calcific tendinitis. Adapted from Speed *et al.*, 2000

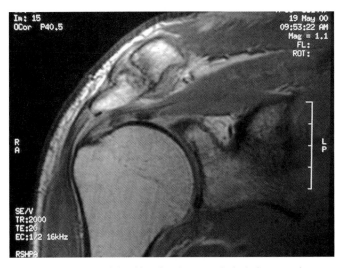

Figure 3.7 MRI scan of shoulder, showing acromioclavicular osteophytes and underlying rotator cuff tendinitis

Treatment—The aims of treatment of rotator cuff disease are to control pain and restore movement and function of the shoulder. Paracetamol is suitable as first-line therapy and may be supplemented by mild opioids such as codeine phosphate if needed. NSAIDs may provide short-term pain relief if there are no contraindications to their use. Initially patients may need to modify their activities and address occupational factors.

Subacromial injection of depot corticosteroid and local anaesthetic may provide rapid relief of pain, but its effect may be small and not maintained beyond a few weeks. If initial response is good, injections may be repeated up to two or three times at six-weekly intervals. Although injections performed under fluoroscopy or ultrasound might increase the accuracy of needle placement, it is not clear whether or not this results in significantly better outcomes.

Physiotherapy comprising a combination of mobilization techniques and directed exercises designed to strengthen and stabilize the cuff and scapular muscles can be used alone or combined with other measures. Global strengthening and proprioception training may reduce instability and minimize impingement in those with glenohumeral joint hypermobility.

Benefits of heat or ice packs, low-power laser, ultrasound and pulsed electromagnetic field therapy are unproven, as trials have yielded conflicting results. There is limited evidence for transitory pain relief following acupuncture, and suprascapular nerve block may also provide short-term pain relief. Trials have failed to establish the efficacy of extracorporeal shock wave therapy (ESWT) for rotator cuff disease.

Surgery may be required when symptoms fail to respond to conservative treatment. Operative treatment involves decompression of the subacromial space, with or without rotator cuff repair. MRI may be useful to plan surgery (Figure 3.7). Observational studies have reported good outcomes of surgery, although three randomized controlled trials found that surgery was not superior to treatment with supervised exercises.

Subacromial steroid injections, needling of the calcific deposits under fluoroscopic guidance and percutaneous needle aspiration and lavage by ultrasound guidance have each been advocated to relieve pain in calcific tendinitis, although no data are available from controlled trials. Ultrasound may provide short-term pain relief and, like ESWT, may improve the radiological appearance of calcific deposits. Surgical removal of calcific deposits may be of benefit if conservative treatments fail.

Adhesive capsulitis

Adhesive capsulitis ("frozen shoulder", or painful stiff shoulder) affects 2–5% of the population, women slightly more often than men, and 10–36% of people with diabetes, in whom it is more severe. It occurs most commonly in the fifth and sixth decades of life and is rare before the age of 40 years. The cause is poorly understood. It is usually idiopathic, although it may occur in the context of prolonged shoulder immobility (e.g. following a stroke or cardiac, breast or shoulder surgery).

Three phases have been described: initial gradual development of diffuse and severe shoulder pain, typically worse at night with inability to lie on the affected side, lasting between 2 and 9 months; a stiff phase with less severe pain present at the end range of movement, characterized by global stiffness and severe loss of shoulder movement, lasting about 4 and 12 months; and finally a recovery phase characterized by a gradual return of movement over 5 and 24 months. Severe disability may result in absence from work and inability to perform leisure activities. Although generally thought to run a self-limiting course over 2 to 3 years, some studies have found that up to 40% of patients have persistent symptoms and restricted movement beyond 3 years.

Diagnosis—The diagnosis can be made clinically, as the restriction of both active and passive movement in all planes of movement, especially external rotation, distinguishes it from other causes of shoulder pain. Plain radiographs are not necessary in primary care unless glenohumeral arthritis is suspected. Likewise, MRI is seldom necessary to establish the diagnosis, even in specialist care.

Treatment—Treatment is needed to control severe pain, improve range of movement and promote function. Patients should be informed of the generally favourable prognosis.

Treatment with analgesia and NSAIDS is the same as for rotator cuff disease.

Intra-articular injection of corticosteroid combined with local anaesthetic using either an anterior or posterior approach may provide rapid pain relief, but the effect may not be sustained beyond 6–7 weeks. There are limited data to provide guidance about frequency, dose and type of corticosteroid for adhesive capsulitis.

Arthrographic distension of the glenohumeral joint (or hydrodilatation) is performed under radiological guidance, usually using a combination of local anaesthetic, corticosteroid and saline to a mean volume of 20–45 ml. It has recently been demonstrated to have a sustained beneficial effect on pain, function and range of movement and is the standard of care in some settings. It may be more effective in the intermediate (stiff) and recovery stages and may also be repeated if the effect wanes over time.

Physiotherapy in the early, painful phase of the condition may aggravate the pain. However, gentle mobilization and strengthening exercises can improve mobility and reduce the duration of disability in the later phases. There is also evidence that mobilization and strengthening exercises following either steroid injection or arthrographic distension provide additional benefits over these treatments alone.

A short course of oral glucocorticoids, prescribed by a specialist, may provide rapid pain relief, although the effect may diminish beyond 6 weeks. Although treatment may be more effective in the very early phase of the condition, benefit has been demonstrated in patients with an average duration of symptoms of 5 to 6 months.

Suprascapular nerve blocks may provide short-term pain relief.

Manipulation under anaesthesia, possibly combined with intra-articular steroid injection and/or arthroscopic debridement of adhesions, may be helpful if conservative options have failed. Manipulation under anaesthesia can however, cause iatrogenic damage such as fractures, haemarthroses and tears of the labrum, tendons or ligaments.

Other shoulder disorders

Acromioclavicular and sternoclavicular joint disorders—Osteoarthritis of the acromioclavicular joint is common and presents with well-localized pain and tenderness over the joint. It can be managed symptomatically with analgesics, and local corticosteroid injections may provide relief. Surgery can be effective in resistant cases. The acromioclavicular joint can be strained or dislocated as a result of traumatic or sports injuries. Examination may find a superior painful arc of abduction (Figure 3.5) and restriction of passive horizontal adduction (flexion) of the shoulder, with the elbow extended across the body. This can be managed with taping and analgesia, and in severe cases, surgery may be required.

The sternoclavicular joint can be the presenting site of an inflammatory arthritis, but it is frequently overlooked. Rarely the sternoclavicular and/or acromioclavicular joints can be involved in the rare SAPHO syndrome (synovitis, acne, pustulosis, hyperostosis, osteomyelitis).

Glenohumeral joint arthritides—Isolated osteoarthritis of the shoulder is rare but may occur following fractures of the humeral head or neck or large rotator cuff tears, or as the end result of rheumatoid arthritis. It may be suspected, particularly in the older age group, if there is a limited range of painful movement sometimes accompanied by crepitus. Plain radiographs are useful in this instance. New onset of bilateral shoulder pain and stiffness should prompt consideration of polymyalgia rheumatica in those over 50 years of age and in rheumatoid arthritis. Milwaukee shoulder, which mainly affects elderly women, is a severe destructive apatite-associated arthropathy that presents with shoulder pain, limited movements and large joint effusion. Aspiration reveals a large amount of blood-tinged synovial fluid, which contains calcium phosphate crystals.

Biceps tendinitis/rupture—The long head of the biceps tendon passes through the bicipital groove of the anterior proximal humerus and is often involved in rotator cuff disease but can present as an isolated problem. It presents with anterior shoulder pain, aggravated by lifting, carrying objects and overhead reaching. Sudden onset of worsening symptoms, which may occur after heavy lifting or be spontaneously accompanied by a swelling just above the antecubital fossa and sometimes bruising, suggests an acute rupture. In most instances proximal tendon rupture is cosmetic and does not require repair. However, distal biceps tendon rupture should be referred urgently for consideration of surgical repair.

Shoulder instability—General glenohumeral instability or looseness may be seen in young women with weak shoulder muscles, in young athletes (especially swimmers and throwers) and following large rotator cuff tendon tears. There may be diffuse shoulder pain, and instability may be multi- or unidirectional.

Glenoid labrum (cartilage) injuries—These can cause persistent shoulder pain and instability, and they usually occur after an episode of trauma or dislocation or with overuse. Diagnosis can be difficult, requiring magnetic resonance arthrography or arthroscopy. Management involves pain control and rehabilitation, which is followed by surgery if necessary.

Neurological causes—Shoulder pain may result from neurological causes, including nerve root entrapment at the neck, brachial plexus lesions or peripheral nerve lesions, including the axillary, long thoracic, suprascapular, radial or musculocutaneous nerves. Brachial neuritis can affect one or more components of the brachial plexus. Often idiopathic, some cases occur after a viral infection, immunizations or mechanical trauma. A sudden onset of diffuse pain in the shoulder, upper arm and occasionally forearm is accompanied by weakness, wasting, scapular winging and variable sensory loss of the affected neuromuscular structures. Electromyographic studies may be confirmatory. Tricyclic agents, carbamazepine, gabapentin or pregabalin may be helpful. Rehabilitation is started early to prevent stiffness and improve function.

Thoracic outlet syndrome—Compression of the neurovascular structures of the thoracic outlet, brachial plexus and subclavian artery may occur due to local masses, a high first or cervical rib or fibrous bands. Symptoms depend on the structures compressed, but they are usually exacerbated by heavy manual work. Neurogenic symptoms usually predominate, including aching in the arm, paraesthesia and weakness. Vascular symptoms are usually intermittent cyanosis; trophic skin changes can occur. A causative structure is rarely identified, and management is symptomatic.

Elbow and forearm pain

Lateral and medial epicondylitis

The 12-month period prevalence of elbow pain has been estimated to be 11.2%. Box 3.4 displays a list of differential diagnoses of elbow pain. Most complaints of elbow pain are due to lateral epicondylitis ("tennis elbow" or lateral elbow pain), which has an estimated annual incidence in general practice of 4–7 per 1000 patients. People aged between 40 and 50 years are most commonly affected. Lateral epicondylitis is thought to be an overload injury at the origin of the common extensors at the lateral epicondyle, and typically follows minor and often unrecognized trauma of the extensor muscles of the forearm. In spite of the title "tennis elbow", tennis is a direct cause in only 5% of cases. Risk factors include repetitive wrist turning or hand gripping. Medial epicondylitis, or "golfer's elbow", is a similar but less common condition involving the common flexors at their origin at the medial epicondyle.

Both conditions are characterized by pain and tenderness over the respective epicondyle, and pain on resisted movements: resisted dorsiflexion of the wrist, middle finger, or both, in lateral epicondylitis (Figure 3.8), and resisted flexion of the wrist in medial epicondylitis. Both may be aggravated by repetitive movements and lifting. There may be night pain, early morning stiffness and stiffness after periods of inactivity. Pain referred from the neck or shoulder is distinguishable by less localized symptoms, associated neurological symptoms and the lack of local signs. Pain arising from the elbow joint is usually more posterior and less well localized and may be associated with an elbow effusion and difficulty straightening the elbow because of restriction.

Lateral and medial epicondylitis are generally self-limiting and patients should be informed of the generally favourable prognosis. In a general practice trial, 80% of patients with elbow pain of already greater than 4 weeks' duration were recovered after 1 year, simply following an expectant policy without any specific treatment. Prognostic factors found to be at least moderately associated with a poorer outcome at 1 year include previous occurrence, high physical strain at work, manual jobs, high baseline levels of pain and/or distress, passive coping and less social support.

Treatment—Interventions have mainly been tested for lateral epicondylitis, but the results are probably generalizable to medial epicondylitis. Treatment in the acute stage involves relative rest and avoidance of specific activities that aggravate the discomfort. Ice may be applied, but there are no data about its effects. Use of a tennis elbow brace or strap is common and may provide short-term pain relief while worn, allowing some return to activity.

Topical and oral NSAIDs may provide short-term relief of pain, although evidence is limited. Local skin reactions may occur with topical treatment.

Stretching and strengthening exercises may be helpful. Most studies have assessed their effect as part of multimodal interventions involving mobilization techniques at the elbow other physical therapies, with mixed results.

Corticosteroid injection with local anaesthetic may provide short-term pain relief (less than 3 months), although over the long term may be less effective than no treatment or physiotherapy (consisting of ultrasound, deep friction massage and an exercise programme). After an initial favourable response lasting 6 or more weeks, there may be a recurrence of symptoms. It is important to consider the close proximity of the ulnar nerve when performing

---

Box 3.4 **Differential diagnosis of elbow pain**

- Lateral epicondylitis ("tennis elbow" or lateral elbow pain)
- Medial epicondylitis ("golfer's elbow" or medial elbow pain)
- Olecranon bursitis
- Elbow joint
  - Rheumatoid arthritis
  - Septic arthritis
  - Osteoarthritis (rare)
- Cervical radiculopathy
- Tendinopathies
  - Biceps tendinopathy (anterior elbow pain)
  - Triceps tendinopathy, avulsion (posterior elbow pain)
- Nerve compression, entrapment
  - Ulnar neuropathy
  - Median nerve
  - Anterior interosseous nerve
  - Cubital tunnel syndrome

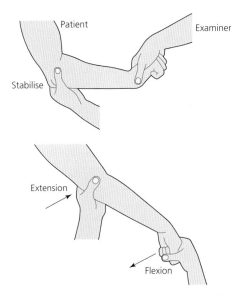

Figure 3.8 Provocation tests for lateral epicondylitis. Resisted extension of the middle finger also elicits pain

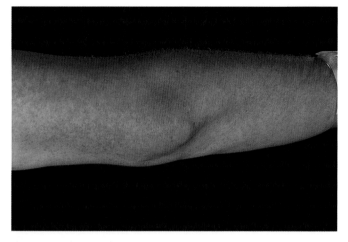

Figure 3.9 Olecranon bursitis—e.g. tophaceous gout at the elbow

steroid injection for medial epicondylitis. Adverse effects of injection are generally mild and transient and include post-injection pain, depigmentation and local skin and subcutaneous atrophy.

Trials of ultrasound have been conflicting but have generally reported marginal or no benefit, while laser therapy trials and trials of various other physical therapies have consistently been negative. There is no strong and consistent evidence that ESWT provides benefits in terms of pain and function in lateral epicondylitis. Acupuncture (needle, laser or electro-acupuncture) may provide short-term pain relief. Botulinum toxin injection and topical glyceryl trinitrate have recently been proposed as treatments for lateral epicondylitis, but further research is required before these therapies can be recommended.

Surgery is reserved for patients with recalcitrant, limiting symptoms, although evidence of benefit from controlled trials is limited. The most common operations are open excision, debridement and release and/or repair of the extensor or flexor tendon origins at the lateral or medial epicondyle. Percutaneous and arthroscopic procedures have also been described.

Other elbow disorders

Arthritis of the elbow joint may be due to systemic inflammatory arthritides, including rheumatoid and seronegative arthritis, crystal-induced synovitis (gout or pseudogout) and, rarely, septic arthritis. Neisseria gonococcus arthritis should be suspected in at-risk individuals. Osteoarthritis of the elbow is rare and usually relates to prior fractures or trauma.

Olecranon bursitis ("student's elbow") presents with discrete swelling, pain and inflammation at the posterior point of the elbow and may be caused by acute or repetitive trauma, crystals or sepsis (Figure 3.9, Box 3.5). The presence of nodules suggests either rheumatoid arthritis (seen in active disease or as a side effect of methotrexate) or gout (tophi). Infection may follow an abrasion or initial cellulitis and the most common causative organism is *Staphylococcus aureus*. Systemic symptoms such as fever, leucocytosis and elevated inflammatory markers occur with sepsis and

crystals. When olecranon bursitis is suspected, blood cultures and aspiration for crystals, Gram stain, and culture are essential.

Steroid injection is often helpful for olecranon bursitis due to inflammatory or crystal arthritis. Broad-spectrum antibiotics and possibly open drainage and lavage are used when there is sepsis.

Entrapment or inflammation of the ulnar, radial and median nerves can cause neurological disturbances involving the elbow and forearm. Paraesthesia and numbness involving the fourth and fifth fingers accompanied by weakness of the interossei may be caused by ulnar neuropathy, the most common compression neuropathy affecting the elbow. Tapping over the ulnar groove (Tinel's sign) may reproduce pain or numbness in the fourth and fifth fingers. Nerve conduction studies are helpful in diagnosis. Management depends on the severity and cause.

Reference

Speed C, Hazleman B, Dalton S. *Fast Facts: Soft Tissue Rheumatology*. Health Press, Oxford, UK, 2000.

Further reading

Arthritis Research Campaign. *The Painful Shoulder*. An information booklet. Arthritis Research Campaign, York, UK, 2009. Available online at http://www.arc.org.uk/arthinfo/patpubs/6039/6039.asp

Binder A. Neck pain. *Clinical Evidence* 2006; **15**: 1654–1675.

Bjelle A. Epidemiology of shoulder problems. *Baillière's Clinical Rheumatology* 1989; **3**: 437–451.

Buchbinder R, Green S, Struijs P. Tennis elbow. *Clinical Evidence* 2008. Available online at http://clinicalevidence.bmj.com

Dalton S. Clinical examination of the painful shoulder. *Baillière's Clin Rheumatol* 1989; **3**: 453–474.

Hadler NM. Coping with arm pain in the workplace. *Clinical Orthopaedics and Related Research* 1998; **351**: 57–62.

McClune T, Burton AK, Waddell G. Whiplash associated disorders: a review of the literature to guide patient information and advice. *Emergency Medicine Journal* 2002; **19**: 499–506.

Mitchell C, Adebajo AO, Hay E, Carr A. Shoulder pain: diagnosis and management in primary care. *British Medical Journal* 2005; **331**: 1124–1128.

Royal College of Radiologists. *Making the Best Use of a Department of Clinical Radiology: Guidelines for Doctors*. Royal College of Radiologists, London, 1999.

Speed C. Shoulder pain. *Clinical Evidence* 2005; **14**: 1543–1560.

CHAPTER 4

Low Back Pain

Rajiv K Dixit[1] and D John Dickson[2]

[1]University of California, San Francisco, USA
[2]Redcar & Cleveland Primary Care Trust, Redcar, UK

OVERVIEW

- Most patients with low back pain improve within 4 weeks.
- Degenerative change in the lumbar spine is the most common cause of pain.
- Imaging studies are rarely indicated, unless symptoms persist beyond 4 weeks.
- Imaging abnormalities should be carefully interpreted as they are frequently present in asymptomatic people.
- Most patients respond to a programme that includes analgesia, education, back exercises, aerobic conditioning and weight control. Surgery is rarely needed.

Low back pain (LBP) is the most common musculoskeletal symptom and poses a major socio-economic burden. An estimated 80% of the population will experience back pain during their lifetime; 90% of these patients will have resolution of their symptoms within 4 weeks.

Sciatica is the result of nerve root impingement and occurs in <1% of patients. The pain is radicular (and almost invariably radiates below the level of the knee) in the distribution of a lumbosacral nerve root, sometimes accompanied by sensory and motor deficits. Sciatica should be differentiated from non-neurogenic sclerotomal pain, which arises from pathology within the disc, facet joint or paraspinal muscles and ligaments. Sclerotomal pain is non-dermatomal in distribution and often radiates into the lower extremities but not below the knee or with associated paraesthesiae as with sciatica.

Causes of LBP

LBP usually originates from the lumbar spine (Figure 4.1); pain is rarely referred to the spine from other structures (Box 4.1). Over 95% of LBP is mechanical. Mechanical pain is generally due to an anatomical abnormality that increases with physical activity and is relieved by rest and recumbency. Systemic disease (infection, neoplasm and spondyloarthropathy) accounts for only 1–2% of LBP.

ABC of Rheumatology, 4th edn. Edited by Ade Adebajo.
©2010 Blackwell Publishing Ltd. 9781405170680.

Box 4.1 **Causes of LBP**

Mechanical
- Lumbar spondylosis*
- Disc herniation*
- Spondylolisthesis*
- Spinal stenosis*
- Fractures (mostly osteoporotic)
- Idiopathic ("non-specific")

Neoplastic
- Primary
- Metastatic

Inflammatory
- Spondyloarthropathies

Infectious
- Vertebral osteomyelitis
- Epidural abscess
- Septic discitis

Metabolic
- Osteoporotic compression fractures
- Paget's disease

Referred pain to spine
- From major viscera, retroperitoneal structures, urogenital system, aorta, or hip

*Related to degenerative changes

Lumbar spondylosis

The most common cause of mechanical LBP is degenerative change. In lumbar spondylosis (lumbar osteoarthritis) degenerative changes occur in the intervertebral disc and facet joint. Imaging evidence of lumbar spondylosis (disc space and facet-joint narrowing, osteophytes and subchondral sclerosis) is common, increases with age and is often asymptomatic.

Disc herniation

The nucleus pulposus in a degenerated disc may prolapse and push out the weakened annulus, usually posterolaterally. Imaging evidence of disc herniation is common even in asymptomatic adults. Occasionally, disc herniation may result in nerve root impingement (Figure 4.2), causing sciatica. Of all clinically significant

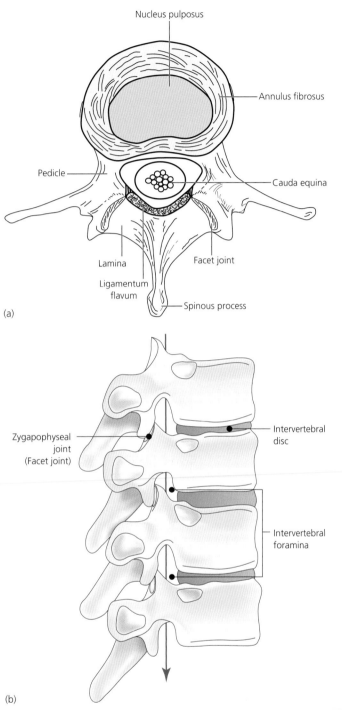

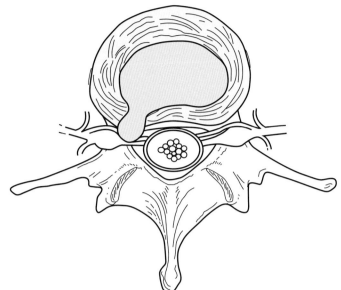

Figure 4.2 Posterolateral disc herniation resulting in nerve root impingement

Box 4.2 **Common symptoms of cauda equina syndrome**

The patient will develop some or all of the following:
- Altered saddle or/and urinary sensation
- Rectal/perineal pain
- Change/reduced awareness of bladder filling
- Need to strain to maintain urine flow
- Difficulty in walking or the legs just "do not feel right" (very early symptoms)
- Urinary retention with overflow incontinence and faecal incontinence (late manifestations of the full syndrome)

Figure 4.1 Basic anatomy of the lumbar spine; (a) cross-sectional view through a normal lumbar vertebra; (b) lateral view of the lumbar spine

herniations, 95% involve the L4-5 or L5-S1 disc. Generally, the more caudal nerve root is impinged; that is, the L5 nerve root with L4-5 herniation and S1 nerve root with L5-S1 herniation. In most patients the sciatic pain resolves over a period of weeks.

Rarely, a large midline disc herniation compresses the cauda equina. This is a surgical emergency. The full cauda equina syndrome usually presents with bilateral sciatica and motor deficits. It

needs to be recognized and treated before urinary retention and/ or incontinence occur for a completely successful outcome. Common symptoms are presented in Box 4.2.

Spondylolisthesis

Spondylolisthesis is the anterior displacement of a vertebra on the one beneath it. It is usually secondary to degenerative changes in the disc and facet joints (degenerative spondylolisthesis) but may result from a developmental defect in the pars interarticularis of the vertebral arch (spondylolysis), which produces isthmic spondy-lolisthesis (Figure 4.3). Patients with minor degrees of spondy-lolisthesis are usually asymptomatic, although some may have mechanical LBP. Greater degrees of spondylolisthesis occasionally cause sciatica or spinal stenosis.

Spinal stenosis

Spinal stenosis (ST) is defined as a narrowing of the spinal canal and its lateral recesses and neural foramina, which may result in a

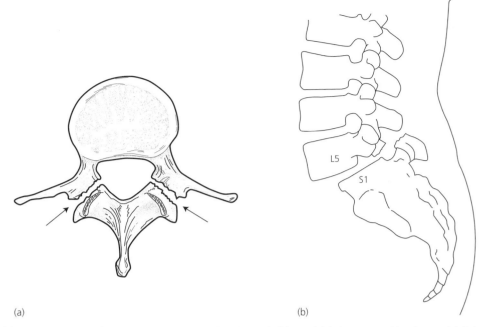

(a)   (b)

Figure 4.3 (a) Spondylolysis with bilateral defects in the pars interarticularis (arrows); (b) spondylolysis at L5 resulting in spondylolisthesis at L5-S1

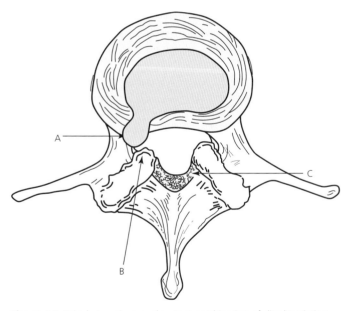

Figure 4.4 Spinal stenosis secondary to a combination of disc herniation (A), facet-joint hypertrophy (B) and hypertrophy of the ligamentum flavum (C)

compression of lumbosacral nerve roots (20% of adults over age 60 have imaging evidence of ST but are asymptomatic). Degenerative changes (leading to disc herniation, facet joint osteophytes and ligamentum flavum hypertrophy) are the causes of ST in most patients (Figure 4.4).

The hallmark of ST is pseudoclaudication (neurogenic claudication). Symptoms are often bilateral with pain, weakness and some-times paraesthesiae in the buttocks, thighs and legs. Symptoms are induced by standing or walking and relieved by sitting or flexing forward. Forward flexion increases the canal diameter and may lead to the adoption of a simian stance. Unsteadiness of gait is common. Physical examination is usually unremarkable, and severe neurologic deficits are rarely seen. The diagnosis is best confirmed by magnetic resonance imaging (MRI).

Idiopathic low back pain

A definitive pathoanatomical diagnosis with precise identification of the pain generator cannot be made in 80% of patients. Non-specific terms such as lumbago, strain and sprain (which have never been anatomically or histologically characterized) have come into use for this mostly self-limited syndrome of LBP.

Assessment

A major focus of the evaluation is to identify the few patients with an underlying systemic disease (infection, neoplasm or spondy-loarthropathy) or significant neurologic involvement that may require urgent and/or specific intervention. It is essential to take a full history and perform a comprehensive physical examination.

History

The patient's back pain should be characterized. Severe mechanical LBP with an acute onset in a slender postmenopausal woman is suspicious for a vertebral compression fracture secondary to oste-oporosis. Non-mechanical LBP, especially when accompanied by nocturnal pain, suggests the possibility of underlying infection or neoplasm. Inflammatory LBP, as seen in the spondyloarthropa-thies, is accompanied by night-time waking with pain and stiffness and/or prolonged morning stiffness that improves with exercise but not with rest. The radicular pain of sciatica suggests nerve root impingement. It should be differentiated from non-neurogenic sclerotomal pain. Pseudoclaudication is seen with spinal stenosis.

Physical examination

This rarely leads to a specific diagnosis. Inspection may reveal a structural or functional scoliosis. Structural scoliosis is secondary to structural changes of the vertebral column. Functional scoliosis

is usually the result of paravertebral muscle spasm or leg-length discrepancy. Functional scoliosis disappears with spinal flexion, whereas structural scoliosis persists.

Paravertebral muscle spasm often leads to loss of the normal lumbar lordosis. Point tenderness on percussion over the spine has sensitivity but not specificity for vertebral osteomyelitis. A palpable step-off between adjacent spinous processes indicates spondylolisthesis.

Limited spinal motion is not associated with any specific diagnosis, because LBP due to any cause may limit motion. Range-of-motion measurements can help in monitoring treatment. Examine the hip for arthritis: this normally causes groin pain, and occasionally referred back pain.

A straight leg raise test (Figure 4.5) should be performed on all patients with back pain that radiates into the lower extremities. This test places tension on the sciatic nerve and stretches the sciatic nerve roots (L4, L5, S1, S2 and S3). Patients with existing nerve root irritation, e.g. impingement from a herniated disc, will experience radicular pain that extends below the knee. This test is very sensitive (95%) but not specific (40%) for clinically significant disc herniation at the L4-5 or L5-S1 level. The straight leg raise test is usually negative in patients with spinal stenosis.

For lower extremities, neurologic evaluation should include motor testing, determination of knee and ankle deep tendon reflexes, and dermatomal sensory loss tests (Figure 4.6). This can help identify the specific nerve root involved (Table 4.1), e.g. a significant left-sided L5-S1 posterolateral disc herniation often impinges upon the left S1 nerve root. Patients will have left-sided sciatica in the distribution of the S1 dermatome and may develop left plantar flexion weakness, diminished light touch and pinprick sensation over the lateral aspect of the foot, and a diminished or absent left ankle jerk.

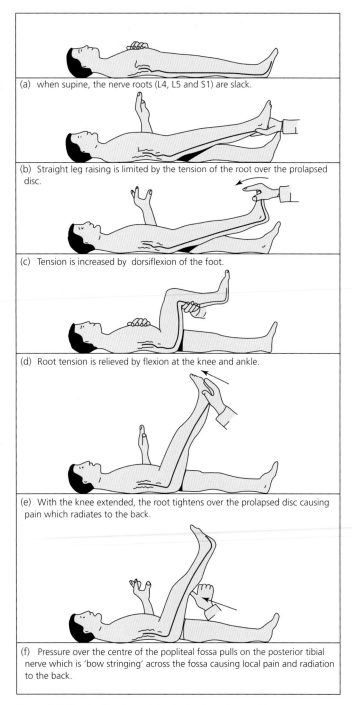

(a) when supine, the nerve roots (L4, L5 and S1) are slack.

(b) Straight leg raising is limited by the tension of the root over the prolapsed disc.

(c) Tension is increased by dorsiflexion of the foot.

(d) Root tension is relieved by flexion at the knee and ankle.

(e) With the knee extended, the root tightens over the prolapsed disc causing pain which radiates to the back.

(f) Pressure over the centre of the popliteal fossa pulls on the posterior tibial nerve which is 'bow stringing' across the fossa causing local pain and radiation to the back.

Figure 4.5 Examination for pain in the back: supine position

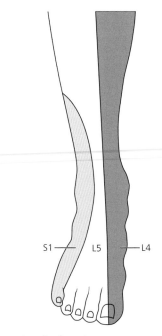

S1   L5   L4

Figure 4.6 Lower-extremity dermatomes

Table 4.1 Neurological features of lumbrosacral radiculopathy

Disc herniation	Nerve root	Motor	Sensory (light touch)	Reflex
L3-4	L4	Dorsiflexion of foot	Medial foot	Knee
L4-5	L5	Dorsiflexion of great toe	Dorsal foot	None
L5-S1	S1	Plantar flexion of foot	Lateral foot	Ankle

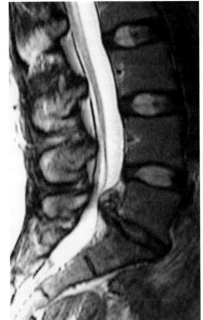

Figure 4.7 MRI showing a posterolateral disc prolapse

Box 4.3 **"Red flags" that indicate need for early diagnostic testing**

Spinal fracture
- Significant trauma
- Prolonged glucocorticoid use
- Age >50 years

Infection or cancer
- History of cancer
- Unexplained weight loss
- Immunosuppression
- Injection drug use
- Nocturnal pain
- Age >50 years

Cauda equina syndrome
- Urinary retention
- Overflow incontinence
- Faecal incontinence
- Bilateral or progressive motor deficit
- Saddle anaesthesia

Spondyloarthropathy
- Night-time waking with pain and stiffness
- Morning stiffness in the back
- Low back pain that improves with activity
- Age <40 years

Imaging studies

Diagnostic testing is rarely indicated unless symptoms persist beyond 4 weeks, as 90% of patients will have recovered within this time, thus avoiding unnecessary testing. "Red flags" indicate early investigations, e.g. underlying systemic disease or patients with a significant neurologic deficit (Box 4.3).

A major problem with all imaging studies is that many of the anatomical abnormalities (often the result of age-related degenerative changes) are common in asymptomatic people. Abnormalities such as single disc degeneration, facet-joint degeneration, Schmorl's nodes, spondylolysis, mild spondylolisthesis, transitional vertebrae (lumbarization of S1 or sacralization of L5), spina bifida occulta

and mild scoliosis are equally prevalent in people with and without LBP. Plain radiographs are usually unhelpful in determining the cause of LBP and should be limited to patients with findings suggestive of systemic disease (infection, neoplasm, spondyloarthropathy) or trauma, or those with continued LBP after 4–6 weeks of conservative care.

Computed tomography and MRI (Figure 4.7) should be reserved for patients in whom underlying infection or cancer is suspected, or for patients with significant or progressive neurologic deficits. MRI is the preferred modality for the detection of spinal infection, neoplasm, herniated discs and spinal stenosis. Bone scanning is used primarily to detect bony metastases, occult fractures and infection.

Treatment

Most patients, regardless of the cause, respond to a general programme that includes analgesia, education, back exercises, aerobic conditioning and weight control. Specific treatment is available only for the small number of patients with major neurologic compression or underlying systemic disease.

For treatment purposes, patients are considered to have acute LBP (duration <3 months), chronic LBP (duration >3 months) or a nerve root compression syndrome.

Acute LBP

Patients are advised to stay active, and bed rest is discouraged. Acetaminophen/paracetamol and non-steroidal anti-inflammatory drugs (NSAIDs) offer symptomatic relief; some people will need short-term narcotic analgesics, and muscle relaxants used for a few days will help others.

Once the acute episode of pain has subsided, a programme of regular back exercises (including stretching), aerobic conditioning and loss of excess weight is used to prevent recurrences. Back exercises help to stabilize the spine. Flexion exercises strengthen the abdominal muscles and extension exercises the paraspinal muscles. Educational booklets that include back exercises and safe lifting techniques are helpful.

Many patients ask about chiropratic and osteopathy treatments. There is no evidence that spinal manipulative therapy is superior to standard treatment for back pain.

Chiropractic focuses on the diagnosis, treatment and prevention of mechanical disorders of the musculoskeletal system, and on the effects of these disorders on the nervous system and on general health. It was founded in the USA by DD Palmer in 1895 who based it on his belief that disorders are caused by misaligned vertebrae which cause nerve compression (subluxations) and dysfunction. The primary chiropractic technique being adjustment of the spine. Chiropractors may specialize in low back pain problems, or they may combine chiropractic with manipulation of the extremities, physiotherapy, nutrition or exercise to improve the strength of the spine.

The General Chiropractic Council (www.gcc-uk.org) has regulated the chiropractic profession since 1994.

Osteopathy is a manual therapy that is primarily focused on the treatment of musculoskeletal conditions. It was founded by Andrew Still in the USA in 1886, who believed that disease was caused when the flow of nerve impulses was disrupted when a person's bones were out of place. He concluded that manipulating bones back into place would restore the interrupted flow of nerve impulses and cure disease.

Underpinning osteopathy is the idea that the body has self-regulatory mechanisms and therefore that it has the capacity to heal itself, that the structure and function of the body are closely inter-related, and that the somatic aspects of disease aren't just manifestations of disease but also contribute to maintenance of the disease state. Osteopaths will commonly treat back pain by manipulation, but may also use soft, tissue massage or advise exercise.

Osteopathy was established in the UK in 1917, and has been subject to statutory regulation since 1993. It is regulated by the General Osteopathic Council (www.osteopathy.org.uk).

There is limited evidence supporting the use of epidural glucocorticoid injections for short-term relief of radicular pain. Nerve-root blocks and injection of anaesthetic agents or glucocorticoid into trigger points, ligaments, sacroiliac joints and facet joints are of unproven efficacy.

Ultrasound, shortwave diathermy, transcutaneous electrical nerve stimulation and other treatments such as lumbar braces, traction, acupuncture and biofeedback are ineffective.

Chronic LBP

Treatment of chronic LBP is focused on relief of pain and restoration of function. Complete relief of pain is an unrealistic goal for most. Acetaminophen/paracetamol and NSAIDs may provide some degree of analgesia. Long-term use of narcotic analgesics should be avoided. Low-dose tricyclic antidepressants may help some patients.

Back exercises, aerobic conditioning, loss of excess weight and patient education are effective in managing chronic LBP. A multi-disciplinary approach focusing on functional restoration through an intensive rehabilitation programme based on cognitive behavioural therapy is often helpful.

The results of back surgery are disappointing when the goal is relief of back pain (such as by spinal fusion or artificial discs) rather than relief of radicular symptoms from neurologic compression.

Nerve root compression syndromes

Disc herniation—Patients with radicular pain secondary to nerve-root compression should be treated conservatively, as described for acute LBP, for the first 6 weeks unless there is severe or progressive neurologic deficit: approximately 90% will improve. Elective surgery may be considered in a few patients among those who have a significant persistent neurologic deficit or severe sciatica after 6 weeks of conservative care. Laminotomy with limited discectomy is generally the procedure of choice.

Spinal stenosis—The symptoms remain stable for years in most patients. Analgesics, NSAIDs, loss of excess weight, exercises (including those that reduce lumbar lordosis) and epidural glucocorticoids may provide symptomatic relief. Surgical treatment, aimed at decompression of the neural elements, is offered to patients with either disabling pseudoclaudication or significant neurologic deficit.

Further reading

Carragee EJ. Persistent low back pain. *New England Journal of Medicine* 2005; **352**: 1891–1898.

Critchley D, Hurley M. *Management of Back Pain in Primary Care*. Reports on the Rheumatic Diseases Series 5, no. 13. Arthritis Research Campaign, York, UK, 2007. Available online at http://www.arc.org.uk/arthinfo/medpubs/6533/6533.asp

Deyo, RA, Weinstein JN. Low back pain. *New England Journal of Medicine* 2001; **344**: 363–370.

HMSO. *The Back Book*. The Stationery Office, London, 2000.

Imboden J, Hellmann D, Stone J. *Current Diagnosis and Treatment in Rheumatology*, 2nd edn. McGraw-Hill, New York, 2007.

Jarvik JG, Deyo RA. Diagnostic evaluation of low back pain with emphasis on imaging. *Annals of Internal Medicine* 2002; **137**: 586–597.

Shapiro S. Medical realities of Cauda equine syndrome secondary to lumbar disc herniation. *Spine* 2000; **25**: 348–351.

Acknowledgements

Table 4.1 and Box 4.3, and Figures 4.1, 4.2, 4.3, 4.4 and 4.6 are taken from Imboden *et al.*, 2007, with permission. Figure 4.5 is taken from *Standards in Rheumatology: a Suggested Management Plan for Some Common Conditions in Rheumatology*. The Medicine Group, 1987.

CHAPTER 5

Pain in the Hip

Andrew J Hamer[1] and Jeffrey N Katz[2]

[1]Northern General Hospital, Sheffield, UK
[2]Case Western Reserve University, Cleveland, USA

OVERVIEW

- Osteoarthritis of the hip is common in adults, and osteoporotic hip fractures are epidemic in the elderly.
- Always examine the hip in patients presenting with knee pain, as referred pain from the hip is common.
- Childhood hip conditions require prompt treatment to reduce the risk of problems in later life.

Box 5.1 **Important causes of childhood hip pain**

- Congenital dislocation of the hip
- Perthes' disease
- Slipped upper femoral epiphysis
- Septic arthritis
- Transient synovitis or "irritable hip"
- Other arthritides

Hip pain in children

A child with hip disease may not present with pain or a history of trauma but with an unexplained limp. Unexplained thigh or knee pain should also raise the suspicion of hip abnormality. See Box 5.1 for a summary of important causes of childhood hip pain.

Congenital dislocation of the hip

Physical examination and/or ultrasound screening should detect at-risk cases (Figure 5.1), but missed cases may present as a delay in walking, a limp or discrepancy in leg length. Children usually present before 5 years of age. Missed cases may lead to a non-congruent joint and early osteoarthritic degeneration in adulthood.

Perthes' disease

Perthes' disease—disintegration of the femoral head, with subsequent healing and deformity of the hip—usually occurs in boys aged 5–10 years. The precise cause is unclear, but segmental avascular necrosis of the femoral head is probably responsible. A limp, hip pain or knee pain may result. Treatment aims to contain the femoral head in the acetabulum to reduce the risks of future osteoarthritis.

Slipped upper femoral epiphysis

This condition is typically seen in overweight, hypogonadal boys, who often present with pain referred to the knee, although girls

may also experience this condition. The diagnosis may be difficult, but a "frog lateral" X-ray radiograph will show the deformity (Figure 5.2).

Surgical stabilization is needed as a matter of urgency to prevent further slippage of the epiphysis. The contralateral hip is at high risk of slippage, and patients and parents should be warned to return if any knee or hip pain occurs.

Septic arthritis

This is relatively uncommon, but it should be suspected in a child who is ill, toxic and unable to walk. Movement of the affected joint is not possible because of pain. Diagnosis is confirmed by raised white cell count and erythrocyte sedimentation rate and perhaps by effusion on ultrasound images. No test is perfectly sensitive or specific, so expert clinical judgement is required. Urgent surgical drainage is vital to reduce the risk of late osteoarthritis. Diagnosis may be particularly difficult in neonates. *Staphylococcus aureus* is the usual infective organism.

Transient synovitis or "irritable hip"

A reactive effusion may occur in the hip in association with a systemic viral illness. Affected children are not acutely ill and can move the hip, but with some degree of stiffness. An effusion may be seen on ultrasound images and the condition is usually self-limiting and responsive to non-steroidal anti-inflammatory drugs. Distinguishing this condition from septic arthritis can be a challenge, and occasionally these children must undergo aspiration to exclude a septic hip. Perthes' disease may present in the early stages with an effusion without changes visible on X-ray examination.

ABC of Rheumatology, 4th edn. Edited by Ade Adebajo.
©2010 Blackwell Publishing Ltd. 9781405170680.

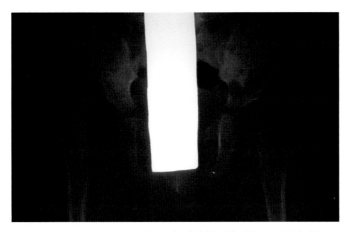

Figure 5.1 Anteroposterior radiograph of child with dislocated right hip. Note the lateral displacement of the femur and the poorly developed ossific nucleus of the hip

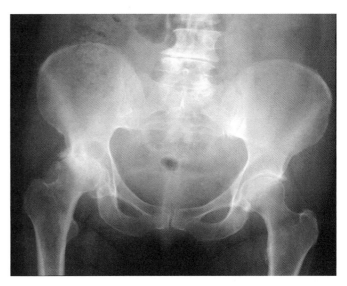

Figure 5.3 Osteoarthritis of the right hip, with joint space loss, subarticular cysts, peripheral osteophytes and subchondral sclerosis

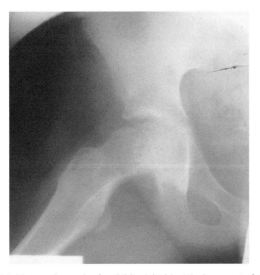

Figure 5.2 X-ray radiograph of a child's right hip. Displacement of the epiphysis relative to the femoral neck is easily seen

Box 5.2 **Causes of hip pain in adults**

- Osteoarthritis
- Other arthritides
  - Rheumatoid arthritis
  - Psoriatic arthritis
  - Ankylosing spondylitis
- Hip fracture
- Paget's disease
- Avascular necrosis
- Malignancy
- Infection
- Painful soft-tissue conditions around the hip
  - Trochanteric bursitis
  - Iliopsoas bursitis
  - Ischial bursitis
  - Meralgia paraesthetica
  - Snapping iliopsoas tendon
  - Torn acetabular labrum

Other arthritides

Juvenile chronic arthritis may present with hip pain. General management of the arthritic process is important, with physiotherapy to prevent joint contracture. Systemic therapy with disease-modifying agents (such as methotrexate, tumour necrosis inhibitor agents) can be very effective. These therapies have important potential toxicities and must be prescribed knowledgeably.

Hip pain in adults

Pain from the hip is usually felt in the groin or lateral or anterior thigh. Hip pain may also be referred to the knee; this may confuse the unwary! Although buttock pain may originate from the hip, the lumbar spine is the usual source. Hip disorders often produce a limp, a reduction in the distance that can be walked, and stiffness.

These functional limitations may prevent activities of daily living, such as getting in and out of baths, putting on shoes, and foot care. See Box 5.2 for a summary of the causes of hip pain in adults.

Osteoarthritis

Osteoarthritis is one of the most common causes of hip pain in adults (Figure 5.3). Although patients with osteoarthritis of the hips usually present in their 60s or even 70s, the problem can present earlier, especially in patients with prior hip trauma or congenital abnormalities (see previous sections on hip pain in children). Rest, simple analgesia, prescribed range-of-motion and

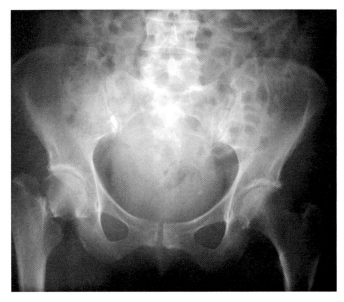

Figure 5.4 Subcapital fracture of the right hip

strengthening exercises and a walking stick often relieve the pain. A limp may develop, with associated stiffness. As hip abductors weaken, the patient may develop a Trendelenburg gait. In extreme situations, leg length is lost, and the hip adopts a fixed flexion and adduction deformity. Total hip replacement is extremely effective at relieving pain and improving functional status in osteoarthritis.

Other arthritides

Rheumatoid arthritis, psoriatic arthritis and ankylosing spondylitis can also produce hip pain. The latter is particularly associated with stiffness. Total hip replacement is often needed.

Hip fracture

Osteoporotic hip fracture in elderly women is epidemic. A fall followed by inability to bear weight and a short externally rotated leg are diagnostic. An undisplaced fracture may not stop the patient from bearing weight, and it may not be visible on initial X-ray examination. Repeat films are usually required, including a bone scan (Figure 5.4) or magnetic resonance imaging (MRI) if there is doubt. Treatment is typically surgical and includes stabilization with plates and/or screws, or by replacement of the femoral head (hemiarthroplasty) or total hip replacement.

Paget's disease

The pelvis is often involved in Paget's disease, and can cause hip pain. Treatment of the disease with bisphosphonates can reduce pain, but coexistent osteoarthritis of the hip can also occur.

Avascular necrosis

Segmental avascular necrosis of the weight-bearing portion of the femoral head can occur. This produces progressive pain, limp and late secondary osteoarthritis. An MRI gives a diagnosis in the early stages, but if radiological evidence is established, surgical treatment to arrest the disease is less successful. Hip replacement may ultimately be required. See Box 5.3 for a summary of the causes of avascular necrosis.

Malignancy

Metastases in the pelvis or proximal femur will produce hip pain. Treatment with local radiotherapy or bisphosphonates, or both, may slow the disease progress. Surgical stabilization of impending fractures may be required. Primary bone tumours as a cause of hip pain are extremely rare.

Infection

Primary septic arthritis is rare in adults. Risk factors include immuncompromise, prior hip joint disease and infection elsewhere. Plain X-ray examination may miss the diagnosis. Ultrasound scanning may show the presence of an effusion. Aspiration under fluoroscopic guidance is generally necessary to establish the diagnosis. Surgical drainage is usually necessary, along with prolonged intravenous antibiotics.

Painful soft-tissue conditions around the hip

Trochanteric bursitis—This is a usually self-limiting inflammation of the bursa between the greater trochanter and fascia lata. It is characterized by pain over the trochanter (not in the groin). This condition frequently accompanies other musculoskeletal problems, such as spinal stenosis, that alter gait and attendant muscle forces across the greater trochanter. Local physiotherapy, anti-inflammatories, rest, and occasionally local anaesthetic and steroid injections, can help.

Iliopsoas bursitis—The iliopsoas bursa is deep to the psoas muscle and anterior to the hip joint. Pain occurs in the groin and anterior thigh and can be exacerbated by resisted hip flexion and passive hip extension. This syndrome occasionally has an infectious aetiology. Thus, when the presentation is acute, especially painful and accompanied by systemic features, the work-up should be aggressive and include imaging-guided aspiration.

Snapping iliopsoas tendon—This causes a painful "clunk" in the groin when the hip goes from extension to flexion. The hip is otherwise normal. The psoas tendon impinges on the capsule of the hip anteriorly to produce discomfort. Diagnosis is made if movement of fluoroscopic X-ray contrast agent injected into the psoas tendon is abnormal. Surgical release may be needed.

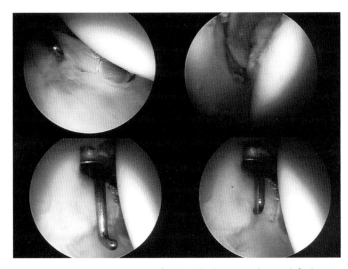

Figure 5.5 Arthroscopic images of a hip. The image at the top left shows a small acetabular labral tear

Ischial bursitis—The ischial bursa separates the gluteus maximus from the ischial tuberosity. Bursitis can arise from prolonged sitting or trauma to the bursa (hence the name "weaver's bottom"). Use of a cushion and local corticosteroid injection may be useful.

Meralgia paraesthetica—This condition refers to local compression of the lateral cutaneous femoral nerve (L2-3 distribution) at the inguinal ligament. Patients experience numbness and burning pain in the anterior thigh. The syndrome is felt to arise from direct compression of the nerve; hence, obesity, pregnancy, tight-fitting belts and waistbands and hip extension (as can occur with high heels) are risk factors, as is diabetes mellitus. The syndrome generally improves with conservative measures such as weight loss, and changes in clothing and shoes.

Torn acetabular labrum—This produces pain in the groin on rotatory movements of the hip, and the hip may feel unstable or give way. Labral tears can be associated with deformity of the femoral head or acetabulum. An MRI shows the abnormality, and the torn labrum can be removed arthroscopically (Figure 5.5).

Management of hip pain

The most important step in management of the painful hip is to establish the underlying aetiology and to treat it as specifically as possible. Thus infection of the hip should be diagnosed expeditiously and treated with surgical drainage and prolonged parenteral antibiotics. Fractures should be diagnosed and stabilized. Inflammatory arthritis can be treated with systemic therapy.

Here we present a few general principles that apply to the management of hip pain due to any number of aetiologies. First, a cane can be extremely helpful in unloading the painful hip and relieving pain. Patients must be shown the proper use of the cane in the contralateral hand.

Second, as with most other joints, the hip can become stiff with disuse and develop flexion contractures. This can be avoided with gentle range-of-motion exercises. If patients are losing motion, referral to a physiotherapist can be helpful.

Finally, it is important to recognize that one musculoskeletal problem can lead to another. Patients with spinal stenosis frequently develop trochanteric bursitis, for example. So while it is tempting to make a single, fully encompassing diagnosis in patients with musculoskeletal pain, the reality is that more than one condition could be present. While a patient's underlying problem may lie in the back, injection of a secondarily involved trochanteric bursa may provide dramatic benefit.

Further reading

McRae R. *Clinical Orthopaedic Examination*. Churchill Livingstone, Edinburgh, 1997.
Miller MD, ed. *Review of Orthopaedics*. WB Saunders, Philadelphia, 2000.
Solomon L, Nayagam D, Warwick D. *Apley's System of Orthopaedics and Fractures*. 8th edn. Arnold, London, 2001.

CHAPTER 6

Pain in the Knee

Adrian Dunbar[1] and Mark Wilkinson[2]

[1]Skipton, North Yorkshire, UK
[2]University of Sheffield, Sheffield, UK

OVERVIEW

- Knee pain is a frequent presenting complaint in primary care.
- Knee pain may arise from overuse injuries, trauma, degenerative change and inflammatory conditions.
- Osteoarthritis and rheumatoid arthritis affect the knee commonly.
- In most cases knee pain responds to simple measures such as lifestyle modification, simple analgesia and physiotherapy.
- Pain poorly controlled by simple measures, mechanical symptoms such as instability and locking, and progressive disability are indications for referral to secondary care.
- Where infection or tumour are suspected as a cause of knee pain, urgent referral to secondary care is required.

The knee is the largest joint in the body. It is a complex hinge that is made up of two separate articulations: the tibio-femoral joint and the patello-femoral joint. Knee motion occurs in a complex manner involving three planes, although the vast majority of its motion occurs in the sagittal plane (from full extension through to 140° of flexion).

Pain in the knee joint is one of the most common musculoskeletal complaints that presents to primary care physicians, and may arise from a broad range of pathologies. In the younger patient, pain most commonly arises from sporting or overuse injuries, which may affect the intra-articular or extra-articular structures of the knee. The knee is also a common site for inflammatory and infective pathologies. In the older patient, the most common cause is degenerative disease. Knee pain arising from osteoarthritis is a major cause of disability in the older patient, the prevalence and health-care costs of which continue to rise as the population ages.

The evaluation of knee pain centres on a thorough history and physical examination supplemented, where necessary, with appropriate imaging and laboratory tests (Figure 6.1).

ABC of Rheumatology, 4th edn. Edited by Ade Adebajo.
©2010 Blackwell Publishing Ltd. 9781405170680.

Traumatic causes of knee pain

Injuries are a common cause of knee pain. Most knee injuries in sport occur as a result of indirect trauma, such as a twisting moment to the knee. The structures most commonly injured by this mechanism are the menisci, the collateral ligaments and the cruciate ligaments. These structures may be damaged in isolation, or may occur in combination (for example the anterior cruciate ligament, medial collateral ligament and medial meniscus may be injured in O'Donoghue's triad). Direct trauma to the knee (such as during contact sport, an industrial accident or a motor-vehicle collision) most commonly causes bone contusions, fracture or dislocation that may affect the patello-femoral or tibio-femoral joint. Dislocation of the tibio-femoral joint indicates high-energy trauma, and is commonly associated with neurovascular damage.

Meniscus injury

Meniscus injury in young people can present as an acute injury or as a chronic condition with an insidious onset. The majority of meniscus tears in young people occur after mild- to moderate-energy twisting injuries and are typically isolated injuries or associated with a collateral ligament strain. The medial meniscus is damaged three times more commonly than the lateral meniscus (Figure 6.2). Higher-energy twisting injuries are commonly associated with an anterior cruciate ligament injury, an acute haemarthrosis and inability to bear weight. Patients with meniscus tears have focal tenderness over the joint line and may experience mechanical catching and locking symptoms in the knee in addition to joint effusion and pain. Magnetic resonance imaging (MRI) can aid in establishing the diagnosis in cases where the history and physical examination are equivocal. Acute tears that occur in the well-vascularized peripheral portion of the meniscus are amenable to arthroscopic repair, which preserves meniscus function. Where an anterior cruciate ligament injury is also present this is reconstructed concurrently. Chronic meniscal tears are typically avascular with degenerative characteristics and will not heal if repaired. Arthroscopic resection is confined to the torn and degenerate portions of meniscus, as early-onset osteoarthritis of the knee commonly follows complete meniscal resection.

Articular cartilage injury

Articular cartilage injury is often the result of a traumatic episode

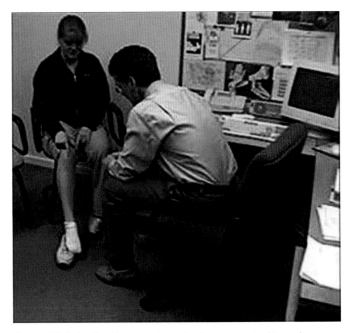

Figure 6.1 A detailed history and examination are required to make an accurate clinical diagnosis in the patient presenting with knee pain

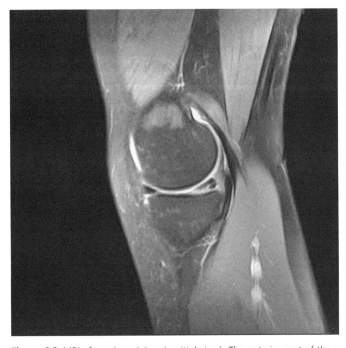

Figure 6.2 MRI of meniscus injury (sagittal view). The anterior part of the medial meniscus can be seen as a black triangle on the left side of the joint line; the black triangle of the posterior part of the meniscus has a white line running through it, representing an oblique tear

Table 6.1 Post-traumatic knee swelling and the most common associated diagnoses

Immediate haemarthrosis	Delayed effusion	Minimal effusion
Anterior cruciate ligament tear	Meniscus tear	Collateral ligament tear
Osteochondral fracture	Posterior cruciate ligament tear	
Patellar dislocation		

removal for displaced osteochondral fragments. Occult episodes of trauma to the knee may result in separation of cartilage from the subchondral bone, termed osteochondritis dissecans. Patients complain of poorly localized pain. The diagnosis is made from plain radiographs or MRI scans, and treatment commonly involves arthroscopic resection of loose cartilage.

A detailed history of the mechanism of injury and physical examination provide valuable information to differentiate between the various traumatic causes of knee pain. Knee pain from injury has a sudden onset at the time of the injury episode and is often accompanied by local soft-tissue swelling and an effusion. Certain fractures and dislocations may exhibit gross deformity; however, the majority of knee and patellar dislocations spontaneously reduce before presentation. A haemarthrosis develops quickly (over a period of minutes to a few hours) and indicates significant intra-articular injury, such as an anterior cruciate ligament tear, intra-articular fracture or osteochondral injury, or patellar dislocation. Effusions, which develop over several hours, tend to be associated with meniscal injuries (Table 6.1).

Radiographs should be obtained when evaluating any knee injury to exclude a fracture, dislocation or other significant abnormality. After obtaining radiographs, additional diagnostic tests may be indicated, including a computed tomography scan in the case of intra-articular fractures, or MRI when a soft-tissue or osteochondral injury is suspected. In the absence of neurovascular compromise or gross deformity, initial treatment of traumatic knee pain should consist of restricted weight bearing, ice and elevation. Severe injuries require immediate referral for orthopaedic surgical evaluation.

Knee pain in younger people and athletes

Knee pain in younger people and athletes can be caused by overuse syndromes, meniscus injury or articular cartilage abnormality. Common overuse syndromes include patellar tendonopathy, anterior knee pain syndrome, pes anserine bursitis and iliotibial band friction syndrome (Table 6.2).

Patellar tendonopathy

Patellar tendonopathy is caused by repetitive activity, particularly "explosive" athletics such as jumping. Patients complain of pain and soft-tissue swelling about the patellar tendon, usually at its

that involves an impact injury to the cartilage surface. Articular cartilage injuries can result in focal pain, joint effusion and mechanical catching symptoms. Treatment comprises graduated physiotherapy for undisplaced injuries and arthroscopic repair or

Table 6.2 Symptoms associated with overuse injuries

Symptom	Likely diagnosis
Pain adjacent to patella Pain ascending/descending stairs Pain when sitting for prolonged periods ("movie theatre sign")	Anterior knee pain syndrome
Pain in patellar tendon Pain with jumping	Patellar tendonopathy
Lateral knee pain with repetitive activity	Iliotibial band friction syndrome
Medial knee pain distal to joint line	Pes anserine bursitis

Box 6.1 Diagnosis of osteoarthritis

- Osteoarthritis is diagnosed clinically by the presence of:
  - Chronic knee pain
  - Morning stiffness lasting less than 30 minutes
  - Joint crepitus
  - Range of movement restricted by pain
  - Presence of osteophytes

Box 6.2 Non-pharmacological treatments

- Non-pharmacological treatments with an evidence base include:
  - Weight loss
  - Aerobic exercise
  - Specific knee-strengthening exercise
  - Patellar taping
  - Acupuncture
  - Knee bracing

proximal attachment to the patella. Treatment consists of ice, pain-relieving medication, activity modification and strengthening exercises focusing on eccentric loading of the tendon.

Anterior knee pain syndrome

Anterior knee pain syndrome occurs in patients who engage in repetitive athletic activity, in those with abnormalities in extensor mechanism alignment and in those who are overweight. Patients with anterior knee pain syndrome complain of pain in the front of the knee, which is accentuated by ascending and descending stairs, squatting, kneeling and by sitting for long periods of time. The pain may be located directly behind the patella or in the medial or lateral retinaculum. Treatment should include activity modification, weight control if necessary, physiotherapy to strengthen the quadriceps muscles (particularly vastus medialis) and core musculature, and appropriate pain-relieving medication.

Pes anserine bursitis

Pes anserine bursitis is an inflammation of the bursa overlying the insertion site of the semitendinosus, gracilis and sartorius tendons in the anteromedial aspect of the proximal tibia. Patients complain of medial knee pain distal to the medial joint line. Treatment can include activity modification, strengthening exercises and anti-inflammatory medication. Chronic symptoms may respond to local corticosteroid injection.

Iliotibial band friction syndrome

Iliotibial band friction syndrome is an inflammation of the iliotibial band, the distal portion of the tensor fascia lata muscle that inserts into the anterolateral aspect of the proximal tibia. Patients are usually runners or cyclists who complain of activity-related lateral knee pain. This condition responds well to activity modification, stretching and strengthening exercises, ice and anti-inflammatory medications.

Knee pain in older people

Twenty-five percent of people over the age of 50 report chronic knee pain, and degenerative arthritis of the knee is common in this age group (Box 6.1). However, clinical symptoms and radiological severity of arthritis are poorly correlated. Many older people with knee pain have minor radiological evidence of arthritic change. Conversely, many people with advanced radiological changes are pain-free. Arthritis of the knee is often associated with periarticular soft-tissue problems, and indeed these can often be a major source of knee pain. Pes anserine bursitis is a common example. Plain radiographic imaging is not always helpful in the assessment of patients with knee pain, and the diagnosis of osteoarthritis is often a clinical one. An MRI scan may assist in the diagnosis of an occult degenerate meniscal tear.

The management of osteoarthritis is, for most people, the management of their knee pain and lifestyle modification (Box 6.2). The high prevalence of knee pain in the community means that such treatments should be simple, safe, cost-effective and, ideally, self-administered. Initial treatments consist of simple analgesia, such as paracetamol, that is safe and effective. The place of oral glucosamine and similar nutraceuticals is still debated in the presence of conflicting reports from different studies, and none have yet been convincingly shown to alter the course of osteoarthritis.

Oral non-steroidal anti-inflammatory drugs (NSAIDs) are prescribed commonly; however, there is little evidence of benefit over simple analgesia, and they are associated with significant risk of serious adverse effects in the older patient. Their use should be considered after failure of simple measures such as weight loss, exercise regimes and use of simple analgesics.

Local treatments, such as topical non-steroidal anti-inflammatory gels are effective in the short term, particularly in the setting of acute symptomatic flares. Injected treatments include corticosteroids and hyaluronans. Intra-articular steroids can be very effec-

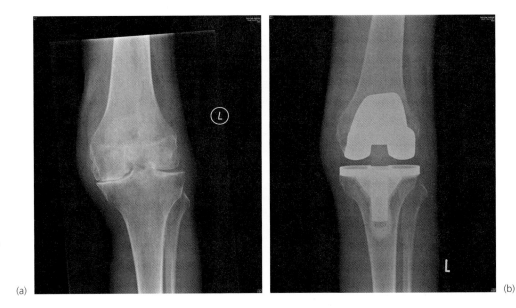

Figure 6.3 Radiograph showing the typical features of knee osteoarthritis, joint-space narrowing, subchondral sclerosis and osteophyte formation (a), and following treatment with total knee replacement (b)

(a)

(b)

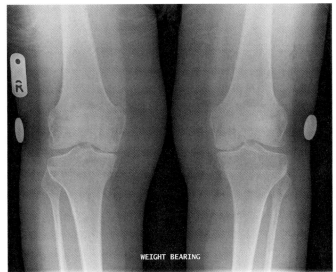

(a)

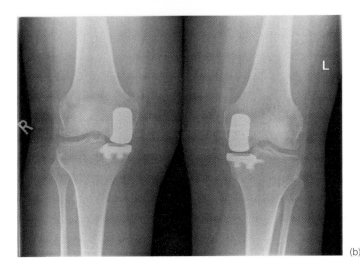

(b)

Figure 6.4 Radiographs showing bilateral isolated osteoarthritis of the medial compartment of the knee (a), and following treatment with bilateral unicompartmental knee replacement (b)

tive in relieving knee pain for several weeks or months. Hyaluronans have a longer-lasting effect, but are very much more expensive and require a series of injections over time. Both have good safety profiles, although certain hyaluronans can cause pseudoseptic joint inflammation and effusion.

Arthroscopic surgical treatment for arthritis of the knee is reserved for the treatment of mechanical symptoms such as joint catching, locking or instability due to a loose body or meniscal tear. In the absence of mechanical symptoms, arthroscopic interventions are no more effective than placebo.

In up to 40% of patients, disease does not progress significantly after initial presentation, or does so very slowly. In these patients use of simple, safe, cost-effective treatments is essential for effective and economic management. Joint replacement surgery is indicated in those patients whose disease progresses such that their symptoms become poorly controlled despite the treatment measures outlined above. In most patients this entails total knee replacement (Figure 6.3). In a small proportion of patients the arthritis is limited to one compartment of knee, in which case a unicompartmental joint replacement is an effective alternative to total knee replacement, and is associated with good functional outcomes in suitable patients (Figure 6.4). The results of joint-replacement surgery are excellent in over 90% of patients in terms of improvement in health-related quality of life.

Knee pain in systemic disease

Pain and swelling in the knee may be a feature of systemic illness. Patients should be asked about pain in other joints, previously painful, swollen joints and a family history of joint disease. Systemic symptoms such as malaise, pyrexia, anorexia and weight loss may provide clues to the origin of the knee pain. Symptoms affecting other organs, such as the skin, bowel, eyes or genito-urinary tract, may also be of diagnostic relevance.

The knee is the most commonly affected large joint in rheumatoid arthritis. The knees are usually affected bilaterally, and symptom onset usually occurs early in the course of the disease. The knee is also commonly affected in the other chronic inflammatory arthritides, including psoriatic arthritis and ankylosing spondylitis. The treatment of the knee pain in these conditions is considered along with the management of the systemic disease and includes lifestyle modification, physiotherapy, disease-modifying agents, NSAIDs, novel biological agents and total joint-replacement surgery.

The knee is the most commonly infected joint. Joint infection presents with a red, swollen, hot knee, difficulty in weight bearing and a limitation in the range of passive motion. Occasionally, the infection may originate in the metaphyseal region of the tibia or femur, rather than the knee joint itself (Figure 6.5). A suspected infection of the knee requires immediate referral to secondary care for assessment and treatment. The most common infecting organism is *Staphylococcus aureus*. Less common infections include *Streptococcus*, *Gonococcus*, *Brucella* and, rarely, tuberculosis. Infective arthritis should always be considered in the immunocompromised and other patients with increased infective risk, e.g. intravenous drug users.

Aspiration of the joint for microbiological culture is the most important investigation for the accurate diagnosis of infection. This must be carried out at initial assessment, and before the administration of antibiotics. Aspiration of the knee made after antibiotic administration often results in a false-negative microbiological culture result and a missed diagnosis. Other useful diagnostic tests include concurrent aspirate microscopy for crystals, and

serological measurement of white cell count, erythrocyte sedimentation rate and C-reactive protein. The treatment of the infected knee includes initiation of systemic antibiotics immediately after knee aspiration, typically using an agent with broad Gram-positive antimicrobial activity, and serial joint aspiration or arthroscopic-assisted washout. The choice of antibiotic is adjusted as indicated by the aspirate microbiological culture sensitivities, and may be continued for up to 6 weeks orally, although specialist microbiological advice should be taken where infection is confirmed from aspirate culture.

The differential diagnosis of the hot, swollen, painful knee includes systemic inflammatory conditions such as calcium pyrophosphate arthropathy, gout, Reiter's disease and pre-patellar bursitis. Aspiration of joint fluid for crystal microscopy and culture is important, as are appropriate serological investigations, both in confirming the correct diagnosis and in excluding joint infection. Rarely, infections of the genito-urinary tract and viral infections may present with bilateral swollen, tender knees with a large effusion of sympathetic origin. Radiographs are frequently of limited diagnostic utility in such cases.

Other causes of knee pain

Hip pain may occasionally refer to the anterior distal thigh or the knee. A complete examination of the patient with knee pain includes an examination of the hip to exclude this cause of knee pain. Knee pain may also present as part of a chronic widespread pain syndrome. An adequate general musculoskeletal assessment is essential if appropriate treatment of the knee pain is to be effected. In the presence of polyarthralgia, or symptoms suggestive of a fibromyalgia syndrome, the knee pain is unlikely to be adequately managed by focusing on the knee alone. Attention should be paid to management of the global pain problem.

"Red flags"

Although primary bone tumours are rare, the knee is one of the most commonly affected sites for benign tumours, including osteoid osteoma, enchondroma and chondroblastoma, and malignant tumours, including osteosarcoma and chondrosarcoma. Ewing's sarcomas also commonly affect the knee. In children and young adults who are very active, knee pain may be related to recent activity. Unexplained pain, pain that is worse at night, unexplained swelling and systemic symptoms are all "red flag" features that may indicate a bone tumour. Patients in whom a bone tumour is suspected should be referred early to a centre specializing in their management.

Further reading

Brukner P, Khan K. Lateral, medial and posterior knee pain. In: Brukner P & Khan K, eds. *Clinical Sports Medicine*, 3rd edn. McGraw Hill, London, 2007. Available online at http://www.clinicalsportsmedicine.com/chapters/index.htm

Brukner P, Khan K, Cooper R, Morris H, Arendt, L. Acute knee injuries. In: Brukner P & Khan K, eds. *Clinical Sports Medicine*, 3rd edn. McGraw Hill,

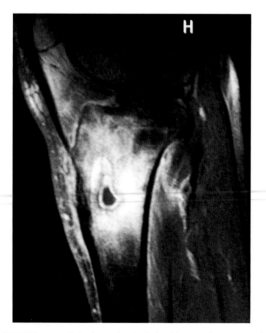

Figure 6.5 MRI scan of the knee (sagittal view) in a patient presenting with an acute, red knee. In this case the diagnosis was acute *Staphylococcal* osteomyelitis of the proximal tibial metaphysis

London, 2007. Available online at http://www.clinicalsportsmedicine.com/chapters/index.htm

Brukner P, Khan K, Crossley K, Cook J, Cowan S, McConnell J. Anterior knee pain. In: Brukner P & Khan K, eds. *Clinical Sports Medicine*, 3rd edn. McGraw Hill, London, 2007. Available online at http://www.clinicalsports-medicine.com/chapters/index.htm

Panayi G, Dickson DJ. *Clinical Practice Series: Arthritis*. Churchill Livingston, London, 2004.

Underwood M. *Chronic Knee Pain in the Elderly*. Reports on the Rheumatic Diseases Series 5, no. 5. Arthritis Research Campaign, York, UK, 2005. Available online at http://www.arc.org.uk/arthinfo/medpubs/6525/6525.asp

CHAPTER 7

Pain in the Foot

James Woodburn[1] and Philip S Helliwell[2]

[1]Glasgow Caledonian University, Glasgow, UK
[2]University of Leeds, Leeds, UK

OVERVIEW

- Foot pain is common and can be associated with a number of local or generalized conditions.
- Clinical examination and simple investigations can usually identify the cause of the pain.
- Foot pain is a common feature in most rheumatic diseases, including rheumatoid arthritis and osteoarthritis.
- Podiatrists, general practitioners, rheumatologists and orthopaedic surgeons are involved in the management of foot pain.

Foot pain is common. It may be caused by local disease, be associated with systemic disease or be a reflection of chronic widespread pain. In general, a multidisciplinary approach to treatment is preferable. This is reflected in increasingly close liaison between podiatry, rheumatology and orthopaedic departments. State-registered podiatrists offer a range of treatments, from skin lesion care to orthoses and, more recently, ambulatory forefoot surgery. To understand dysfunction, clinicians should be familiar with the normal development and anatomical variants of the foot (Figures 7.1 and 7.2; Boxes 7.1 and 7.2).

Foot pain in children

Foot pain may be associated with congenital abnormalities, such as equinovarus deformity. Such structural abnormalities may reflect underlying neurological diseases, such as cerebral palsy. A rigid pronated foot in the early teens may be the first symptom of a tarsal coalition (Figure 7.3). Gait abnormalities, such as intoeing, may be of concern to parents, but they are seldom treated actively.

Juvenile chronic arthritis

The knee and ankle joints are most often affected in all subtypes of juvenile chronic arthritis. Children may present with a limp or reluctance to walk. In the hind foot, pain and reflex muscle spasm can lead to valgus deformity (in two-thirds of cases) or varus deformity (in one-third of cases). In some patients, this may

progress to bony ankylosis. The child may be reluctant to push off with the forefoot during walking, and pressure studies show poor contact of the foot to the floor. Lack of use can lead to delayed maturation of bone or soft tissue, and, in such cases, discrepancy in leg length should be sought carefully.

Box 7.1 **Characteristics of the adult foot**

Three main types of foot
- Normal
- Pronated (flat)
- Supinated (high arch)

Examination
- Examine the foot when bearing weight and when unloaded and be sure to look at the plantar surface of the foot for callus formation (often associated with high pressure)
- Inspect the patient's shoes for abnormal or uneven wear
- Consult a podiatrist if a structural or mechanical abnormality is suspected—many can be treated with orthoses

Box 7.2 **Characteristics of children's feet**

Normal foot
- Flexible foot structure (may look flat with a valgus heel)
- Medial longitudinal arch forms when child stands on tiptoe
- Heel-to-toe walking
- Forefoot in line with rear foot
- Mobile joints with painless motion and no swelling
- Adopts adult morphology by about 8 years of age

Abnormal foot
- Inflexible
- Lesser toe deformities
- Rigid valgus (pronated) foot with everted heel position
- High-arch foot with toe retraction and tight extensor tendons
- Toe walking
- Delay or difficulty in walking or running
- Abducted or adducted forefoot relative to heel
- Pain, swelling or stiffness of joints
- Hallux deformity

ABC of Rheumatology, 4th edn. Edited by Ade Adebajo.
©2010 Blackwell Publishing Ltd. 9781405170680.

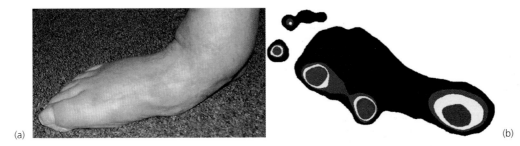

Figure 7.1 Abnormally pronated foot (a), with pressure profile showing large weight-bearing surface and higher pressures medially (b)

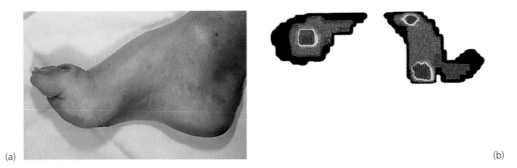

Figure 7.2 Abnormally supinated foot (a), with pressure profile showing small weight-bearing surface and high pressures over first and fifth metatarsal heads (b)

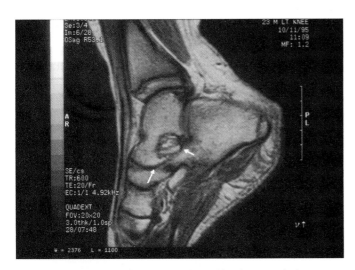

Figure 7.3 Tarsal coalition. MRI in a patient with calcaneonavicular coalition. Note synostosis between the calcaneus and navicular bones (arrows)

Pain in the forefoot (metatarsalgia)

Morton's metatarsalgia (interdigital neuroma)

This normally affects the proximal part of the plantar digital nerve and accompanying plantar digital artery. Trauma to these structures leads to histological changes, including inflammatory oedema, microscopic changes in the neurolemma, fibrosis and, later, degeneration of the nerve. Morton's neuroma is the result of an entrapment lesion of the interdigital nerve.

Clinical features—Clinical features include a gradual onset, with sudden attacks of neuralgic pain or paraesthesia during walking—often in the third and fourth toe. Examination may show lesser toe deformities, slight splaying of the forefoot, abnormal pronation and hallux valgus. These often occur in women who wear court shoes. Compression of the cleft or laterally across the metatarsal heads may produce acute pain and the characteristic "Mulder's click."

Treatment—Patients should be given advice about suitable footwear and possibly should be given orthoses to control abnormal pronation. Injections of local anaesthetic and hydrocortisone around the nerve, or surgical excision, can be helpful.

Stress fracture (march fracture)

Stress fractures are associated with increased activity, and lesions can affect any of the metatarsal shafts, often along the line of the surgical neck. They can occasionally be seen in patients with osteoporosis as a pathological fracture.

Clinical features—Patients have a history of a change in the amount of activity, change in occupation or footwear, or sudden weight gain. The symptom is a dull ache along the affected metatarsal shaft, which changes to a sharp ache just behind the metatarsal head. The pain is exacerbated by exercise and is more acute at "toe off." Tenderness and swelling is felt over the dorsal surface of the shaft. Pain is produced by compression of the metatarsal head or traction of the toe. X-ray examination may not show the fracture for 2–4 weeks, but if it is important to confirm the diagnosis—e.g. for an athlete who needs advice on whether to continue playing sport—a bone scan can reveal it earlier.

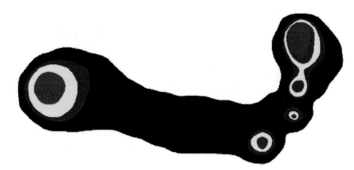

Figure 7.4 Pressure profile of the right foot of a 54-year-old patient with rheumatoid arthritis. Note absent lesser toe contact and high pressure (hot colours) over central metatarsal heads

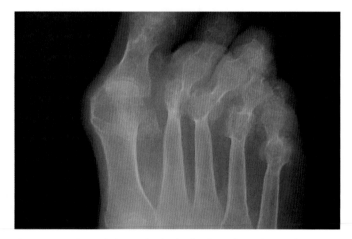

Figure 7.5 Advanced destruction in the forefoot of a patient with rheumatoid arthritis

Treatment—Rest and local protective padding with partial immobilization are usually enough. These fractures rarely require casting.

Acute synovitis

This condition is normally associated with acute trauma, which leads to inflammation of the synovial membrane and effusion. Freiberg's disease may also contribute. Systemic causes of acute synovitis, such as rheumatoid arthritis (Figures 7.4 and 7.5) or infection, should be excluded when making a diagnosis.

Clinical features—It is rare in children but often affects young adults. Patients complain of a sudden onset of painful throbbing that is made worse by movement. The patient may have experienced trauma or have a systemic inflammatory disorder. Any movement of the joint produces pain. Fusiform swelling is present around the distended joint, and crepitus may be felt.

Treatment—Rest, immobilization and ultrasound treatment may help if trauma is the cause. Anti-inflammatory drugs sometimes help. Previously unsuspected systemic arthritis should be investigated.

Acute inflammation of anterior metatarsal soft tissue

This common condition is generally found in middle-aged women. It affects the soft tissues of the plantar aspect of the forefoot and is associated with increased shear forces, such as occur when wearing "slip-on" and high-heeled court shoes.

Clinical features—Patients present with a burning or throbbing pain localized to the soft tissues anterior to the metatarsal heads. The pain usually develops over a few weeks, is often associated with walking in a particular pair of shoes, and is usually relieved by rest. The tissues are inflamed, warm and congested. Direct palpation, rotation and simulation of shear forces on the foot exacerbate the pain. Examination of patients' shoes may reveal a worn insole, with a depression under the metatarsal heads.

Management—Advice on footwear, with adequate support or cushioning, should be given. Associated abnormal pronation or lesser toe deformities should be corrected with orthoses.

Osteochondritis (Freiberg's infraction)

This quite common condition generally affects the second or third metatarsal heads. It is an aseptic necrosis or epiphyseal infraction associated with trauma and localized minute thrombosis of the epiphysis.

Clinical features—Osteochondritis affects teenagers and is associated with increased sporting activity. The presenting complaint is often a limp, with dull pain associated with movement of the metatarsal phalangeal joint, exacerbated at "toe off". The long-term result is a flattened metatarsal head, which can progress to arthritis. The affected joint may be slightly swollen, with a disparity in toe length and width. Traction causes pain. Restricted movement may be due to muscle spasm in the early stages and later to arthritis. Radiographs show distortion of the metatarsal head.

Treatment—In the early stages, rest and immobilization are enough, but sometimes patients eventually need corrective surgery.

Plantar metatarsal bursitis

This condition may affect the deep anatomical or superficial adventitious bursae. In the acute form—such as in dancers, squash players or skiers—the first metatarsal is usually affected, while the second to fourth metatarsals are affected in chronic inflammatory arthritis (Figure 7.6).

Clinical features—Patients present with a throbbing pain under a metatarsal head that usually persists at rest and is exacerbated when the area is first loaded. The acute condition affects men and women equally, usually in younger adults. If a superficial bursa is affected, there will be signs of acute inflammation, with fluctuant swelling and warmth. With deep bursitis, the tissues are tight and congested. Direct pressure or compression produces pain, as does dorsiflexion of the associated digit.

Treatment—Anti-inflammatory drugs are useful; in practice, local gels and systemic oral drugs help. Injections of corticosteroid may

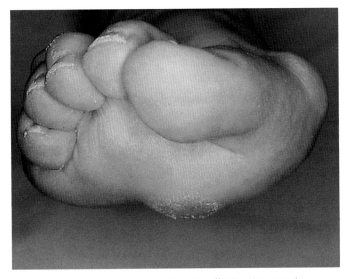

Figure 7.6 Severe plantar metatarsal bursitis affecting the second metatarsal head of a patient with rheumatoid arthritis. The overlying callus suggests that this is a high-pressure site during normal gait

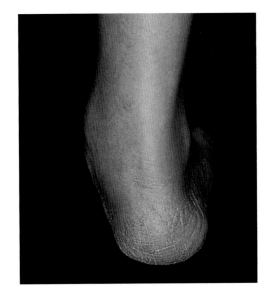

Figure 7.7 Valgus heel with bulging of the talar head medially

---

Box 7.3 **Causes of pain in the forefoot**

Primary
• Functional and structural forefoot pathologies

Secondary
• Rheumatoid disease
• Stress lesions
• Post-traumatic syndromes
• Diabetes
• Gout
• Paralytic deformity
• Sesamoid pathology
• Osteoarthritis

Unrelated to weight distribution
• Nerve-root pathology
• Tarsal tunnel nerve compression syndrome
  ○ Analogous to carpal tunnel syndrome
  ○ Often misdiagnosed as foot strain or plantar fasciitis
  ○ Primary symptom is burning feeling on sole of foot in the dermatome served by the medial plantar nerve

---

be indicated in severe cases. Patients must rest the affected part; this may be achieved by protective padding. Any underlying deformity or foot type with abnormal function should be assessed and treated.

A summary of causes of pain in the forefoot is presented in Box 7.3.

Plantar fascia affections

Pain along the medial longitudinal arch is quite common. Most affected patients have abnormal foot mechanics, such as abnormal pronation, valgus heel (Figure 7.7) or flat foot. Mechanical dys-

function and change in medial arch posture can place strain on soft tissues, which results in localized or more diffuse pain—the foot's equivalent to low back pain syndrome. Other conditions include true plantar fasciitis, which is characterized by a few fast-growing nodules in the fascia, and plantar fibromatosis, which is characterized by fibrous nodules and contracture of the fascia.

Treatment of true plantar fascial strain requires rest, control of abnormal function with orthoses, and stretching exercises. Ultrasound treatment seems helpful, but controlled trials are lacking.

Painful heel

Sever's disease (calcaneal apophysitis)

This was thought to be an avascular necrosis of growing bone but is now interpreted as a chronic strain at the attachment of the posterior apophysis of the calcaneus to the main body of the bone, possibly from pull of the Achilles tendon. It is analogous, therefore, to Osgood-Schlatter disease of the tibial tuberosity.

Clinical features—The condition usually affects boys aged 8–13 years, who complain of a dull ache behind the heel of gradual onset that is exacerbated by jumping or occurs just before "heel lift". A limp is usually seen with early heel lift. Rest normally relieves the pain. Tenderness is seen over the lower posterior part of the tuberosity of the calcaneus. Radiographs are usually normal.

Treatment—In most cases, reassurance and advice about reducing activities will suffice: the condition usually subsides spontaneously. In some cases, heel lifts help; occasionally, if the pain is severe, a below knee walking cast is needed.

Plantar calcaneal bursitis ("policeman's heel")

This is inflammation of the adventitious bursa beneath the plantar aspect of the calcaneal tuberosities (Figure 7.8). It is associated with shearing stress caused by an altered angle of heel strike.

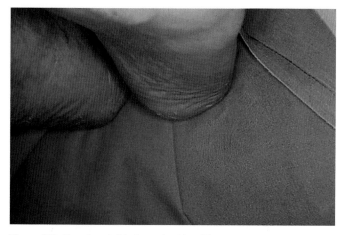

Figure 7.8 Chronic painful plantar heel bursitis

Clinical features—The condition is characterized by an increasingly severe burning, aching and throbbing pain on the plantar surface of the heel. A history of increased activity or weight gain is usual. The heel seems normal but may feel warm. Direct pressure or sideways compression causes pain. The tissues may feel tight and congested.

Treatment—Rest and anti-inflammatory drugs may be useful. Heel cushions and medial arch supports are also used. Stretching exercises (such as rolling a bottle under the foot) can help. Little evidence supports ultrasound treatment, local steroid injections or shortwave diathermy.

Chronic inflammation of the heel pad

This is a distinct clinical condition that usually results from trauma or heavy heel strike. It is sometimes seen in elderly people as their fat pads atrophy or in those who suddenly become more active.

Clinical features—A generalized warm, dull throbbing pain is felt over the weight-bearing area of the heel; this develops over a few months. The pain is most intense typically on first rising. Tenderness is experienced over the heel, which feels tight and distended.

Treatment—Normally, this condition improves with time and rest. Soft heel cushions and medial arch fillers sometimes help. Ultrasound treatment and shortwave diathermy are often used, but controlled trials are few. Steroid injections have an early effect but do not influence the condition's favourable natural history. Steroid injections can be more painful than the condition unless they are done carefully, with adequate slow infiltration of local anaesthetic (or an ankle tibial nerve block) before injection.

Achilles tendon affections

Inflammation of the Achilles tendon and surrounding soft tissue may be associated with overuse or systemic inflammatory disorders (Box 7.4). Inflammation of the tendon, peritendon tissues and bursae give slightly different clinical pictures. Conditions such as xanthoma can also affect the Achilles tendon and produce fusiform swelling in the tendon. In such cases, cholesterol concentrations

---

Box 7.4 **Achilles tendon affections**

Tendinitis
- Presents as painful local swelling of the tendon, which moves with the tendon as the foot is dorsiflexed and plantar flexed
- Important to check the tendon for evidence of partial or complete rupture, which is often missed because of inflammation
- Note recent use of quinolone antibiotics (e.g. ciprofloxacin)

Peritendinitis
- Presents as large diffuse swelling of tissues surrounding the tendon that remains static as the tendon is stretched
- Patients experience pain and crepitus on palpation

Achilles tendon bursitis
- Presents as diffuse fusiform swelling inferior to the Achilles tendon that fills the normal indentation seen below the malleoli and deep to the Achilles tendon

---

Box 7.5 **Common causes of painful heel**

Pain within heel
- Disease of calcaneus-osteomyelitis, tumours, Paget's disease
- Arthritis of subtalar joint complex

Pain behind heel
- Haglund's deformity ("pump bumps", "heel bumps")
- Rupture of Achilles tendon
- Achilles paratendinitis
- Posterior tibial paratendinitis or tenosynovitis
- Peroneal paratendinitis or tenosynovitis
- Posterior calcaneal bursitis
- Calcaneal apophysitis

Pain beneath heel
- Tender heel pad
- Plantar fasciitis

---

should be checked and treated if raised. Rheumatoid nodules, and occasionally gouty tophi, can also be found within the substance of the Achilles tendon.

Clinical features—Clinical features vary according to the tissues affected. Increased activity leading to an overuse syndrome may be a feature in younger, active patients.

Treatment—Treatment depends on the primary cause. Partial or complete ruptures of the tendon need immobilization and surgical repair. For inflammatory conditions, non-steroidal anti-inflammatory drugs may help, as may ultrasound treatment, friction, rest and shock-absorbing heel lifts. Inflammation may be triggered by overuse through poor foot mechanics; in such cases, orthoses may control the pronation. Hydrocortisone injections may be useful if the bursa or peritendons are affected, but they are contraindicated for the tendon itself. Ultrasound imaging may be useful.

A summary of common causes of painful heel is presented in Box 7.5.

Arthropathies that affect the foot

Osteoarthritis
Osteoarthritis in the foot may be asymptomatic, but it can lead to pain, joint stiffness, functional loss and disability. The most common sites are the first metatarsophalangeal joint (hallux rigidus) and the tarsus joints. Biomechanical factors are often involved in the development of degenerative joint changes (for example, compensatory foot pronation in subtalar osteoarthritis). Trauma, recurrent urate gout, and the demands of fashion—such as inappropriate footwear—are other factors; however, the broad style of modern shoes may be beneficial.

Rheumatoid arthritis
Rheumatoid arthritis often starts in the foot, particularly at the metatarsophalangeal joints. The forefoot is painful and stiff, and direct transverse pressure to the forefoot or squeezing a single metatarsophalangeal joint is painful. Non-specific metatarsalgia is often diagnosed. In the early stages of the disease, the hind foot, particularly the subtalar joint, may also be painful. Synovitis of tendon sheaths around the ankle may also occur. In chronic rheumatoid feet, severe pain in the forefoot may continue, with a sensation of walking on pebbles. Gross deformity causes dysfunction and disability (Figures 7.9–7.12).

Seronegative spondyloarthritis
This group includes ankylosing spondylitis (Figure 7.13), psoriatic arthritis (Figure 7.14), undifferentiated seronegative arthropathy and reactive arthritis. Achilles peritendinitis and retrocalcaneal bursitis can be seen. In radiographs, inflammatory spurs may be seen on the calcaneum at the insertion points of the Achilles tendon and plantar fascia. Asymmetrical heel pain may result from a plantar calcaneal enthesopathy.

The pattern of articular involvement in the foot may vary from a single "sausage toe" (dactylitis) (Figure 7.15) to a very destructive arthritis. Painful stiff interphalangeal and metatarsophalangeal joints, often in an asymmetrical pattern, are common. Claw toe

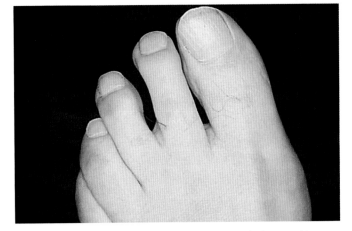
Figure 7.10 Metatarsophalangeal joint synovitis in early rheumatoid arthritis: note a widening of the first and second cleft—the "daylight sign"

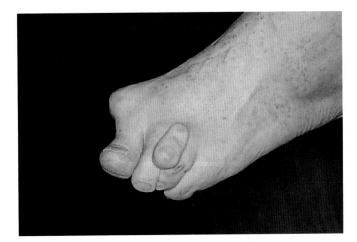
Figure 7.11 Extensive foot deformity

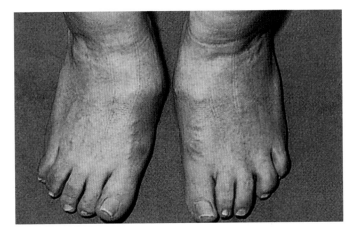
Figure 7.9 Midtarsal osteoarthritis

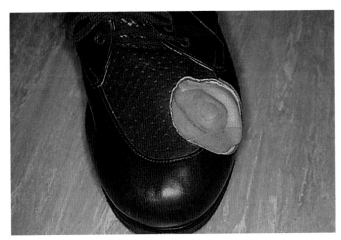
Figure 7.12 Drastic self-adjustment of surgical shoes to gain pain relief

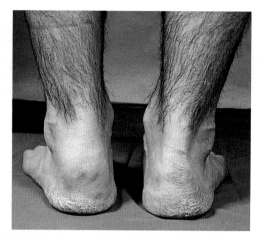

Figure 7.13 Ankylosing spondylitis of the feet: the hind foot is predominantly affected

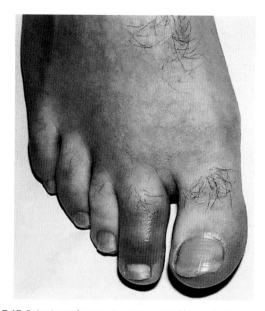

Figure 7.15 Reiter's syndrome—"sausage toe" (this is also found with psoriatic arthropathy)

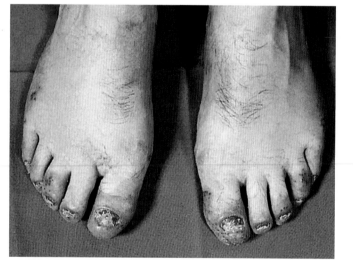

Figure 7.14 Psoriatic arthropathy

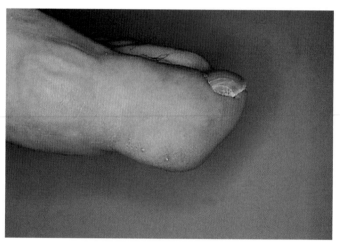

Figure 7.16 Large painful tophi over the interphalangeal joint of the hallux

and hallux valgus deformity are more obvious. Nail dystrophy may be seen, with typical psoriatic pitting, onycholysis, subungual hyperkeratosis, discoloration and transverse ridging.

Pustular psoriasis and keratoderma blennorrhagica on the plantar aspect of the foot may contribute to pain when walking.

The diabetic foot—In the presence of neuropathy, the diabetic foot is vulnerable to developing an acute progressive Charcot-like arthropathy. Patients complain of (paradoxically) pain and swelling in the foot, often after minor trauma. The rear and midfoot areas are most often involved. Untreated this will rapidly deteriorate, leaving a disorganized and dysfunctional foot. Treatment must be early and intensive with immobilization of the foot and intravenous bisphosphonates. Early referral is recommended.

Sudeck's atrophy—A similar condition can develop in the non-diabetic foot following trauma. Sudeck's atrophy ("reflex sympathetic dystrophy", or "complex regional pain syndrome type I") is a painful condition of the foot and ankle associated with regional bone loss, tissue inflammation and vascular abnormalities. This may be mediated by abnormalities of the autonomic nervous system. The foot may look blue and swollen and is painful at rest and exercise. Plain X-ray may show widespread osteoporosis in the affected area. Treatment is effective pain control and physiotherapy. Sympathetic blockade and intravenous bisphosphonates are sometimes used.

Gout

Chapter 10 discusses the manifestations of acute gout in the foot. In the chronic state, tophi in the foot (Figure 7.16) may ulcerate if they act as pressure points. Permanent destructive joint damage and deformity may result and lead to painful dysfunction in the foot.

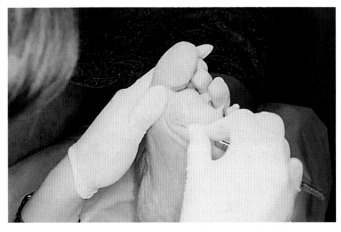

Figure 7.17 Scalpel debridement of plantar lesions provides effective pain relief

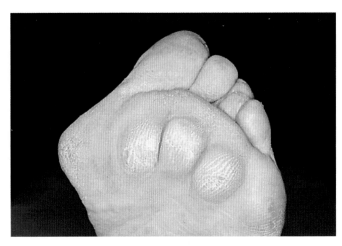

Figure 7.18 "Walking on pebbles"—metatarsophalangeal callosities in rheumatoid arthritis

---

Box 7.6 **Common abnormalities in the rheumatoid foot**

- Hallux valgus
- Lesser toe deformities—e.g. hammer toes and claw toes
- Prominent metatarsal heads with overlying painful callosities or ulceration
- Pronation of foot with valgus heel deformity and collapse of midtarsal joint, giving a flat-footed appearance
- Tenosynovitis, especially of tibialis posterior and peroneal tendons, plantar heel bursitis, calcaneal spur and tendo-Achilles bursitis
- Tarsal tunnel nerve compression syndrome

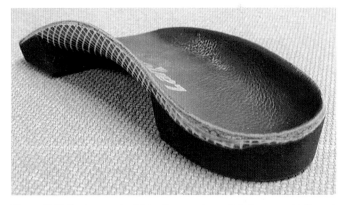

Figure 7.19 Custom-made rigid orthoses act as splints to support inflamed joints in early rheumatoid arthritis

Management of rheumatic foot conditions

Patients with rheumatic foot problems (Box 7.6) are best managed by a team that includes a physician, a surgeon and therapists. Podiatrists have a particular role in several aspects of care (Figure 7.17).

Use of orthoses for rheumatic foot problem needs suitable footwear. Podiatrists and orthotists should liaise when extra-depth shoes or surgical shoes are needed

---

Tissue viability

Joint deformity causes pressure lesions such as callosities (Figure 7.18), corns or ulceration and may be compounded by other factors, such as ingrowing toenails, peripheral neuropathy or the effects of systemic corticosteroids. Podiatrists undertake proce-

dures such as scalpel reduction, design and manufacture of insoles and orthoses, and surgery under local anaesthesia to relieve pain and restore or maintain tissue viability.

Foot function and joint protection

Foot dysfunction due to arthritis can be improved with orthoses, which can be ready-made or individually designed from casts. Orthoses may be used to control deformities—such as the valgus heel seen in rheumatoid arthritis—but they also have a major role in maintaining tissue viability and relieving pain (be it joint, soft tissue or skin lesion in origin) (Figure 7.19). Training towards gait modification may be necessary, and pressure-relieving orthoses of a total contact design may serve to reduce pressures at painful joint sites.

Foot health promotion

Patients will often need advice on daily care of feet. Family members may be involved when patients cannot reach their feet or are unable

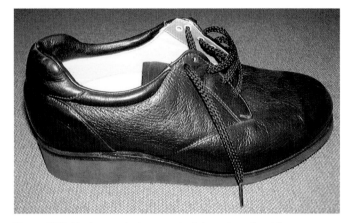

Figure 7.20 Modern stock shoes can be light and comfortable

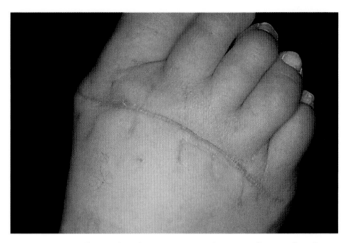

Figure 7.21 Forefoot arthroplasty is necessary in cases of severe fore foot pain and deformity

to perform tasks on the feet because of other disability. Advice may be needed on splints, walking aids, footwear (Figure 7.20), insoles, foot hygiene and exercise.

Foot surgery

Many rheumatic patients have conditions of the toenails that need surgery under local anaesthetic; they are best dealt with by an experienced clinician such as a podiatrist. Foot surgery may be effective for relieving pain and improving deformity when conservative measures have failed (Figure 7.21).

Further reading

Fam AG. The ankle and foot: regional pain problems. In: Klippel JH, Dieppe PA, eds. *Rheumatology*. Mosby, London, 1998.

Hintermann B, Nigg BM, Hames MR, Cooper PS, Sammarco GJ, Renstrom PAFH, *et al*. Foot and ankle. In: Nordin M, Anderson GBJ, Pope MH, eds. *Musculoskeletal Disorders in the Workplace: principles and practice*. Mosby, St Louis, 1997: 537–595.

Jayson MIV, Smidt LA, eds. *The Foot in Arthritis*. Baillière Tindall, London, 1987.

Helliwell PS, Woodburn J, Redmond AC, Turner DE, Davys HJ. *The Foot and Ankle in Rheumatoid Arthritis*. Churchill Livingstone Elsevier, Oxford, 2007.

Rana NA. Rheumatoid arthritis, other collagen diseases, and psoriasis of the foot. In: Jahss MH, ed. *Disorders of the Foot and Ankle: medical and surgical management*. WB Saunders, Philadelphia, 1991: 1719–1751.

CHAPTER 8

Fibromyalgia Syndrome

Sarah Ryan[1] and Anita Campbell[2]

[1]Haywood Hospital, Stoke on Trent Community Health Service, Stoke-on-Trent, UK
[2]Richmond Medical Centre, Sheffield, UK

OVERVIEW

- Acknowledge and validate patients' experience of symptoms.
- Offer explanations linking psychological factors with physical symptoms.
- Adopt a biopsychosocial approach.
- Help patients manage their symptoms and optimize functioning.
- Use a combination of treatments such a tricyclics and graded exercise.

Fibromyalgia syndrome describes widespread musculoskeletal pain and hyperalgesic tender spots with no single identifiable organic cause. Some papers refer to chronic widespread pain, but we will concentrate on fibromyalgia, which represents one end of a spectrum (Figure 8.1). Fibromyalgia is not simply related to pain, and patients often have stiffness, fatigue and sleep disturbance among other physical and psychological symptoms.

The concept of fibromyalgia is useful for patients and doctors as a starting point for management; and this management, described later, has an evidence base.

Doctors will meet patients with fibromyalgia in a variety of settings, and commonly so, as the prevalence is about 2% of the population. Chronic widespread pain can affect up to 12% of the population. There are similarities between patients with fibromyalgia, chronic fatigue syndrome/myalgic encephalopathy (ME), multiple chemical sensitivities and depression. A common approach to treatment will be found with each of these conditions. It is important for all doctors to understand these conditions so that patients may receive appropriate evidence-based treatment in order to avoid the significant functional impairment and high use of health services seen in the past. Although patients may present in a variety of settings, the most appropriate setting for diagnosis and ongoing management is primary care. Recent evidence has shown that general practitioners may not be labelling patients with either fibromyalgia or chronic widespread pain. Nevertheless they may be using a holistic approach to these patients, which is similar to the management we describe in this chapter.

Diagnosis

In 1990 the American College of Rheumatology developed criteria in order to define the condition of fibromyalgia for research purposes (Box 8.1). Clinicians tend to look at these criteria in addition to their own assessment of the history and examination findings. It is important not to use these criteria too literally. However, the history will be of at least 3 months and the pain will be widespread. The story given and the objective findings are often in discordance. The main finding on examination will be multiple hyperalgesic tender sites (Figure 8.2). Patients without fibromyalgia may find pressure on these sites uncomfortable, but in general will not wince or withdraw in the manner that a patient with fibromyalgia will.

Box 8.1 **American College of Rheumatology diagnosis of fibromyalgia (1990)**

- Widespread musculoskeletal pain in all four quadrants of the body and some axial pain (cervical spine, anterior chest, thoracic spine or low back)
- Present for at least 3 months
- Hyperalgesic points positive on digital pressure of 4 kg in 11 out of 18 points on the figure (hyperalgesia is absent in other control areas of the body, e.g. forehead)
- The points are all bilateral and situated in:
  - suboccipital muscle insertions at the base of the skull
  - low cervical spine C5-7 interspinous ligaments
  - trapezius muscles at the midpoint of the upper border
  - supraspinatus origins above the scapulae spines
  - second costochondral junctions on upper surface lateral to junction
  - 2 cm distal to lateral epicondyles
  - upper outer quadrants of buttocks in anterior fold of gluteus medius
  - greater trochanters posterior to trochanteric prominence
  - medial fat pads of knee proximal to the joint line

ABC of Rheumatology, 4th edn. Edited by Ade Adebajo.
©2010 Blackwell Publishing Ltd. 9781405170680.

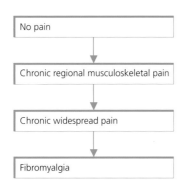

Figure 8.1 The pain spectrum

No pain

↓

Chronic regional musculoskeletal pain

↓

Chronic widespread pain

↓

Fibromyalgia

Table 8.1 Physical and psychological associations with fibromyalgia

Physical	Psychological
Irritable bladder	Panic attacks
Irritable bowel	Anxiety
Migraine	Depression
Muscle spasm	Irritability
Dizziness	Memory lapses
Perception of swelling	Word mix-ups
Paraesthesiae	Reduced concentration
Temperature changes	
Fatigue	

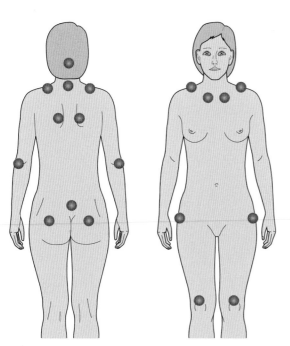

Figure 8.2 Distribution of hyperalgesic tender spots

Fibromyalgia occurs as a stand-alone condition or can occur as a consequence of other rheumatological conditions, e.g. rheumatoid arthritis, systemic lupus erythematosus and Sjögren's syndrome. The term "secondary fibromyalgia" is sometimes used in these situations.

Some of the more common physical and psychological symptoms associated with fibromyalgia syndrome are listed in Table 8.1.

A full examination must therefore be undertaken at presentation or at referral. There should be no "red flags" (such as unexplained weight loss) potentially signalling serious underlying conditions. There may well be "yellow flags", which suggest psychosocial problems, although they may not be apparent initially.

Limited investigations to exclude other causes of widespread pain are usually undertaken at presentation (thyroid function tests, full blood count, inflammatory markers, serum calcium and alkaline phosphatase, biochemical profile, creatine kinase, random blood glucose). The emphasis has to be on the biopsychosocial perspective, and any subsequent tests may well increase levels of anxiety. It is important to make a positive diagnosis of fibromyalgia after initial examination of the patient and explain to the patient that the blood tests are simply to ensure there is no underlying condition. They need to know there is no diagnostic test for fibromyalgia. It is useful at this stage to discuss what fibromyalgia is and possible models for causation with the patient in order to prepare them for the normal results of investigations. A well-informed patient will then not feel rejected.

Clinical picture

The typical patient will tend to be female, aged 30–50 years, with long-standing diffuse pain. She will often have a history of physical or psychological trauma, and this may have been related to previous abuse. She will describe a fatigue on waking. The symptoms are always present but are exacerbated by other stressors in her life. She may have experienced rejection by other doctors who investigated but did not find an organic cause of the symptoms. This rejection can lead to more anxiety and hence intensification of the symptoms. The patient may have also become depressed if her symptoms have not been helped by previous interventions.

The examination of such a patient reveals tender hyperalgesic sites and the patient visibly winces when they are pressed.

Cause

No single pathophysiological causative mechanism has been identified (Box 8.2), and the evidence to date suggests that fibromyalgia is a multifactorial syndrome characterized by abnormal processing of pain, known as central sensitization. In this process neuronal pain pathways originally activated from an identifiable noxious source later become activated in the absence of a clear stimuli. Neuroendocrine abnormalities have also been identified, but their clinical significance is not understood.

Box 8.2 **Theories regarding causation**

- Neuroendocrine disturbance
- Neurohormonal dysfunctions
- Abnormal pain processing
- Autonomic nervous system dysfunction
- Genetic predisposition to pain sensitivity
- Sleep physiology
- Lack of stage 4 sleep
- Muscle pathology
- Changes in regulation of intramuscular microcirculation
- Decrease in energy-rich phosphates
- Allergy, infection, toxicity and nutritional deficiency
- Psychosomatic
- Trauma-whiplash
- Neurotransmitter regulation

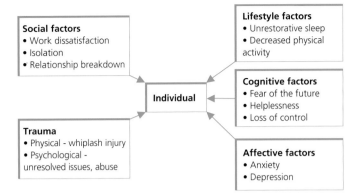

Figure 8.3 Factors that may influence pain perception

Management of fibromyalgia

The experience of pain is influenced by physical, psychological and social factors, which may mitigate or enhance the pain experience (Figures 8.3 and 8.4). Therefore as part of the assessment process it is important to identify any psychological (emotional distress, anxiety, difficult life predicaments, identifiable stressors) or social (family history, work issues) influences on the pain, as these will need to be addressed as quickly as possible to facilitate behavioural change.

The goals of management are twofold to assist the patient in the development of self-management skills and to improve the patient's physical and psychological function.

Education

The patient will often need guidance, support and motivation from a health professional before feeling able to take an active role in the management of their symptoms. Physical inactivity, unrestorative sleep and emotional stress can increase the intensity of pain, and these areas need to be addressed. Patient-centred management goals need to be realistic to prevent failure and increased feelings of helplessness. A review of the evidence from multidisciplinary rehabilitation in fibromyalgia advocates the use of behavioural strategies (graded exercise, pacing, cognitive behavioural therapy, goal setting and relaxation) and stress-management techniques. Some of these strategies are covered in chronic-disease-management programmes such as the Expert Patient Programme.

Graded exercise

Many patients become physically de-conditioned and are fearful that exercise will induce damage to the joints or increase the pain and fatigue. The aim of graded exercise (that is, gradually increasing activity over a period of time) is to improve the patient's general level of physical fitness by increasing muscle strength, stamina and flexibility. Through improving fitness levels the patient will be able to increase their general level of activity and experience a positive effect on well-being and sleep. Several sessions of super-

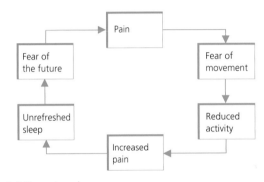

Figure 8.4 The pain cycle

vised exercise may be needed at first to provide reassurance and feedback.

Pacing activities

Pacing involves breaking down everyday activities into achievable components. Patients tend to exert themselves on a "good day" and under-exert on a "poor day". Pacing removes the "all-or-nothing" mentality that is not helpful in this condition. If patients can plan their activities, e.g. cleaning one room in the house a day instead of doing all the rooms in one go, they will still achieve the desired outcome and be able to remain active every day instead of continually entering the "boom-and-bust" cycle. Patients should be encouraged to remain in the workplace and where possible apply the principles of pacing in their work situation.

Relaxation

Relaxation can reduce muscle tension, muscle pain, general feelings of anxiety, improve sleep and foster a sense of control over the condition.

Developing a sleep routine

Patients often develop an erratic sleep pattern and feel unrefreshed on waking. This increases the perception of pain, leads to poor cognitive functioning and low mood state and reduces the ability to cope with everyday events. Self-help measures can improve the quality of a person's sleep. These include avoiding daytime sleeping, going to bed at the same time each night, carrying out relaxation techniques to clear the mind prior to settling, avoiding stimulants such as coffee and providing a quiet, well-ventilated environment.

Drug therapy

Pharmacological treatments are not particularly successful. Tricyclics such as amitriptyline may be helpful in improving sleep disturbance. Amitriptyline is prescribed in small incremental doses in general ranging from 10–50 mg (some patients are sensitive to side effects and need only 5 mg) and should be taken 2 hours prior to settling at night. The decision to increase the dose will be based on efficacy and side effects. Even with low doses side effects are common, albeit usually minor. Tricyclics should help improve sleep within 2 weeks, but a longer trial of 3–4 months is required to assess efficacy on pain. Serotonin-uptake inhibitors can improve energy and provide pain relief but tend to lose their effectiveness over time. Duloxetine has also been shown to reduce pain in women with fibromyalgia. Pregabalin has been shown to be helpful in reducing pain and fatigue and improving sleep. Simple analgesia, such as paracetamol, may be prescribed, but there is little evidence to support the use of strong narcotics.

Complementary/alternative medicine

Although few studies have examined the benefits of complementary/alternative medicine, patients often use numerous types of such treatments, including massage therapy, chiropractic and acupuncture.

In conclusion, a biopsychosocial approach to the assessment and management of patients with fibromyalgia is required, with an emphasis on assisting patients to develop coping strategies.

Further reading

Bird H. Drug treatment for fibromyalgia. *Musculoskeletal Care* 2004; **2**: 90–100.

Rorbeck J, Jordan K, Croft P. The frequency and characteristics of chronic widespread pain in general practice. *British Journal of General Practice* 2007; **57**: 109–115.

Sim J, Adams N. Physical and other non-pharmacological interventions for fibromyalgia. *Bailliere's Best Practice & Research Clinical Rheumatology* 1999; **13**: 507–523.

White KP, Harth M. An analytical review of 24 controlled clinical trials for fibromyalgia syndrome. *Pain* 1996; **64**: 211–219.

Wolfe F. Stop using the American College of Rheumatology criteria in clinic. *Journal of Rheumatology* 2003; **30**: 1671.

CHAPTER 9

Osteoarthritis

Virginia Byers Kraus[1] and Michael Doherty[2]

[1]Duke University Medical Center, Durham, USA
[2]Nottingham City Hospital, Nottingham, UK

OVERVIEW

- Osteoarthritis (OA) is the most common form of arthritis.
- Symptoms of OA are often episodic.
- The goals of treatment are to relieve pain, minimize disability and improve quality of life.
- Non-pharmacologic treatments are as important as pharmacologic treatments for OA.
- Criteria for joint replacement include uncontrolled pain and severe impairment of function despite conservative treatment.

Introduction

Osteoarthritis (OA) is the most common condition to affect synovial joints, the most important cause of locomotor disability, and a major challenge for health-care providers (Figure 9.1a). Because OA increases significantly with age (Figure 9.1b), it was long considered to be a degenerative disease that was an inevitable consequence of ageing and trauma. However, it is viewed now as a metabolically dynamic process characterized by an imbalance of joint breakdown in association with a maladaptive and insufficient repair process.

OA can result from abnormal biomechanical stresses (e.g. severe injury, repetitive excessive loading) superimposed on normal joint physiology. It may also result from normal stresses applied to an inherently compromised joint with abnormal physiology, for example weakened cartilage due to a genetic mutation in collagen II (Figure 9.2). In fact, the genetic contribution to OA is equal to or greater than the genetic contribution to the most common inflammatory arthritis in women—rheumatoid arthritis (RA) (Figure 9.3). Moreover, the relative disability associated with these two forms of arthritis is similar (Figure 9.4). Thus, OA can be considered as the consequence or final common pathway of a number of interacting risk factors and processes, including genetic factors, gender, increasing age, excess weight, injury, joint deformity and occupational exposures. Risk factors may vary in importance according to the site of involvement (Table 9.1), and risk factors for development of OA may differ from risk factors for progression. For example, high bone density is a risk factor for development of knee, hip and hand OA, but low bone density is a risk factor for more rapid radiographic progression of hip and knee OA.

Presentation

OA is traditionally separated into two main categories: primary and secondary. Primary OA typically involves joints in characteristic locations (Figure 9.5a) and is likely to result mainly from genetic predisposition—the case of abnormal joint physiology as described above. Multiple Heberden's nodes (bony enlargement of distal interphalangeal joints of the hand) (Figure 9.6) appear in middle age and are a strong marker for subsequent predisposition to knee OA and OA at other common target sites ("nodal generalized OA"). However, OA can occur in any joint. When OA occurs in atypical joints, such as the ankle, the presentation alone should trigger consideration of secondary OA. Typical aetiologies of secondary OA include joint trauma, previous fracture and preceding inflammatory arthropathy such as gout—the case of abnormal joint stressors as described above. The most common of these, joint trauma, can lead to OA 15–20 years after the joint insult and can be a cause of young-onset mono- or pauciarticular OA (Figure 9.7). When abnormal joint stressors and abnormal joint physiology occur together, the outcome is potentially even more severe. This is illustrated by the fact that severe meniscal damage to the knee is more likely to cause eventual knee OA in patients with hand OA (evidence for a genetic predisposition to OA) compared with patients without hand OA (Englund *et al.*, 2004).

It is useful to contrast the distribution of OA joints with that of RA (Figure 9.5b). RA involves multiple joints in a symmetrical pattern, and spares the distal interphalangeal joints of the fingers. The radiographic manifestations of these two arthritides are distinct and can be used in their differential diagnosis as described below.

Despite the varying aetiologies, the presenting manifestations of OA are pain, loss of joint motion and function, minimal (<30 minutes) morning stiffness and short-lived stiffness after

ABC of Rheumatology, 4th edn. Edited by Ade Adebajo.
©2010 Blackwell Publishing Ltd. 9781405170680.

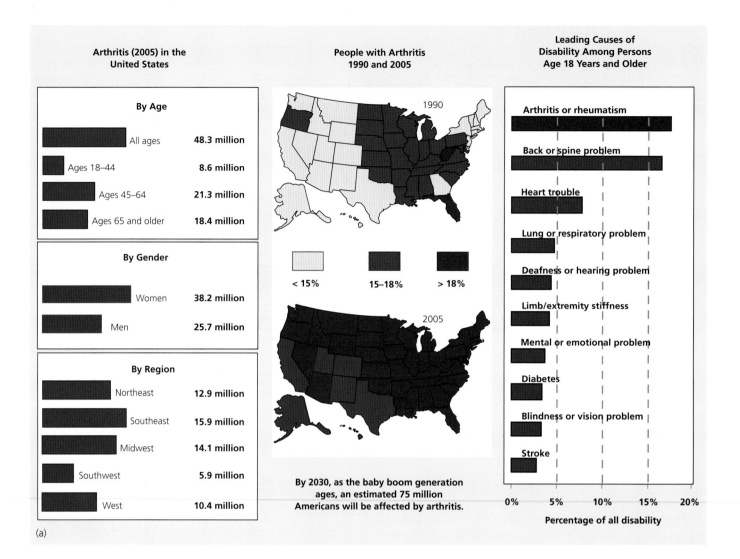

Arthritis (2005) in the United States

By Age

All ages	48.3 million
Ages 18–44	8.6 million
Ages 45–64	21.3 million
Ages 65 and older	18.4 million

By Gender

Women	38.2 million
Men	25.7 million

By Region

Northeast	12.9 million
Southeast	15.9 million
Midwest	14.1 million
Southwest	5.9 million
West	10.4 million

(a)

People with Arthritis 1990 and 2005

1990

< 15%   15–18%   > 18%

2005

By 2030, as the baby boom generation ages, an estimated 75 million Americans will be affected by arthritis.

Leading Causes of Disability Among Persons Age 18 Years and Older

Arthritis or rheumatism
Back or spine problem
Heart trouble
Lung or respiratory problem
Deafness or hearing problem
Limb/extremity stiffness
Mental or emotional problem
Diabetes
Blindness or vision problem
Stroke

0%   5%   10%   15%   20%
Percentage of all disability

Age-specific OA prevalence (%)

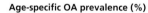
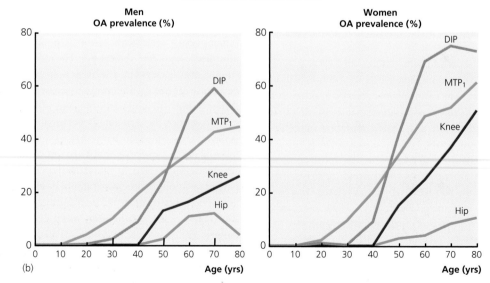

Men
OA prevalence (%)

Women
OA prevalence (%)

(b)   Age (yrs)   Age (yrs)

Figure 9.1 (a) Prevalence of OA in the US and disability figures overall. Data derived from the *Behavioral Risk Factor Surveillance System Survey Data*, *Morbidity and Mortality Weekly Report* and US Census (CDC, 2001, 2005, 2006, 2007). (b) Age-specific OA prevalence by joint site. Adapted from van Saase *et al.*, 1989, with permission of the publisher, BMJ Publishing Group. DIP = distal interphalangeal joint of the hand; MTP$_1$ = first metatarsal phalangeal joint of the foot

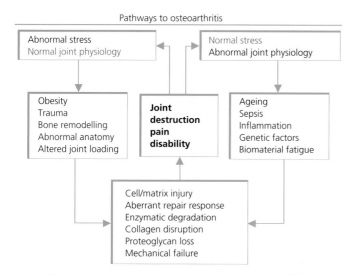

Pathways to osteoarthritis

| Abnormal stress | | Normal stress |
| Normal joint physiology | | Abnormal joint physiology |

Obesity	**Joint**	Ageing
Trauma	**destruction**	Sepsis
Bone remodelling	**pain**	Inflammation
Abnormal anatomy	**disability**	Genetic factors
Altered joint loading		Biomaterial fatigue

Cell/matrix injury
Aberrant repair response
Enzymatic degradation
Collagen disruption
Proteoglycan loss
Mechanical failure

Figure 9.2 Pathways to osteoarthritis. Taken from Poole *et al.* 2007, with permission of Dr Farshid Guilak and the publisher, Lippincott Williams & Wilkins

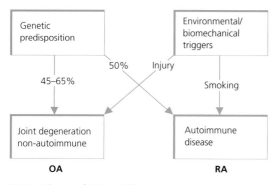

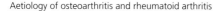

Aetiology of osteoarthritis and rheumatoid arthritis

| Genetic predisposition | | Environmental/ biomechanical triggers |

50%   Injury

45–65%   Smoking

| Joint degeneration non-autoimmune | | Autoimmune disease |

OA   **RA**

Figure 9.3 Aetiologies of OA and RA

Table 9.1 Important risk factors for osteoarthritis

Risk factor	Notes
Genetics	Hand, knee and hip OA show strong heritability (40–60%); this probably results from combinations of multiple common polymorphisms rather than rare single genes with a large individual effect
Race	Knee OA is prevalent across the world, whereas hip OA is particularly prevalent in Caucasians
Age	Although not an inevitable consequence of ageing, OA is strongly age-related; this may reflect the cumulative effect of insults to the joint, aggravated by decline in neuromuscular function, or senescence of homoeostatic repair mechanisms
Sex	Women have a higher prevalence and radiographic severity of OA at all joint sites apart from the hip. Women are also more likely to have symptoms if radiographic OA is present
Obesity	This is an important risk factor for knee OA, but a more modest risk factor for hip and hand OA
Bone density	High density is a risk factor for development of knee, hip and hand OA; low density is a risk factor for more rapid progression of knee and hip OA
Abnormal joint shape and alignment	Acetabular dysplasia is a recognized cause of hip OA, and distal femoral dysplasia (often overlooked) may contribute to knee OA; varus or valgus malalignment may be a risk for development and more rapid progression of knee OA—this can have a major interaction with obesity
Joint trauma and usage	Major joint injury is an important factor at the knee (especially if it causes subchondral fracture, meniscal injury or ligament rupture) and can cause OA at any site; recognized occupational hazards include farming (hip OA), underground mining (knee OA), professional soccer (knee OA) and some heavy manual jobs (hand OA)

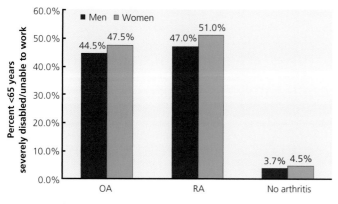

Figure 9.4 Relative work disability for OA and RA. Data taken from Pincus *et al.*, 1989, based on 1978 US Social Security Survey of Disability and Work. In the original paper, OA and RA were referred to by their respective surrogates: asymmetric oligoarthritis and symmetric polyarthritis

resting ("gelling"), in the absence of systemic symptoms (fatigue, fever) or other system involvement. Joint stiffness arises, at least in part, from the accumulation of hyaluronan (a joint lubricant and the most abundant constituent of synovial fluid) and hyaluronan fragments in the deep layers of arthritic synovium during periods of rest, excluding water within the synovial tissue. Joint movement mobilizes hyaluronan from the tissue to the lymphatics and blood with attendant hydration of synovial tissue and improvement in joint stiffness symptoms (Engstrom-Laurent, 1987). The cartilage changes that accompany OA encourage deposition of crystals—both calcium crystals (calcium pyrophosphate and basic calcium phosphates), especially at the knee, and urate crystals. Patients with OA may therefore develop superadded acute pseudogout (mainly knees and wrists), and are at increased risk of secondary gout if they are on long-term diuretics or have chronic renal impairment (see Chapter 10).

Distribution of primary OA and RA

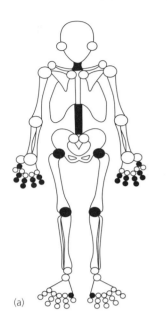
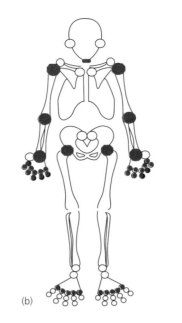

● OA
● RA

(a)   (b)

Figure 9.5 Pattern of joint distribution of primary OA and RA

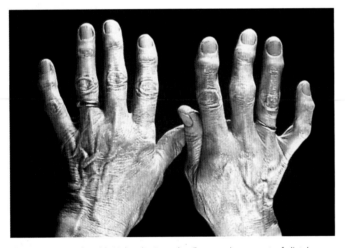

Figure 9.6 Hands with Heberden's nodes (bony enlargement of distal interphalangeal joints) and Bouchard's nodes (bony enlargement of proximal interphalangeal joints)

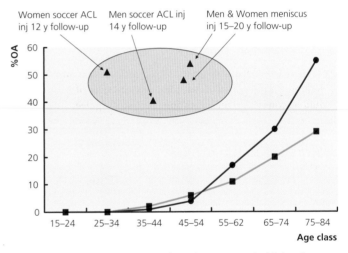

Women soccer ACL inj 12 y follow-up   Men soccer ACL inj 14 y follow-up   Men & Women meniscus inj 15–20 y follow-up

Figure 9.7 Prevalence of knee OA after injury compared with baseline risk. Taken from Roos, 2005, with permission of Dr Ewa Roos and the publisher, Lippincott Williams & Wilkins

Examination

The main clinical features of OA are symptoms, functional impairment and signs. Considerable discordance can exist between these three (Figure 9.8). Pain may arise from several sites in and around an osteoarthritic joint (Table 9.2). Suggested mechanisms include increased intra-capsular and intra-osseous pressure, subchondral microfracture and enthesopathy or bursitis secondary to muscle weakness and structural alteration. Severity of pain and functional impairment are greatly influenced by personality, anxiety, depression, daily activity and reduced muscle strength and proprioception (muscle performs an important proprioceptive role).

Table 9.2 Types of joint pain in OA

Nature of pain	Probable aetiology of pain
Pain with use	Mechanical joint damage, enthesopathy from ligament or ligamentous attachments
Pain at rest	Inflammation with effusion and joint capsule distension
Pain at night	Intra-osseous hypertension
Sudden flare of pain	Crystal synovitis, torn meniscus, exacerbation of cartilage breakdown due to abnormal stressor with secondary synovitis from pro-inflammatory cascade due to release of cartilage matrix fragments; consider sepsis as a rare possibility

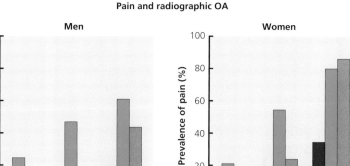

Pain and radiographic OA

Figure 9.8 The discordance between radiographic OA and symptoms in the hands (distal interphalangeal joints, knees and hip). Taken from Arden and Nevitt, 2006, with permission of Drs Nigel Arden and Michael Nevitt and the publisher, Elsevier

Crepitus, bony enlargement, deformity, instability and restricted movement may occur together and predominantly reflect structural changes. Varying degrees of synovitis (warmth, effusion and synovial thickening) may be superimposed, especially noticeable in knees, and muscle weakness or wasting is extremely common.

Assessment aims to establish the source of symptoms in each patient. When diffuse and generalized tender points are identified at tendon insertion sites, then the co-occurrence of fibromyalgia should be considered and attention to improving sleep be included in the management considerations. Only an adequate history and examination can determine how much structural and inflammatory change is present and how much these contribute to a patient's problems.

Diagnosis

Typical OA can be diagnosed by history and examination alone. Currently the main investigation that can help confirm OA is the plain X-ray, with demonstration of characteristic structural abnormalities—focal joint-space narrowing (due to cartilage loss), marginal osteophyte or "spur" formation and subchondral sclerosis of bone (Figure 9.9). It is increasingly recognized that biochemical abnormalities of the joint precede radiographic abnormalities by as much as decades. For this reason, much effort is currently being put into identifying more sensitive imaging modalities, such as magnetic resonance imaging, bone scintigraphy and ultrasound, along with biochemical indicators in blood, urine or synovial fluid, that might identify and quantify OA more precisely and earlier than by X-ray.

Management

The goals of medical management of OA (summarized in Figure 9.10) are to: (a) provide patient education and information access; (b) relieve pain; (c) optimize function; and (d) minimize disease

Box 9.1 **European and US Guidelines for management of OA**

- The management plan must be individualized, taking into account the site and severity of OA symptoms, any co-morbidity, concurrent medications and patient acceptability
- Non-pharmacological treatments are central—drug treatments are adjuncts
- A core and option approach is required—all patients should be offered education, an exercise programme, advice to reduce adverse mechanical factors and paracetamol as the first oral analgesic to try; there is a wide range of other treatment options from which to select additional treatments, as required

progression. See Box 9.1 for European and US guidelines on management of OA.

Symptoms of OA often are episodic. It is therefore advisable to provide the patient with an armamentarium of treatment options to choose from during periods of relative quiescence and relative flare.

Patient education and information access

This is a professional responsibility, but education also improves outcome and is a treatment in its own right. The myth that OA is a progressive wearing-out of joints due to old age still persists; this invariably leads to inappropriate reductions in activity. A major contribution to managing OA has been the finding that a patient's psychological status (anxiety, depression and social support) is an important determinant of symptomatic and functional outcome. Good evidence supports the use of educational programmes to help patients understand OA and develop self-management strategies.

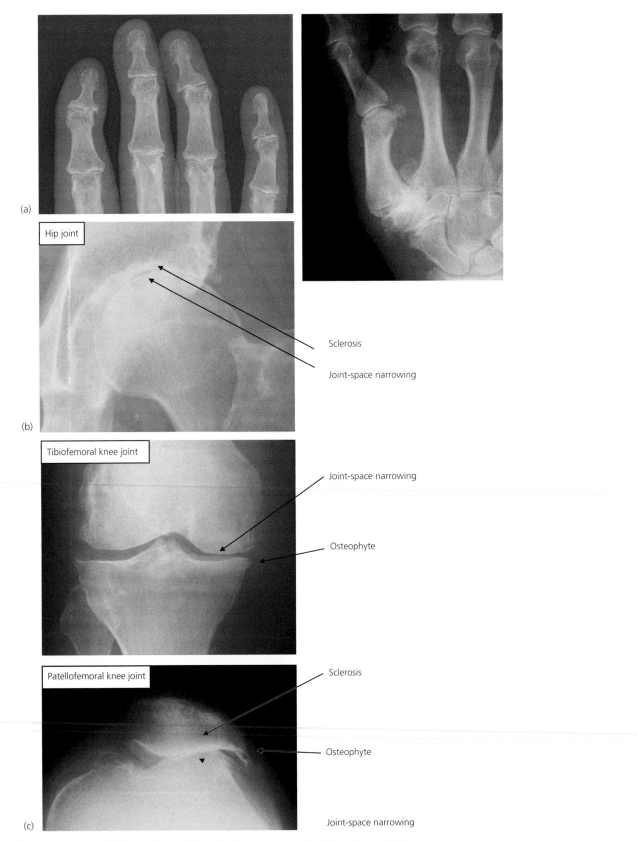

(a)

Hip joint

Sclerosis

Joint-space narrowing

(b)

Tibiofemoral knee joint

Joint-space narrowing

Osteophyte

Patellofemoral knee joint

Sclerosis

Osteophyte

(c)

Joint-space narrowing

Figure 9.9 Radiographic OA: representative images of a hand (a), a hip (b) and a knee (c) with radiographic OA

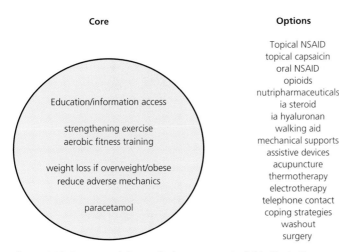

Figure 9.10 Summary of the medical management of OA, illustrating the need for a holistic approach. ia = intra-articular

Core

Education/information access

strengthening exercise
aerobic fitness training

weight loss if overweight/obese
reduce adverse mechanics

paracetamol

Options

Topical NSAID
topical capsaicin
oral NSAID
opioids
nutripharmaceuticals
ia steroid
ia hyaluronan
walking aid
mechanical supports
assistive devices
acupuncture
thermotherapy
electrotherapy
telephone contact
coping strategies
washout
surgery

Exercise

Local quadriceps-strengthening exercise can reduce pain and disability and improve the physiological accompaniments of knee OA (muscle weakness, impaired proprioception and balance, tendency to fall). Aerobic activity also reduces pain and disability from OA, improves well-being and sleep quality, and is beneficial for common co-morbidities. Both forms of exercise need to be prescribed. Increased activity and exercise can be accomplished in a variety of ways (e.g. home exercise, group classes), tailored to the patient's wishes and lifestyle. Pool exercise, wherein people weigh just one-eighth what they weigh on land, can mitigate negative effects of excessive joint loading due to obesity and allow freedom of joint movement and aerobic training for individuals with lower extremity OA.

Reduction of adverse biomechanical factors

Spreading physically hard jobs (e.g. housework, mowing the lawn) at intervals through the day, with breaks in between ("pacing"), can reduce sustained mechanical loading. Weight reduction can improve function and reduce pain in obese and overweight patients and may slow progression of knee and hip OA. Appropriate footwear (thick soft sole, no raised heel, broad forefoot and deep soft uppers) can reduce impact loading in people with knee and hip OA, and wedged insoles can counteract knee varus deformity. Walking sticks and other walking aids reduce loading across OA joints.

Pharmacological treatments

The high prevalence of OA, especially in the elderly, means that co-morbid conditions often exist, and management of OA must take into account these conditions and potential for drug interactions.

Pain is the main reason patients seek help. Long term, the non-pharmacological lifestyle measures mentioned above can all reduce pain, but drugs are often helpful adjuncts to help quickly reduce pain during exacerbations of symptoms. Paracetamol should be the first oral analgesic to try, based on its excellent safety and reasonable efficacy. Topical non-steroidal anti-inflammatory drugs (NSAIDs) and topical capsaicin are also safe and are particularly useful for hand and knee OA.

Oral NSAIDs, including highly selective COX inhibitors, and weak opioids (e.g. codeine, tramadol) may be considered for those patients who obtain insufficient relief from paracetamol and/or topical agents. The increased risk of gastrointestinal ulceration and bleeding from traditional NSAIDs can be decreased by concomitant prescription of a proton pump inhibitor or misoprostol. The highly selective COX inhibitors, although safer on the gut, may increase the risk of myocardial infarction and stroke, as indeed may many of the traditional NSAIDs. Traditional NSAIDs also cause adverse effects on renal function, especially in the elderly, and have multiple potential drug interactions. Oral NSAIDs and selective COX inhibitors therefore should be given at the lowest effective dose on an as-required, rather than regular, basis. Weak opioids, either alone or in combination with paracetamol, may provide good pain relief, but central nervous system side effects (e.g. constipation, headache, confusion) often limit their usefulness.

Nutraceuticals provide an alternative in older, high-risk patients with co-morbidity because they have no associated renal or gastrointestinal side effects and are very popular with patients. Glucosamine is contraindicated in patients with shellfish allergy. The initiation and use of either glucosamine or chondroitin sulphate requires monitoring of glucose in diabetics, as these agents are associated with mild insulin resistance in animals.

Intra-articular corticosteroid injection is a valuable treatment that often gives quick effective relief of pain that may last just a few weeks to a few months. It is particularly useful to tide a patient over an important event (e.g. family wedding, holiday) and to improve pain during initiation of other interventions such as an exercise programme. A variety of hyaluronan preparations are also available, given as a single injection or a course of one per week for 3–5 weeks. Although a modest, relatively prolonged (several months) improvement in pain may result, the cost and logistics of this treatment are limiting.

Surgical

The success of prosthetic joint replacements has greatly advanced management of end-stage hip and knee OA. Surgery is also used increasingly now at the shoulder, elbow, and thumb base. Although issues of funding, waiting times, choice of prosthesis and revision have to be faced, there is no doubt that such surgery can transform a patient's life. Other surgical approaches (osteotomy, arthrodesis or joint fusion) may also be useful in specific circumstances. Arthroscopic debridement and lavage is indicated if a patient with OA describes mechanical locking. Symptomatic improvement following joint lavage alone can last several months.

The criteria for referral for consideration of joint replacement are not universally agreed upon, but include uncontrolled pain and severe impairment of function despite conservative treatment. Age, in itself, is not a contraindication. Autologous chondrocyte transplantation is a procedure that is currently typically reserved for young patients with severe chondral defects.

In summary, OA is a condition of increasing prevalence characterized by a phasic progression with periods of relative quiescence and flare. An individualized and holistic approach to management is essential as the best means for relieving pain, minimizing disability and improving quality of life.

References

Arden N, Nevitt M. Osteoarthritis: epidemiology. *Best Practice and Research Clinical Rheumatology* 2006; 20: 3–25.

CDC (Centers for Disease Control and Prevention). *Morbidity and Mortality Weekly Report*, vol. 50, no. 7. US Department of Health and Human Services, CDC, Atlanta, Georgia. February 23, 2001: 123.

CDC (Centers for Disease Control and Prevention). *Behavioral Risk Factor Surveillance System Survey Data*. US Department of Health and Human Services, CDC, Atlanta, Georgia, 2005.

CDC (Centers for Disease Control and Prevention). *Morbidity and Mortality Weekly Report*, vol. 55, no. 40. US Department of Health and Human Services, CDC, Atlanta, Georgia. October 13, 2006: 1091.

CDC (Centers for Disease Control and Prevention). *Morbidity and Mortality Weekly Report*, vol. 56, no. 17. US Department of Health and Human Services, CDC, Atlanta, Georgia. May 4, 2007: 424.

Englund M, Paradowski PT, Lohmander LS. Association of radiographic hand osteoarthritis with radiographic knee osteoarthritis after meniscectomy. *Arthritis and Rheumatism* 2004; 50: 469–475.

Engstrom-Laurent A, Hallgren R. Circulating hyaluronic acid levels vary with physical activity in healthy subjects and in rheumatoid arthritis patients. Relationship to synovitis mass and morning stiffness. *Arthritis and Rheumatism* 1987; 30: 1333–1338.

Pincus T, Mitchell JM, Burkhauser RV. Substantial work disability and earnings losses in individuals less than age 65 with osteoarthritis: comparisons with rheumatoid arthritis. *Journal of Clinical Epidemiology* 1989; 42: 449–457.

Poole AR, Guilak F, Abramson SB. Etiopathogenesis of osteoarthritis. In: Moskowitz RW, Altman RD, Hochberg MC, Buckwalter JA, Goldberg VM, eds. *Osteoarthritis: diagnosis and medical/surgical management*, 4ᵗʰ edn. Lippincott Williams and Wilkins, Philadelphia, PA, 2007: 27–49.

Roos EM. Joint injury causes knee osteoarthritis in young adults. *Current Opinion in Rheumatology* 2005; 17: 195–200.

van Saase JL, van Romunde LK, Cats A, Vandenbroucke JP, Valkenburg HA. Epidemiology of osteoarthritis: Zoetermeer survey. Comparison of radiological osteoarthritis in a Dutch population with that in 10 other populations. *Annals of the Rheumatic Diseases* 1989; 48: 271–280.

Further reading

American College of Rheumatology. Recommendations for the medical management of osteoarthritis of the hip and knee. *Arthritis and Rheumatism* 2000; 43: 1905–1915.

Arden N, Nevitt MC. Osteoarthritis: epidemiology. *Best Practice and Research. Clinical Rheumatology* 2006; 20: 3–25.

Brandy KD, Doherty M, Lohmander LS, eds. *Osteoarthritis*, 2ᵗʰ edn. Oxford University Press, Oxford, UK, 2003.

Felson DT, Lawrence RC, Dieppe PA *et al.* Osteoarthritis: new insights. Part 1: the disease and its risk factors. *Annals of Internal Medicine* 2000; 133: 635–646.

Jordan KM, Arden N, Doherty M *et al.* EULAR recommendations: an evidence based medicine approach to the management of knee osteoarthritis. *Annals of the Rheumatic Diseases* 2003; 62: 1145–1155.

Moskowitz RW, Altman RD, Hochberg MC, Buckwalter JA, Goldberg VM, eds. *Osteoarthritis: diagnosis and medical/surgical management*, 4ᵗʰ edn. Lippincott Williams and Wilkins, Philadelphia, PA, 2007.

Zhang W, Doherty M, Arden N *et al.* EULAR recommendations: an evidence-based medicine approach to the management of hip osteoarthritis. *Annals of the Rheumatic Diseases* 2005; 64: 669–681.

Zhang W, Doherty M, Leeb BF *et al.* EULAR evidence-based recommendations for the management of hand osteoarthritis. *Annals of the Rheumatic Diseases* 2007; 66: 377–388.

Acknowledgements

We would like to express sincere appreciation to Shelby Addison for her invaluable assistance with graphics and permissions for figures.

CHAPTER 10

Gout, Hyperuricaemia and Crystal Arthritis

Martin Underwood[1] and Ade Adebajo[2]

[1]University of Warwick, Coventry, UK
[2]University of Sheffield, Sheffield, UK

OVERVIEW

- Asymptomatic hyperuricaemia does not need treating.
- Steroids, non-steroidal anti-inflammatory drugs (NSAIDs), or colchicine can be used to treat acute gout; oral steroids might provide the best balance of risks and benefits.
- Patients with recurrent gout twice or more a year should be offered urea-lowering medication.
- Target serum urate for patients on urate-lowering drugs is <0.30 or <0.36 mmol/l.
- Dose of urate-lowering medication should be titrated according to response; many patients with recurrent gout get inadequate doses of urate-lowering drugs.

Gout and hyperuricaemia

Gout is a common metabolic disorder, typically presenting as an acute monoarthritis, most commonly of the first metatarsal phalangeal joint. The term "gout" includes an acute attack, the propensity for repeated episodes and also for chronic gouty arthritis. The underlying problem is a build-up of urate, a purine breakdown product. Humans, and some primates, lack uricase, which in other mammals oxidizes urate to allantoin, which is readily soluble. Both an increased dietary purine intake and an increased breakdown of endogenous proteins (e.g. cancer treatment or haematological malignancy) can increase urate levels.

Urate excretion is mainly renal. The rate of renal excretion is affected by urine flow, pH and competition for renal tubular exchange (e.g. diuretics). Patients whose problems are primarily due to increased purine turnover will have a high urinary urate, and those whose problems are primarily renal will have a low urinary urate. This distinction is rarely of clinical importance. For uric acid crystals to form, the serum needs to be saturated with urate, i.e. >0.42 mmol/l (>7.0 g/dl). This is, coincidentally, the upper limit of the normal range in men and postmenopausal women in many laboratories. For premenopausal women, the upper limit of the normal range for serum urate is 0.36 mmol/l (>6.0 mg/dl).

ABC of Rheumatology, 4th edn. Edited by Ade Adebajo.
©2010 Blackwell Publishing Ltd. 9781405170680.

Epidemiology

Prevalence is probably around 1% in white populations. Gout is rare in premenopausal women. However, there are few reliable data on how many people are affected each year, or how many people are taking prophylactic drugs. As gout is associated with increasing age and obesity, it is likely to become commoner. Some non-white populations are more prone to gout/hyperuricaemia; e.g. the prevalence of gout is 6.4% and 3.6%, respectively, in New Zealanders of Maori and European origin. There is generally a higher prevalence of gout in indigenous ethnic groups around the Pacific Rim. In Malaysia, the three largest ethnic groups are Malay, Chinese and Tamil. All have higher mean levels of uric acid in serum than most white populations. Environmental factors also play a part; for example, changes to from a traditional island lifestyle to a more Westernized diet increased prevalence of gout 9-fold, to Maori levels, in Tokelauan islanders who migrated to New Zealand. The prevalence of gout may also be higher in black Afro-Caribbean ethnic groups. In sub-Saharan Africa gout is particularly associated with high alcohol intake in all socio-economic groups. A particular problem for some groups in sub-Saharan Africa is saturnine gout due to the effects of lead, absorbed from containers used for homemade alcoholic drinks, on renal tubular function.

Risk factors

Age and sex—Gout becomes commoner with increasing age (Figure 10.1). In men the reported prevalence ranges from <0.5% in those aged under 35 to over 7% in those aged over 75. It is rare in premenopausal women but increases to 2.5–3.0% in those aged over 75. The later age of onset in women may relate to the uricosuric effects of oestrogens.

Obesity—Relative risk of gout increases with increasing body mass index (BMI). Compared to people with a BMI of 21–25, those with BMI of >35 are four times as likely to develop gout (Figure 10.2).

Diet—Each additional daily portion of meat per day increases the risk of gout by 20%. Purine-rich vegetables do not appear to increase the risk of gout, while consuming more dairy products reduces the risk of developing the disease (Table 10.1).

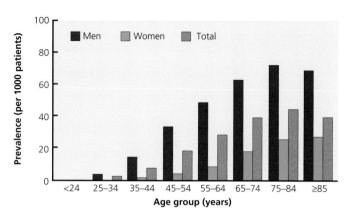

Figure 10.1 Prevalence of gout; data from general practice research database. Reproduced with permission from Underwood (2006)

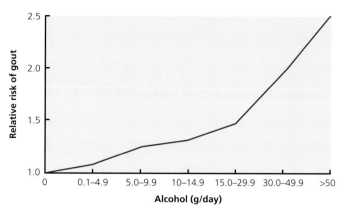

Figure 10.3 Effect of total alcohol intake on the relative risk of a first attack of gout; data from the health professionals follow-up study. Reproduced with permission from Underwood (2006)

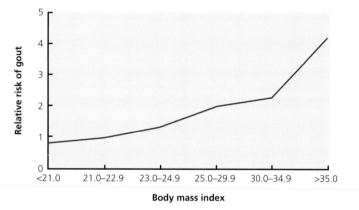

Figure 10.2 Obesity and the incidence of a first attack of gout in men; data from the health professionals follow-up study. Reproduced with permission from Underwood (2006)

Table 10.1 Effect of diet and alcohol on incidence of a first attack of gout in men; data from the health professionals follow-up study. Reproduced with permission from Underwood (2006)

Portion	Relative risk (95% CI)
Alcohol	
Beer 335 ml	1.49 (1.32 to 1.70)
Sprits 44 ml	1.15 (1.04 to 1.20)
Wine 118 ml	1.04 (0.88 to 1.22)
Food:	
Meat	1.21 (1.04 to 1.41)
Seafood (fish)*	1.07 (1.01 to 1.12)
Purine rich vegetables	0.97 (0.79 to 1.19)
Total daily products	0.82 (0.75 to 0.90)
Low-fat daily products	0.79 (0.71 to 0.87)
High-fat daily products	0.99 (0.89 to 1.10)

Data from health professionals follow-up study.
*Calculated from weekly intake.

Dietary fructose may also increase the risk of developing gout. This occurs naturally and is also present in high-fructose corn syrup (HFCS), which is commonly used as a sweetener for soft drinks and other foods in the USA. The use of HFCS is uncommon outside the USA.

Drugs—A number of drugs can increase serum urate; this is most commonly due to diuretics. Aspirin and salicylates at low doses decrease urate excretion, but at high doses (4–6 g/day) they have a uricosuric effect.

Alcohol—Compared to non-drinkers, people consuming >50 g alcohol per day are 2.5 times as likely to develop gout (Figure 10.3). While there is a strong relationship between beer intake and gout, there is only a weak relationship between intake of spirits and gout. There does not appear to be a relationship between wine intake and gout. Alcohol is catabolized to ketones that compete with urate for excretion by the renal tubule. Beer typically contains substantial amounts of purines, from yeast, which are catabolized to urate by gut bacteria. Alcohol may also increase the dose of allopurinol needed by decreasing the conversion of allopurinol to its effective metabolite, oxipurinol.

Relationship between gout and hyperuricaemia

Hyperuricaemia is necessary for the development of gout. Crystal deposition can only occur when the serum is saturated with urate: ≥0.42 mmol/l. This may be different from some laboratories' normal ranges, which are based on population norms. Only a minority of people with hyperuricaemia develop gout. For example, the annual incidence of gout is only 6% in people with a urate of 0.60 mmol/l (Figure 10.4). Serum urate can fall during an acute

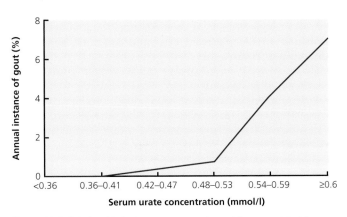

Figure 10.4 Relationship between serum urate and the annual incidence of gout; data from normative ageing study. Reproduced with permission from Underwood (2006)

Table 10.2 Investigation of patients with gout

Diagnosis	Causes	Co-morbidities
Serum urate May fall during an attack	**Full blood count** To exclude myelo- and lymphoproliferative disorders, secondary polycythaemia, haemolytic anaemia, haemoglobinopathies; white count may be slightly raised; if very high consider septic arthritis	**Blood pressure** **Cholesterol** **Blood sugar** **Thyroid function** 15% of patients with gout have hypothyroidism
Joint aspiration Consider if diagnosis uncertain; will enable the alternative diagnosis of pseudogout to be made if pyrophosphate crystals are present; note, however, that both types of crystals can coexist	**Liver enzymes** Possible alcohol abuse Renal function Drug doses might need adjusting if renal function is poor	**Uric acid excretion** Consider if strong family history of gout, if onset under age 25 or if renal stones present
	Review medication Diuretics and some other drugs increase urate	
	Investigations if pseudogout suspected Calcium, magnesium, ferritin, thyroid function	

attack, and patients on urate-lowering medication can still be affected until crystal deposits have cleared from the joints. Thus, demonstrating a raised serum urate is not an essential prerequisite for diagnosing gout.

Hyperuricaemia and cardiovascular disease

There is a well-recognized association between hyperuricaemia and cardiovascular disease. It is not clear whether hyperuricaemia is an independent risk factor for cardiovascular disease. Thus, screening for hyperuricaemia in those with a high cardiovascular risk is not indicated. However, assessing cardiovascular risk in people presenting with gout is worthwhile.

Clinical features

Acute gout

Typically gout presents as a rapid onset of a monoarthritis associated with severe pain and inflammation classically affecting the first metatarsophalangeal joint (podagra) Low-grade fever, general malaise and anorexia may accompany the joint symptoms. Onset may follow a drinking bout, or local trauma. Untreated, acute gout usually resolves spontaneously within 7–10 days but can on occasion last several weeks. The other most commonly affected areas are the other joints in the foot, ankle, knee, wrist, finger and elbow. The affected joint is warm, tender and swollen, and in most cases, the overlying skin is erythematous. The predilection for peripheral joints is probably because crystals are more likely to form in cooler joints. Typically, the attack occurs during the night. After the acute attack patients may be symptom-free for months or years.

Diagnosis—The diagnosis of acute gout is usually clinical. The European League Against Rheumatism (EULAR) recommendations for gout suggest that:

> *'the rapid development of severe pain, swelling and tenderness that reaches its maximum within just 6–12 hours, especially with overlying erythema, is highly suggestive of crystal inflammation though not specific for gout'*

and that:

> *'for typical presentations of gout (such as podagra with hyperuricaemia) a clinical diagnosis alone is reasonably accurate but not definitive without crystal confirmation.'*

The gold standard is demonstrating urate crystals in synovial fluid. However, few generalists (or their patients) will relish aspirating an acutely inflamed first metatarsophalangeal joint. Urate crystals are strongly negatively birefringent on polarizing microscopy. Pyrophosphate crystals, which are weakly positively birefringent under polarized light, are found in pseudogout. Both types of crystals coexist in about 10% of crystal-associated synovial effusions. In the acute situation the important differential diagnosis is septic arthritis. If septic arthritis is suspected, then urgent specialist assessment is needed. Bursitis of the first metatarsophalangeal joint can mimic podagra and is often mislabelled and mistreated as gout, especially in young women.

Investigations—All patients with a suspected first episode of gout should be investigated to obtain some confirmatory evidence to support the diagnosis, to look for underlying causes and to identify associated co-morbidities (Table 10.2). X-rays are not helpful in the diagnosis of acute gout.

Chronic gout

Chronic, poly- or oligoarticular gout can cause inflammatory arthritis in older people, especially those on diuretics. No diagnostic pattern exists, although lower-limb-joint involvement is common. Crystal deposits (tophi) can develop around hands, feet, elbows and ears; they are particularly common in older women with secondary, diuretic-induced gout, in whom they may develop without a history of acute gout. Tophi are chalky deposits of urate embedded in a matrix of lipid, protein and calcific debris. They are usually subcutaneous, but may occur in bone and other organs, including heart valves and the eye. Tophi can contribute to a destructive arthropathy and secondary osteoarthritis. This picture can also develop in patients with recurrent acute gout.

Diagnosis—Urate crystals can be demonstrated in aspirate from tophi. These can be seen radiographically as soft-tissue swellings (occasionally with associated calcification) and there are characteristic X-ray changes of subcortical cysts without erosions and geodes (punched-out type erosions with sclerotic margins and overhanging edges).

Urate stones

One in five patients with gout over-excrete urate and may develop urate stones. Around 5% renal stones are pure urate. However, urinary urate may co-precipitate in calcium oxalate or phosphate stones. Serum urate should be measured in patients with a history of renal colic. Uricosuric drugs should be avoided in patients with history of urate containing renal stones. Patients with ileostomies are prone to urate stones as a consequence of producing concentrated acidic urine.

Inherited metabolic disorders

Gout in childhood may be a manifestation of one of the several rare inherited disorders of metabolism, such as Lesch–Nyhan syndrome and G6PD deficiency and should be investigated in detail. Adults with new onset gout may be heterozygous for one of these conditions, but investigations should be restricted to those with indicative family histories.

Treatment

There are few robust data to inform the management of gout. Recommendations for the treatment are largely based on clinical experience rather than randomized controlled trial evidence. There are now some suggested quality standards for the management of gout/hyperuricaemia that can be used to audit practice (Box 10.1), and the British Society of Rheumatology has produced guidelines for the management of gout.

Acute gout

The choice of drug treatment is dependent on the balance of risks and benefits. Our view, backed by some empirical data, is that for many patients with acute gout a short course of oral steroids often provides the best balance of benefits and risks.

Non-steroidal anti-inflammatory drugs (NSAIDs)—There is one small randomized controlled trial of NSAIDs compared to placebo for acute gout. Decades of clinical experience attest to the efficacy of these drugs for acute gout. Typically, high-dose NSAIDs, e.g. indometacin 50 mg three times a day, are recommended, although there are no empirical data to support this. The only firm conclu-

---

Box 10.1 Suggested quality care indicators for gout management. Reproduced with permission from Underwood (2006)

Treatment of acute gout
- Patients presenting with acute gouty arthritis who do not have significant renal impairment (creatinine clearance ≤50 ml/min or creatinine concentration ≥167 µmol/l) or peptic ulcer disease should be treated with one of the following:
- A non-steroidal anti-inflammatory drug
- A drenocorticotrophic hormone or steroids (systemic or intra-articular)
- Colchicine

Prevention of recurrent gout
- Patients with gout who are obese (body index >28), or who have one or more alcoholic drinks per day, should be advised to lose weight or decrease their alcohol consumption, or both
- When starting allopurinol in patients with major renal impaiment, initially use a low dose (<300 mg/day)
- When coprescribing a xanthine oxidase inhibitor with azothiaprine or 6-mercaptopurine, reduce dose of azothiaprine or 6-mercaptopirine by at least 50%
- When starting a urate-lowering drug in patients with gout who do not have major renal impairment (see definition above) or peptic ulcer disease, coprescribe a non-steroidal anti-inflammatory drug or colchicine to reduce the incidence of rebound gout attacks
- Patients with asymptomatic hyperuricaemia do not need treatment
- Uricosuric drugs should not be used in patients with significant renal impairment (see definition above) or a history of renal stones
- Patients with gout and either tophaceous deposits, gouty erosive changes on rediographs, or more than two attacks per year should be offered urate-lowering treatment
- Patients with gout who are taking axanthine oxidase inhibitor should have their serum urate level checked at least once during the first 6 months of continued use
- Patients taking long term prophylactic oral colchicine who have major renal impairment (see definition above) should have a full blood count and creatine kinase checked least once every 6 months

---

sion from comparative studies of NSAIDs is that pain reduction with indometacin or etoricoxib are equivalent. If NSAIDs or COX-2 inhibitors are used, a co-prescription of a proton pump inhibitor is usually indicated.

Colchicine—There is one small controlled trial of colchicine compared to placebo for acute gout; everyone taking colchicine developed diarrhoea and vomiting, frequently before pain relief. Severe diarrhoea when immobilized with acute gout can be an unpleasant experience. Other adverse reactions include bone marrow and neuromuscular dysfunction. Traditionally high doses of colchicine are recommended; however, a lower dose of 0.5 mg three times a day is less toxic and can be adequately effective.

Steroids/adrenocorticotrophic hormone (ACTH)—There are no controlled trials comparing steroids/ACTH with placebo for acute gout. One trial, in a Hong Kong emergency department, compared indometacin 150 mg/day with prednisolone 30 mg per day for 5 days. Prednisolone was at least as effective as indometacin. Among the patients that received indometacin, 5% had a gastrointestinal haemorrhage and 11% were admitted to hospital for treatment of a serious adverse effect. No one in the control group had a haemorrhage or was admitted to hospital. A second trial, in Dutch primary care, compared naproxen 1 g/day with prednisolone 35 mg per day and found effectiveness to be equivalent and a similar incidence of adverse effects.

Clinical experience supports the use of intra-articular steroids, but septic arthritis must be positively excluded. Intra-articular injections in acute gout can be difficult and very painful, particularly in smaller joints.

Analgesics—Gout is painful. Patients may need potent analgesic in addition to specific treatments. For some frail patients, just using analgesics may be appropriate.

Other treatments—Experience and some controlled trial evidence suggest that some non-drug pain-relief modalities such as the use of ice packs may give additional pain relief.

Intercritical and chronic gout

The mainstay of treatment for prevention of recurrent acute gout and chronic gout is reducing serum urate enough to allow crystals to clear. Different authorities suggest <0.30 mmol/l or <0.36 mmol/l as the therapeutic target. Asymptomatic hyperuricaemia does not require treatment.

Patients with two or more attacks of gout per year should be offered urate-lowering medication. Starting urate-lowering drugs during an attack may delay resolution and should be avoided as lowering serum urate can trigger acute gout. An NSAID, probably with a proton pump inhibitor, or colchicine should be co-prescribed for the first 3 months.

Medication review—Consider stopping diuretics or any other drugs known to increase serum urate.

Lifestyle interventions—Patients should be advised to: lose weight; reduce the amount of meat and fish eaten; reduce alcohol intake and avoid beer; increase intake of low-fat dairy products.

Xanthine oxidase inhibitors—These prevent the purine breakdown products xanthine and hypoxanthine being converted into urate. Allopurinol has been available for over 40 years. A new xanthine oxidase inhibitor, febuxostat, has been developed.

Allopurinol—Allopurinol reduces serum urate, but its effect on recurrent gout is unclear. Only a minority of patients taking the typical dose of 300 mg/day achieve a target urate of 0.36 mmol/l. Its dose should be titrated according to response, up to 900 mg/day. Allopurinol hypersensitivity may occur in up to 2% of patients; this can be severe or even fatal. Desensitizing regimens of allopurinol can be tried in milder cases of hypersensitivity.

Febuxostat—Over half of patients taking febuxostat 80 mg achieve a urate of <0.36 mmol/l compared to one in five of those taking allopurinol 300 mg. However, febuxostat does not appear to be more effective at reducing recurrent gout over 1 year. It may have a role in patients who cannot take allopurinol, either because of intolerance or because it is contraindicated.

Uricosuric drugs—Uricosuric drugs lower serum urate by inhibiting its tubular reabsorption. There is no randomized controlled trial evidence supporting their use for prevention of recurrent gout. Only sulfinpyrazone is generally available for the treatment of gout. Benzbromarone can also be used, but it is not universally available, and there are concerns about it causing liver problems. Historically, probenecid has also been used. One should consider measuring urinary urate before starting uricosurics.

NSAIDs and colchicine—Both regular NSAIDs and colchicine can be used to prevent recurrent gouty attacks but have no effect on serum urate.

Uricase drugs—Uricase drugs work by oxidizing uric acid to the more soluble allantoin. A number of these are currently under investigation. Their role, if any, in the management of gout is unclear.

Other drugs—Several other drugs have, coincidentally, been found to have urate-lowering effects. These include losartan, fenofibrate, atorvastatin and amlodipine. Although they are not licensed for the treatment of gout, they may have a role if other drugs cannot be tolerated or if they are otherwise indicated for patients with multiple pathology.

Pseudogout

Pseudogout, which can be easily confused with gout, is caused by deposition of calcium pyrophosphate crystals. It most commonly affects knees, wrists, shoulders, ankles, elbows or hands. Typically it produces an episodic monoarthritis, but it can also have a clinical picture similar to osteoarthritis or rheumatoid arthritis. Its prevalence increases from 3% in people in their 60s to half of those in their 90s. It can be associated with hypothyroidism, hypercalcaemia, haemochromatosis or hypomagnesaemia.

Diagnosis is based on identifying pyrophosphate crystals or chondrocalcinosis seen on X-ray. Acute episodes can be treated with NSAIDs or intra-articular steroids. Long-term NSAIDs or colchicine can be used to try and prevent recurrence.

Other crystal diseases

A number of other crystals can produce acute musculoskeletal inflammation. Most common are hydroxyapatite crystals, which typically deposit in tendons, periarticular soft tissue and synovium. Hydroxyapatite deposition may be asymptomatic but can on occasion lead to significant joint destruction. Involvement of the shoulder is sometimes called Milwaukee shoulder, but virtually any joint may be affected. Identifying and correcting an underlying cause of hypophosphataemia or hypercalcaemia may reduce the risk of future attacks. Calcium oxalate may also cause acute arthritis. Its identification in joint fluid requires special staining with Alizarin Red dye. Treatments for acute attacks include NSAIDs and intra-articular steroids.

Reference

Underwood M. Diagnosis and management of gout. *British Medical Journal* 2006; **332**: 1315–1319.

Further reading

Baker JF, Krishnan E, Chen L, Schumacher HR. Serum uric acid and cardiovascular disease: recent developments, and where do they leave us? *American Journal of Medicine* 2005; **118**: 816–826.

Janssens HJ, Janssen M, van de Lisdonk EH, van Riel PL, van Weel C. Use of oral prednisolone or naproxen for the treatment of gout arthritis: a double-blind, randomised equivalence trial. *Lancet* 2008; **371**: 1854–1860.

Jordan KM, Stewart Cameron J, Snaith M *et al.* on behalf of the British Society for Rheumatology and British Health Professionals in Rheumatology Standards, Guidelines and Audit Working Group (SGAWG). British Society for Rheumatology and British Health Professionals in Rheumatology Guidelines for the Management of Gout. *Rheumatology* 2007; **46**: 1372–1374.

Underwood M. Gout. *British Medical Journal Clinical Evidence* 2008; **11**: 1120.

CHAPTER 11

Osteoporosis

Eugene McCloskey[1], Nicola Peel[2] and Richard Eastell[2]

[1]University of Sheffield, Sheffield, UK
[2]Northern General Hospital, Sheffield, UK

OVERVIEW

- Osteoporotic fractures cause substantial morbidity and place a significant burden on health-care resources.
- An individual's risk of fracture in the next 10 years can be readily estimated by the FRAX® tool and incorporated into clinical management.
- The measurement of bone mineral density plays an important role in the diagnosis of osteoporosis and contributes to fracture risk assessment as part of the FRAX tool.
- Effective treatments include the bisphosphonates, selective oestrogen receptor modulators, strontium ranelate and parathyroid hormone peptides.
- Falls risk assessment and prevention is an important consideration in patient management.

Osteoporosis is a systemic skeletal disease characterized by low bone mass and micro-architectural deterioration of bone tissue that results in a high risk of fracture. Currently, the diagnosis is generally based on bone mineral density (BMD) thresholds measured by dual X-ray absorptiometry (DXA—see below), whereby an individual's bone mineral density is compared with the mean (peak bone mass) for a young adult, as a standard deviation score (T score) (Table 11.1).

These thresholds were developed for measurements of BMDs of the spine, hip or forearm made with X-ray-based techniques in postmenopausal women. It is probably appropriate to use the same thresholds for BMD measurements made in men and premenopausal women after attainment of peak bone mass, but they should not be used for children or adolescents.

Pathophysiology

The human skeleton is composed of approximately 20% trabecular bone and 80% cortical bone. Bone undergoes a continual process of resorption and formation in discrete bone remodelling units. Approximately 10% of the adult skeleton is remodelled per year.

ABC of Rheumatology, 4th edn. Edited by Ade Adebajo.
©2010 Blackwell Publishing Ltd. 9781405170680.

This turnover prevents fatigue damage and is important in maintaining calcium homeostasis. Irreversible bone loss results from an imbalance between the rates of resorption and formation. Trabecular bone is the more metabolically active type, and osteoporotic fractures are more common at sites that contain more than 50% trabecular bone.

Bone loss leads to thinning, and often perforation, of the trabecular plates (Figure 11.1). Trabecular perforation occurs particularly in situations of increased bone turnover, e.g. after the menopause, and the resulting loss of normal architecture leads to a disproportionate loss of strength for the amount of bone lost. Increased bone turnover is an independent predictor of fracture risk. This may reflect the increase in number of remodelling sites, which can act as a stress riser and increase bone fragility. As a result of accelerated bone loss caused by oestrogen deficiency, postmenopausal osteoporosis initially leads to predominant loss of trabecular bone and frequent trabecular perforation. This typically results in fractures of vertebral bodies and the distal forearm in the sixth and seventh decades of life. In later life, age-related reductions in bone due to remodelling imbalances predominate in both sexes in both cortical and trabecular bone, resulting in the typical manifestation of fracture of the proximal femur.

Epidemiology

The classical osteoporotic fractures are those of the spine, wrist and hip (Figure 11.2) but all fragility fractures in the elderly can be regarded as osteoporotic once pathological fracture (e.g. metastatic disease) has been excluded. Osteoporotic fractures cause considerable morbidity and mortality. Recent estimates suggest that the cost of managing such fractures in the UK is over £1.7 billion a year. One in two women and one in five men are likely to sustain a fracture related to osteoporosis by the age of 90 years. The incidence of osteoporotic fractures is increasing more than expected from the ageing of the population. This may reflect changing patterns of exercise or diet in recent decades.

Classification of osteoporosis

Traditionally, osteoporosis has been classified as primary (includes postmenopausal and age-related bone loss) or secondary (where bone loss is accelerated by the presence of an underlying disease) (Table 11.2). Secondary osteoporosis accounts for up to 40% of cases of osteoporosis in women and 60% of cases in men.

Table 11.1 The World Health Organization's diagnostic thresholds for bone mineral density at the spine, hip or distal forearm

Diagnosis	Bone mineral density T score (SD units)
Normal	≥−1
Osteopaenia (or low bone mass)	<−1 but >−2.5
Osteoporosis	≤−2.5
Severe osteoporosis	≤−2.5 plus one or more fragility fractures

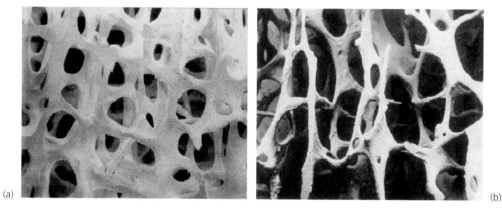

(a)　　　　　(b)

Figure 11.1 Comparison of structure of trabecular bone from healthy (a) and osteoporotic (b) subjects, illustrating the architectural damage resulting from trabecular perforation

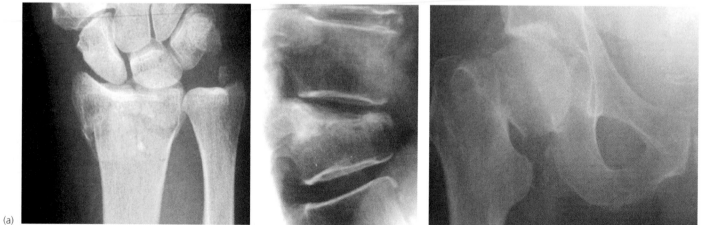

(a)　　　　　(b), (c)

Figure 11.2 Typical sites of osteoporotic fracture: wrist (a), vertebrae (b) and hip (c)

Table 11.2 Relatively common causes of secondary osteoporosis

Endocrine	Gastrointestinal	Rheumatological	Malignancy	Drugs
Thyrotoxicosis	Malabsorption syndrome, e.g. coeliac disease, partial gastrectomy	Rheumatoid arthritis	Multiple myeloma	Glucocorticoids
Primary hyper-parathyroidism		Ankylosing spondylitis	Cancer-treatment-induced bone loss (see drugs)	Anticonvulsants
Cushing's syndrome	Inflammatory bowel disease			Heparin
Hypogonadism, including anorexia nervosa	Liver disease, e.g. primary biliary cirrhosis			Aromatase inhibitors
Diabetes type I				Androgen-deprivation therapy

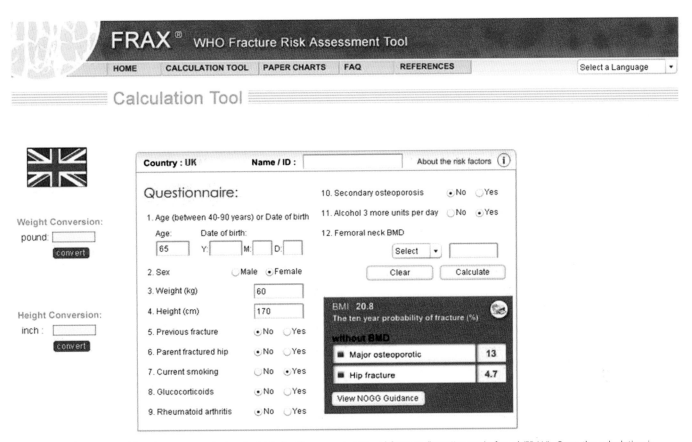

Figure 11.3 The FRAX tool for the assessment of an individual's 10-year probability of fracture (http://www.shef.ac.uk/FRAX). Once the calculation is completed, clicking on the "View NOGG guidance" button will automatically display the individual's probability within the suggested care pathways published by the National Osteoporosis Guideline Group (http://www.shef.ac.uk/NOGG)

Assessment of osteoporosis

This largely comprises the assessment of future fracture risk (determines the need for intervention) and the diagnosis or exclusion of underlying causes of osteoporosis.

Assessment of future fracture risk

Clinical risk factors—Several risk factors for fracture have been well established. Many of these risk factors impact on BMD but also contribute independently to future fracture risk. Clinicians frequently take account of these other risk factors in deciding whether treatment is required, and a number of algorithms have been developed to improve the prediction of fracture risk. Recently, the World Health Organization produced an algorithm (FRAX®) that estimates the probability of a major osteoporotic fracture (clinical vertebral, hip, wrist or proximal humerus) or hip fracture alone in the next 10 years (see http://www.shef.ac.uk/FRAX). The algorithm

incorporates BMD as an additional, measurable risk factor to information gleaned from clinical risk factors and adds value to the prediction of risk. BMD is probably of most value in those deemed to be at intermediate or high risk. A history of prior low trauma fracture in adult life is a very important risk factor to identify and can usually be obtained by a good clinical history. In contrast, the suggestion of prior vertebral fracture requires spinal imaging for confirmation and appropriate management. The National Osteoporosis Guideline Group (NOGG) has recently published a new management guideline (Figure 11.3) that integrates FRAX with clinical management algorithms.

Spinal radiographs—Up to half of vertebral fractures are asymptomatic and may be suspected from height loss and the development of kyphosis. The latter features may also result from degenerative spinal disease, however, and radiographs of the thoracic and lumbar spine are important to differentiate fractures from degenerative changes. The importance of vertebral fractures for future fracture risk cannot be overstated, and strategies in the near future will involve the assessment of patients by low-radiation-imaging DXA scans to identify prevalent fractures. In the absence of fractures, the assessment of bone mass on plain radiographs is unreliable, so radiological reports of osteopaenia require confirmation by bone densitometry prior to any therapeutic decisions.

Bone densitometry—After age and prior fragility fracture, BMD is the next major determinant of a person's risk of fracture. The predictive ability of bone density is comparable with that of blood pressure for determining the risk of cerebrovascular accident and of serum cholesterol for determining the risk of coronary thrombosis. The relative risk of fracture increases approximately 2-fold for each standard deviation decrease in bone density.

BMD is usually measured by DXA—a technique that uses extremely low doses of ionizing radiation to quantify BMD accurately and precisely. DXA of the spine and hip are the optimal clinical measurements for diagnosis. Measurement of bone density in peripheral skeletal sites with techniques such as quantitative ultrasound has useful predictive value for osteoporotic fractures, but appropriate intervention thresholds for these measurements remain uncertain, and they are probably not useful for monitoring responses to treatment.

Currently, no rationale exists for population screening of BMD. If access to bone densitometry is limited, it may be appropriate to treat individuals who have had previous low-trauma fractures or who have other strong risk factors for fracture, such as elderly people who need high-dose corticosteroid therapy. Otherwise, measurements should be targeted to individuals likely to be at increased risk of osteoporosis, where knowledge of BMD will influence management. Traditionally, this has meant the measurement of BMD in all patients with recognized risk factors, an approach encapsulated in the Royal College of Physician Guidelines published in 1999. This guidance has now been updated to incorporate the availability of the FRAX tool for assessing fracture risk (http://www.shef.ac.uk/NOGG). The National Institute for Health and

Clinical Excellence (NICE) has also recently published guidance for the primary and secondary prevention of fracture in post-menopausal women (Table 11.3) (http://www.nice.org.uk).

Identifying or excluding underlying causes of osteoporosis

Individuals with a low-trauma vertebral fracture or low BMD for age should be investigated for underlying causes of osteoporosis. In addition to a good clinical history, a small number of investigations can exclude the most common secondary causes of osteoporosis (Box 11.1). Treating the underlying cause often leads to at least partial recovery of bone mass.

Reducing fracture risk

The ultimate goal of osteoporosis management is to reduce the future risk of fracture. This involves educating the patient about the nature of the disease, their fracture risk, lifestyle modification (Box 11.2) and, if necessary, the different types of therapy available.

Table 11.3 Clinical risk factors used for the assessment of fracture probability

Age	Secondary causes of
Sex	osteoporosis including:
Low body mass index (≤19 kg/m²)	• Rheumatoid arthritis
Previous fragility fracture, particularly of the hip, wrist and spine, including morphometric vertebral fracture	• Untreated hypogonadism in men and women
	• Prolonged immobility
Parental history of hip fracture	• Organ transplantation
Current glucocorticoid treatment (any dose, by mouth for 3 months or more)	• Type I diabetes
	• Hyperthyroidism
Current smoking	• Gastrointestinal disease
Alcohol intake of 3 or more units daily	• Chronic liver disease
	• Chronic obstructive pulmonary disease
	Falls*

*Not presently accommodated in the FRAX algorithm, but an important risk factor to be taken into account in patient management

---

Box 11.1 **Investigations to exclude underlying causes of osteoporosis**

Routine
- History and physical examination
- Blood cell count, sedimentation rate or C-reactive protein, serum calcium, albumin, creatinine, phosphate, alkaline phosphatase and liver transaminases
- Thyroid function tests
- Bone densitometry (DXA)

Other procedures, if indicated
- Lateral radiographs of lumbar and thoracic spine/DXA-based vertebral imaging
- Protein immunoelectrophoresis and urinary Bence Jones proteins
- Serum testosterone, SHBG, FSH, LH (in men)
- Serum prolactin
- 24-hour urinary cortisol/dexamethasone suppression test
- Endomysial and/or tissue transglutaminase antibodies (coeliac disease)
- Isotope bone scan
- Markers of bone turnover, when available
- Urinary calcium excretion

SHBG = sex-hormone binding globulin; FSH = follicle-stimulating hormone, LH = luteinizing hormone

---

Box 11.2 **Lifestyle modification**

Optimizing peak bone mass and reducing bone loss
- Exercise needs to be regular and weight-bearing (such as walking or aerobics); excessive exercise may lead to bone loss
- Dietary calcium may be important, especially during growth
- Avoidance of smoking and excessive alcohol consumption

In some patients, particularly those with recent vertebral fractures, additional approaches aim to reduce pain and improve mobility.

Guidance

In October 2008, NICE published two Technology Appraisal Guidance documents to address the primary (http://www.nice.org.uk/Guidance/TA160) and secondary (http://www.nice.org.uk/Guidance/TA161) prevention of osteoporotic fractures with alendronate, etidronate, risedronate, raloxifene, strontium ranelate and teriparatide (secondary prevention only). While welcome, there a number of challenges to the implementation of these guidelines, particularly with regard to prescribing alternative treatments when generic alendronate is contraindicated or not tolerated. NICE plan to have clinical guidelines that will address some of the limitations with these approaches (such as not giving guidance for glucocorticoid-induced osteoporosis or men). In the meantime, a more pragmatic approach to treatment has been proposed by NOGG with the support of many professional and patient societies. This approach suggests that treatment should be considered when an individual's probability of fracture is comparable to or exceeds that of a woman of the same age who has already sustained a low-trauma fracture.

Antiresorptive agents

Bisphosphonates—Alendronate and risedronate are available as once-weekly preparations with evidence for significant reductions in vertebral and non-vertebral fractures. These drugs have largely replaced the use of cyclical etidronate. Ibandronate, available as a once-monthly tablet or a three-monthly intravenous slow injection reduces vertebral fractures with indirect evidence for a reduction in non-vertebral fractures. More recently, zoledronate has become available as a once-yearly short infusion with good evidence of anti-fracture efficacy at all sites. Both NICE and NOGG recommend the use of generic alendronate as first-line therapy, although this may not be suitable for or tolerated by all. Poor absorption of these agents means they must be taken on an empty stomach before breakfast (30 minutes before for alendronate and risedronate; 60 minutes before for ibandronate) or on an empty stomach in the middle of a 4-hour fast (cyclical etidronate). The move away from oral daily dosing regimens to more convenient, less frequent dosing has improved adherence to the bisphosphonates.

Hormone or oestrogen replacement therapy—The use of hormone replacement therapy is no longer thought to be appropriate in the management of osteoporosis unless it is needed to control climacteric symptoms, or in women under 50 who have undergone an early menopause. The safety profile of oestrogen-only therapy appears somewhat better than combined oestrogen–progestogen therapy.

Selective oestrogen receptor modulators—These synthetic agents act as oestrogen agonists on bone and lipids, but without oestrogen-like stimulation of breast and endometrial tissues. Raloxifene reduces the risk of vertebral fracture but has not been shown to decrease the risk of non-vertebral fractures. Like hormone replacement therapy, raloxifene is associated with small increases in the number of thromboembolic events but conversely is associated with a significant reduction in the number of new cases of breast cancer. Other agents in this class will be available in the near future.

Calcium (1000–1200 mg daily)—This has a less marked effect on fracture reduction than the other antiresorptive agents. Adherence can be problematic, and several preparations are now available to aid patient choice and compliance.

Vitamin D (800 units daily) and calcium (1000–1200 mg daily)—This has been shown to reduce hip fracture risk in the frail elderly and should be considered in all elderly patients who are housebound or in residential care. In patients at higher risk of fracture, it should be used as adjunctive therapy in combination with another antiresorptive agent.

Calcitonin—Calcitonin may be administered as subcutaneous injections or as a nasal preparation, which is associated with fewer side effects. Calcitonin has been shown to reduce the risk of vertebral fracture. This agent has analgesic properties that may be useful in the acute management of vertebral fracture.

Formation-stimulating agents

Teriparatide and parathyroid hormone—These agents have good evidence for their abilities to increase bone formation (and later bone resorption) with an improvement in bone mass and structure, particularly in trabecular bone such as the vertebrae, with reductions in spine fracture risk. A reduction in non-vertebral fractures has also been shown by recombinant teriparatide (PTH 1-34), possibly mediated by improvements in cortical bone width and/or thickness. They are expensive agents and their use is limited to patients with severe, progressive osteoporosis despite exposure to antiresorptive therapy. Teriparatide is licensed for use in men and women, whereas recombinant parathyroid hormone 1-84 is only licensed for postmenopausal women. Treatment is currently limited to 18–24 month durations and most patients will require treatment with antiresorptive agents after discontinuation to maintain the improvements in bone mass. Very recently, teriparatide has been shown to induce greater increases in spine and hip BMD than alendronate in patients with glucocorticoid-induced osteoporosis and is now licensed for use in this setting.

Alternative agents

Strontium ranelate—Strontium ranelate been shown to significantly reduce vertebral and non-vertebral fracture risk in postmenopausal women. The precise mechanism(s) of action remains unclear, but treatment is associated with significant increases in BMD, partly mediated by the presence of strontium in bone, which impacts on the interpretation of changes in BMD. The change in BMD is therefore a potential marker of adherence to therapy, though it may also complicate future estimates of fracture risk.

Pain relief

Pain relief is frequently adequately achieved with analgesics, but physical measures—such as hydrotherapy or transcutaneous nerve stimulators—may be useful adjuncts to treatment. The pain-modulating effects of low-dose antidepressants can be helpful, and many patients benefit from assessment at specialist pain clinics. The pain associated with fractures usually resolves within 6 months, but patients with vertebral fractures may need to be given long-term analgesia because of secondary degenerative disease. NICE has also approved techniques such as vertebroplasty (http://www.nice.org.uk/Guidance/IPG12) and kyphoplasty (http://www.nice.org.uk/Guidance/IPG166) for use in selected patients with recent vertebral fractures and persistent or severe pain. Both techniques give good pain relief. Kyphoplasty may also result in some restoration of vertebral height.

Falls prevention

Predisposing factors, such as postural hypotension or drowsiness due to drugs, should be eliminated where possible. Patients may benefit from physiotherapy to improve their balance and saving reflexes. Patients should be provided with appropriate walking aids, and an environmental assessment should be made of their accommodation to eliminate hazards such as loose rugs and cables. Hip protectors have a limited role to play. Visual assessment and treatment is also important. Assessment via specialized falls clinics may be appropriate, particularly in those individuals with features suggesting a medical cause for falls, such as palpitations or blackouts.

Education

An important part of the management of osteoporosis is education and support of the patient, their carers and their family. Groups such as the National Osteoporosis Society (Box 11.3) have a vital role in this area.

Box 11.3 National Osteoporosis Society (NOS)

Camerton
Bath BA2 0PJ
Tel.: 01761 471771 (for general enquiries); 0845 4500234 (for medical enquiries)

Monitoring of treatment

The rationale for monitoring treatment response is that a proportion of patients fail to respond to treatment, commonly due to non-persistence with therapy, poor dosing compliance or, less commonly, due to underlying disease. The current standard measure used to monitor treatment response is spine DXA at 18–24 months after treatment initiation. Biochemical markers of bone turnover may offer a more rapid assessment of treatment response—within 3–6 months. The decrease in bone turnover in response to antiresorptive agents may be a superior predictor of the decrease in fracture risk.

Further reading

Barlow D, ed. *Osteoporosis: clinical guidelines for prevention and treatment.* Royal College of Physicians, London, 1999.

Kanis JA, McCloskey EV, Johansson H, Strom O, Borgstrom F, Oden A and the National Osteoporosis Guideline Group. Case finding for the management of osteoporosis with FRAX®-assessment and intervention thresholds for the UK. *Osteoporosis International* 2008; **19**: 1395–1408.

Kanis JA, Oden A, Johnell O et al. The use of clinical risk factors enhances the performance of BMD in the prediction of hip and osteoporotic fractures in men and women. *Osteoporosis International* 2007; **18**: 1033–1046.

National Institute for Clinical Excellence. *NICE Interventional Procedure Guidance 12: percutaneous vertebroplasty.* National Institute for Clinical Excellence, London, 2003.

National Institute for Clinical Excellence. *NICE Technology Appraisal Guidance 160: elendronate, etidronate, risedronate, raloxifene and strontium ranelate for the primary prevention of osteoporotic fragility fractures in postmenopausal women.* National Institute for Clinical Excellence, London, 2008.

National Institute for Clinical Excellence. *NICE Technology Appraisal Guidance 161: alendronate, etidronate, risedronate, raloxifene, strontium ranelate and teriparatide for the secondary prevention of osteoporotic fragility fractures in postmenopausal women.* National Institute for Clinical Excellence, London, 2008.

National Institute for Clinical Excellence. *NICE Technology Appraisal Guidance 166: balloon kyphoplasty for vertebral compression fractures.* National Institute for Clinical Excellence, London, 2008.

Royal College of Physicians. *Glucocorticoid-induced osteoporosis: guidelines for prevention and treatment.* Royal College of Physicians, London, 2002.

CHAPTER 12

Rheumatoid Arthritis: Clinical Features and Diagnosis

Kamran Hameed[1] and Mohammed Akil[2]

[1]Aga Khan University Hospital, Pakistan
[2]Royal Hallamshire Hospital, Sheffield, UK

OVERVIEW

- Rheumatoid arthritis (RA) is a chronic disabling inflammatory arthritis, which is associated with a significant morbidity and an increased mortality.

- It has a wide spectrum of disease manifestations, both articular and non-articular. Progressive joint destruction and extra-articular manifestations account for the disability and increased mortality. Early recognition and intervention with disease-modifying therapy is key to preventing the progressive disability.

- It is vital that clinicians develop expertise in identifying early disease and recognizing the spectrum of its manifestations. Geographical variations in disease pattern have been reported and attributed to lifestyle differences in populations; however, genetic differences have also been implicated in the severity of the disease.

- RA occurs with varying prevalence in different parts of the world; the highest incidence is reported in some Native American tribes (5%), but it is far less common in Chinese and Japanese people (0.3%).

- It is three times more common in women than men.

Pathogenesis

The cause of rheumatoid arthritis (RA) is not yet established; however, the postulate that remains popular is that an unknown antigen in a genetically predisposed individual is able to initiate a self-perpetuating immune response. The response has cross-reactivity with host tissue, initiating an autoimmune synovitis and subsequent hypertrophy. Synovial hypertrophy is the key factor that leads to cartilage and bone destruction, causing progressive joint damage and disability. Other tissues are affected through different mechanisms, accounting for the extra-articular manifestations.

Many cellular and chemical markers have been studied; the key effector cell still appears to be the T-cell, which orchestrates the immune response through a host of cytokines. The key cytokines involved in the pathogenesis of RA have been tumour necrosis factor-alpha (TNF-α) and interleukin-1. The advances in knowledge about RA pathogenesis have directed development of targeted therapy, which has led to major advances in the management of this disease.

Knowledge has advanced in genetics, and HLA-DR4 has been established as a marker of prevalence as well as severity in RA. However, other alleles have also been implicated, and this has been ascribed to a "shared epitope" on the hypervariable region of the human leukocyte antigen-DRB1 chain.

Clinical features

The objectives of clinical assessment for RA are mainly to: (a) establish the diagnosis; (b) evaluate the disease activity (is the disease active or quiescent?); (c) assess the disease severity (amount of damage and disability); and (d) look for extra-articular manifestations.

Usually the disease is insidious in nature, rarely occurring in men younger than 30 years, with gradually rising incidence with advancing age. In women the incidence steadily increases from the mid-20s to peak incidence between 45 and 75 years. In the classical presentation, which remains the more common variant, the disease affects the small joints of the hands and feet in a more symmetrical pattern. The joints predominantly affected are the metacarpophalangeal joints, the proximal interphalangeal joints and the wrists (Figure 12.1); in the feet the metatarsophalangeal joints and the forefoot joints are affected.

Less common forms of presentation are acute monoarticular, palindromic rheumatism and asymmetrical large joint arthritis. Theoretically all synovial joints can be affected; however, spine joints other than the cervical spine are very rarely involved in RA.

Extra-articular manifestations (Figure 12.2) are varied and also differ in different populations. They can affect almost any system of the body and are mediated by various mechanisms. Immune responses such as immune complex deposition, cytokine production and direct endothelial injury can produce distant and local effects. Also, mechanical causes such as synovial hypertrophy and subluxation of joints may cause entrapments of the nerves or vessels. The disability leads to disuse and abnormal mechanics, which leads to degenerative changes and osteoporosis.

ABC of Rheumatology, 4th edn. Edited by Ade Adebajo.
©2010 Blackwell Publishing Ltd. 9781405170680.

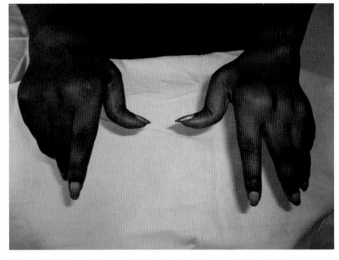

Figure 12.1 Typical changes in the hands in rheumatoid arthritis

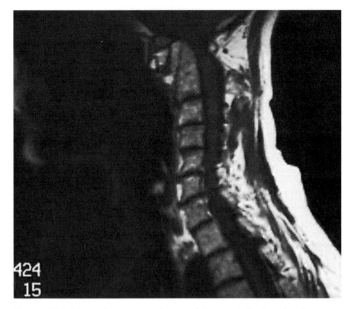

Figure 12.3 Magnetic resonance image of the cervical spine showing atlanto-axial involvement in rheumatoid arthritis

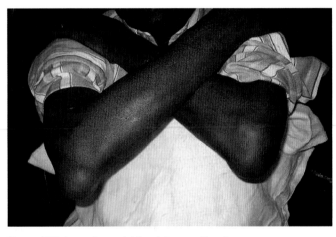

Figure 12.2 Large rheumatoid nodules over the elbows

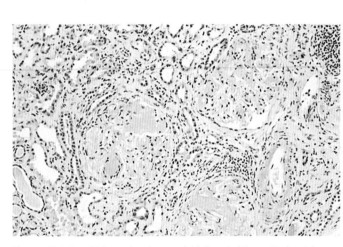

Figure 12.4 Renal biopsy showing amyloid deposit (Congo Red stain)

"Red flags"

A variety of complications of RA or its treatment can occur and require vigilance on the part of clinicians to pick them up early and intervene to prevent severe morbidity, and even mortality in certain cases; some of these are detailed below.

Atlanto-axial subluxation—This results from involvement of the atlanto-axial joint, which may be clinically asymptomatic until the subluxation develops. Development of pain around the occiput, radiating arm pain, numbness or weakness of the limbs and vertigo on neck movement are warning signs; if not picked up this may lead to sudden death, especially if patients undergo neck manipulation for endotracheal entubation during surgical procedures. It is advisable to actively look for it as part of pre-surgical evaluation. It can be picked up easily by doing lateral views of the cervical spine

in flexion (Figure 12.3) and extension and measuring the distance between the posterior margin of the atlas ring and the anterior surface of the odontoid process.

Amyloidosis—Renal deposition of amyloid (Figure 12.4) is a recognized feature of longstanding RA and should be suspected if the patient develops increasing leg oedema, proteinuria and worsening renal functions. Drug-related causes such as gold- or penicillamine-induced proteinuria need to be ruled out. A renal biopsy will conclude the diagnosis.

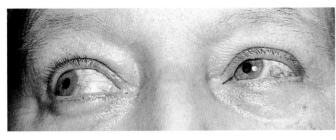

Figure 12.5 Epicleritis in rheumatoid arthritis

Table 12.1 Other manifestations of rheumatoid arthritis

Haematological	Cutaneous
Anaemia	Rheumatoid nodules
Neutrophillia	Peripheral vasculitis
Thrombocytosis	Leg ulcers
Felty's syndrome	Alopecia
Neurological	**Ocular**
Entrapment neuropathies such as carpal tunnel syndrome	Xeropthalmia
Mononeurits multiplex	Scleritis
Peripheral neuropathies	Episcleritis
Pulmonary	**Others**
Pleural effusions	Dry mouth
Interstitial lung disease	Osteoporosis
Bronchiolitis oblitrans	Muscle wasting
Cardiac	
Pericarditis	
Coronary vasculitis (rare)	

Pericarditis—Onset of central chest pain worsened by lying flat, accompanied by a pericardial rub, merits urgent echocardiogram to confirm and urgent initiation of steroid therapy. Infective causes such as tuberculosis need to be ruled out by aspiration and analysis when suspected.

Monoarticular flare—A single joint worsening should always be viewed with suspicion in RA, and septic arthritis needs to be looked for. It is prudent to initiate treatment for possible septic arthritis until the results of the joint aspirate rule it out.

Eye involvement—Sudden onset of eye pain and increased lacrimation should alert the clinician to the possibility of scleritis (Figure 12.5); if left untreated this may lead to full-thickness involvement of the sclera, with thinning and risk of perforation. Called scleromalacia perforans, this sinister condition is thankfully rare but needs to be looked out for.

Other manifestations of RA are given in Table 12.1.

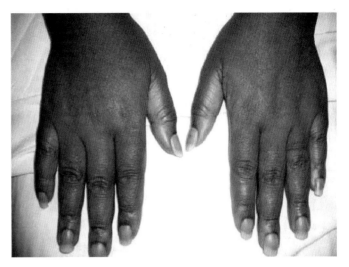

Figure 12.6 Subtle features of synovitis in early rheumatoid arthritis

Diagnosis

The diagnosis of RA is predominantly a clinical one; no diagnostic test has been shown to be foolproof, and both false-positive and false-negative results are seen with varying frequency.

History

A detailed history of the problem, its onset and progression with time, relieving and aggravating factors and the distribution of the symptoms are all important elements in the history. A progressive pattern of joint involvement, stiffness and increased pain after a period of inactivity and a history of joint swellings are indicative of inflammatory joint disorders. A family history of rheumatological disease can raise the suspicion further. The distribution of joint involvement helps in distinguishing other forms of arthritides such as spondyloarthritis and psoriatic arthritis.

Clinical examination

The objective of the clinical assessment is to identify signs of inflammatory arthritis, such as swelling, tenderness and restriction of movement of the joints. A symmetrical involvement of the hands, especially the metacarpophalangeal and proximal interphalangeal joints, with relative sparing of the axial skeleton, are some key elements that support the diagnosis of RA. Clinical evaluation may also pick up extra-articular findings that can support the diagnosis or refute it—for example, the presence of rheumatoid nodules and psoriatic skin patches, respectively. In early disease the classical signs of structural changes may be missing and subtle synovitis (Figure 12.6) may escape notice; however, tenderness and restriction without history of trauma should arouse suspicion.

Laboratory evidence

Active RA is associated with a variety of haematological responses. Acute-phase responses such as a high erythrocyte sedimentation rate or C-reactive protein, a high platelet count and high serum ferritin can be seen in most patients. Anaemia of chronic disease may be present in many patients with chronic conditions. A very high leucocyte response is uncommon and usually indicative of an infection, which should be looked for in such situations.

The traditional test of rheumatoid factor that detects immunoglobulin M (IgM) antibodies directed against IgG can be used as supporting evidence in establishing the diagnosis, but is neither conclusive nor universal in patients with RA. A number of conditions are associated with the presence of rheumatoid factor in serum (Box 12.1).

A new test that seems more promising, called anti-cyclic citrullinated peptide (anti-CCP), is now commercially available. This test seems to be more specific (95–98%) for the diagnosis of RA and it is sensitive (50–60%) in early rheumatoid disease. It is also a marker of erosive disease and can predict eventual development of RA in undifferentiated arthritis.

Radiology

Radiological features of classical periarticular erosions (Figure 12.7) are characteristic and may appear within the first 3 years of disease in the majority of the patients; more subtle changes, such as juxta-articular osteopenia and early joint-space narrowing, are less specific and can be misleading. Conventional radiology can still be useful in monitoring progression of the disease in established diagnosis and to plan corrective surgeries when there is significant disability. Newer modalities such as magnetic resonance imaging are now increasingly employed to detect early synovitis and bone oedema and can be utilized effectively in picking up early disease. Ultrasonography may be useful in picking up joint effusions, a Baker's cyst and pleural disease. High-resolution computed tomography is the modality of choice in picking up interstitial lung disease and pulmonary fibrosis. It should be carried out in patients with progressive loss of lung function.

Synovial fluid analysis

This test is rarely required to establish diagnosis in a typical presentation; however, in atypical presentations with large joint involvement, especially monoarticular, it is vital to rule out infective aetiology and crystal arthropathy. The fluid would typically show a high protein and leucocyte count and the absence of crystals and organisms on Gram stain.

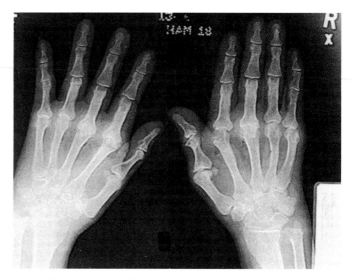

Figure 12.7 Radiograph of the hands, showing erosions at the metacarpophalangeal and proximal interphalangeal joints

The American College of Rheumatology has formulated and modified classification criteria to aid in diagnosis of RA (Box 12.2); however, these criteria have poor sensitivity in picking up early rheumatoid disease.

Differential diagnosis

Other arthritides can be distinguished on the basis of joint-involvement pattern; however, atypical presentations may prove

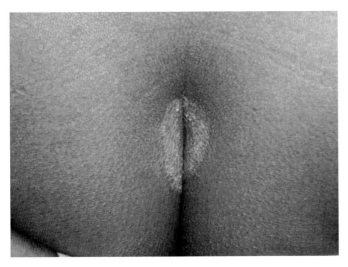

Figure 12.8 Psoriatic rash at the natal cleft

challenging to rule out. A careful search for evidence of nail pitting or skin lesions may clinch the diagnosis in psoriatic disease (Figure 12.8), but joint aspiration for crystals may be needed to exclude

polyarticular gout. Malignant conditions such as leukaemias and lymphomas should be sought, especially in acute presentations in younger patients. In areas of high incidence, conditions such as hepatitis B and C and HIV need to be borne in mind.

As RA is a chronic disease that leads to significant morbidity and disability, the clinician has the vital responsibility of making an early diagnosis and commencing treatment early to prevent these problems from occurring. No laboratory tests are diagnostic, and ultimately the diagnosis relies on a clinical evaluation by the practitioner.

Further reading

Firestein GS, Panayi G & Wollheim F, eds. *Rheumatoid Arthritis*, 2nd edn. Oxford University Press, Oxford, 2006.

Isaacs J, Moreland LW. *Fast Facts: rheumatoid arthritis*. Health Press, Oxford, 2002.

Isenberg D, Maddison P, Woo P, Glass D, Breedveld F, eds. *Oxford Textbook of Rheumatology*. Oxford University Press, Oxford, 2004.

Taylor P. *Rheumatoid Arthritis in Practice*. Royal Society of Medicine Press, London, 2006.

CHAPTER 13

Treatment of Rheumatoid Arthritis

Edwin S L Chan[1], Anthony G Wilson[2] and Bruce N Cronstein[1]

[1]New York University School of Medicine, New York, USA
[2]University of Sheffield, Sheffield, UK

OVERVIEW

- Rheumatoid arthritis (RA) is a disease requiring life-long treatment.
- Treatment should begin early because radiological damage can occur much earlier than previously thought.
- Disease-modifying antirheumatic drugs (DMARDs) and biological-response modifiers have been proven to retard disease progression.
- Combination therapy is often more efficacious than monotherapy.
- Inadequately treated rheumatoid arthritis is associated with increased mortality.

Remarkable strides have been made in controlling clinical and radiological progression of rheumatoid arthritis (RA) in recent years. However, the usefulness of small molecules such as methotrexate has not been overshadowed by the current interest in biological-response modification. Our understanding of the molecular mechanisms responsible for the pathogenesis of RA has heralded a shift from empiricism to selective molecular targeting in immunomodulatory pharmacotherapeutics. While symptomatic control and reduction of the clinical signs of synovitis have been the foremost considerations in the past, modern pharmacotherapy has emphasized the need to slow down, if not halt, disease progression as well as to prevent the development of potential complications. It is now recognized that significant documented radiological damage can occur in this disease much earlier than previously thought, certainly within the first 2 years of disease onset. Disease-modifying therapy is therefore introduced early following confirmation of diagnosis, particularly in those with poor prognostic indicators, such as severe disease activity, radiological damage or anti-cyclic citrullinated peptide positivity. Some favour a more aggressive combination of drugs in early disease, with a possible "step-down" approach once the disease comes under control. The old "pyramidal" treatment approach has therefore been called into question, and new advances have dramatically improved the disease outlook for the RA patient.

Non-steroidal anti-inflammatory drugs

Non-steroidal anti-inflammatory drugs (NSAIDs) are inhibitors of cyclooxygenase, an enzyme that catalyses the conversion of arachidonic acid to prostanoids. The enzyme exists in two isoforms. Cyclooxygenase-1 is constitutively expressed in many tissues including platelets, blood vessels and the upper gastrointestinal (GI) mucosa, where production of prostaglandin E_2 mediates a protective mucosal effect that includes mucus secretion and diminution of acid production. Expression of cyclooxygenase-2 is induced at sites of inflammation, particularly on polymorphonuclear cells and macrophages. Thus, non-selective inhibition of both isoforms by traditional NSAIDs may ameliorate desirable gastroprotective effects mediated by cyclooxygenase-1, and reported hospitalization of RA patients as a result of upper GI complications may exceed 1% of patients treated per year. Selective inhibition of cyclooxygenase-2, however, has met with concerns over potential cardiovascular risks, although recent evidence suggests that this problem is also associated with several traditional NSAIDs. Despite these concerns, NSAIDs continue to be used for symptomatic control in RA, but it must be emphasized that they have little effect in limiting joint damage or radiological progression.

Corticosteroids

The demonstration of the anti-inflammatory efficacy of corticosteroids in RA resulted in the first Nobel Prize awarded for a clinical observation, and 70 years hence, these potent anti-inflammatory agents continue to have an important place in the management of RA. Furthermore, multiple routes of administration, including depot injections (methylprednisolone and triamcinolone acetonide) and local intra-articular injections offer a variety of therapeutic options. Given orally, the onset of action is quick and is therefore useful in relieving symptoms while awaiting the onset of DMARD activity. Lower oral doses have been favoured (prednisolone up to 10 mg/day) owing to fear of suppression of the hypothalamus–pituitary–adrenal axis, and prevention of corticosteroid-induced osteoporosis must be considered in patients receiving these medications long term.

ABC of Rheumatology, 4th edn. Edited by Ade Adebajo.
©2010 Blackwell Publishing Ltd. 9781405170680.

Disease-modifying antirheumatic drugs

Gold—Originally intended for the treatment of infectious diseases, gold is one of the oldest of the disease-modifying antirheumatic drugs (DMARDs) and has been in use for almost a century for the treatment of RA. An intramuscular drug of proven efficacy, radiological improvement with decrease in radiological damage bore evidence of its disease-modifying capacity. However, weekly injections may be cumbersome, and an oral form proved inefficacious. This, together with the fact that over half of drug discontinuations were reported to be the result of toxicity (such as severe skin rash and nephrotoxicity), heralded a decline in its popularity over the years.

Methotrexate—A dihydrofolate reductase inhibitor originally used for its anti-proliferative effects in the treatment of cancer, methotrexate is now an anchor drug among DMARDs and a gold standard against which all emerging therapies are compared. An oral drug administered on a weekly basis, its anti-inflammatory mechanisms of action are thought to differ from its anti-malignant effects, and are largely related to its induction of adenosine release to the inflammatory environment. Compared with gold it has an excellent side-effect profile, the only frequent problem being post-dosage nausea, which frequently responds to folic acid (Box 13.1).

Sulfasalazine—Sulfasalazine, the first drug developed specifically for the treatment of RA, was first synthesized in the 1940s. It is composed of sulfapyridine and 5-aminosalicylic acid moieties and should be avoided in patients allergic to sulfa medications. Plasma half-life is greatly influenced by acetylation status, and slow acetylators are more likely to develop serious toxicities. While minor upper GI side effects and rashes are common, drug-induced hepatitis, cytopenias and Stevens–Johnson syndrome may also occur.

Hydroxychloroquine—Hydroxychloroquine is an antimalarial with proven efficacy in the treatment of RA, particularly in early and mild disease. Unlike its sister drug, chloroquine, occurrence of retinopathy is extremely rare. However, evidence for radiological protection has been unconvincing, and this benign medication in most often used in conjunction with other DMARDs in combination therapy rather than alone.

Leflunomide—The youngest member among the DMARDs, leflunomide inhibits the *de novo* synthesis of pyrimidines by inhibiting dihydroorotate dehydrogenase, and this action principally affects lymphocytes which lack salvage pathways for pyrimidine synthesis. It may be useful in patients who have failed to respond to methotrexate, but can also be administered together with methotrexate to improve response. It has a long half-life, requiring a loading dose for 1–3 days. As a long washout period of up to 2 years is suggested prior to conception, careful planning is needed in premenopausal women.

Some of the other DMARDs in use are listed in Box 13.2.

Combination therapy

Although DMARDs represent a marked improvement over previous symptom-oriented therapies, response to monotherapy is often partial at best, and discontinuation, whether due to toxicity or lack of response, is commonplace. It has been suggested that using these medications with different but complementary mechanisms of action in combination not only allows for greater efficacy, but also limits effective required dosage and hence toxicity. Various combinations, including step-up and step-down regimens have been tried, often with the inclusion of methotrexate.

Biological-response modifiers

A major development in the treatment of RA in the last decade was the emergence of biological-response-modifying therapy. Previous attempts at drug development have largely been empirical efforts. Understanding of the molecular and cellular mechanisms that contribute to the generation and maintenance of the inflammatory processes that culminate in synovial inflammation and joint destruction has escalated astronomically in recent decades. These fundamental elements of the inflammatory cascade, whether it be a cytokine or an inflammatory cell subset, have become the targets of new treatment modalities. These drugs are administered parenterally, and the onset of action, unlike DMARDs, is rapid.

Tumour necrosis factor antagonists

Tumour necrosis factor (TNF) is a pivotal cytokine released in excess in RA, and is a major contributor to synovial inflammation and cartilage destruction. Blockade of its actions by the human TNF receptor 2–immunoglobulin constant region fusion protein, etanercept, resulted in the first success of biological-response-modifying therapy in RA. Since then, monoclonal antibodies to human TNF have come into use, whether chimeric (infliximab) or fully humanized (adalimumab). These agents have been demonstrated to be efficacious in the treatment of RA on clinical, radiological and laboratory measures, particularly when used in combination with methotrexate.

Anakinra

The next cytokine to be targeted for therapeutic use was interleukin-1 (IL-1) and anakinra is a recombinant human IL-1 receptor antagonist. Its short half-life means that subcutaneous injections have to be given on a daily basis. Used alone or in combination with methotrexate, anakinra produces significant if modest clinical improvement in RA. Radiological improvement, including rates of progression of joint-space narrowing and erosion, have been more striking, however.

Rituximab

The B-lymphocyte is not only the source of inflammatory cytokines and antibodies important to the pathogenesis of the disease such as rheumatoid factor and anti-cyclic citrullinated peptide; B-cell help is a vital contributor to T-cell activation and antigen presentation. It is therefore little surprise that the B-lymphocyte may be a suitable target for RA therapy, despite previous dogma that RA is predominantly a T-cell-mediated disease. Rituximab targets the B-cell surface marker, CD20, which is expressed from the pre-B-cell stage through to the mature memory B-cell. Binding of this chimeric monoclonal antibody depletes CD20$^+$ B-cells in a transient manner. Rituximab, whether alone or in combination with methotrexate, is effective at suppressing inflammatory parameters and limiting structural joint damage in RA, although seronegative patients have responded less well. While the risk of infection remains a concern with B-cell depletion, this has not been a problem based on available clinical trial data. However, clinicians should be alerted to reports of rare neurological diseases, such as progressive multifocal leukoencephalopathy, caused by infection with the JC polyoma virus.

Abatacept

T-lymphocyte activation and proliferation requires a dual stimulatory signal that involves both the T-cell and the antigen-presenting cell. Interruption of any individual part of this signalling complex, such as CTLA-4, the target of abatacept, disrupts T-cell contributions to the inflammatory environment. Abatacept has proven benefits in slowing disease activity and joint damage in RA, including in patients who have failed to respond to anti-TNF therapy, although it has not been recommended for use in Britain in a preliminary judgment by the National Institute for Health and Clinical Excellence.

Identification of coexisting problems

RA has long been regarded as an indolent disease, until recently when it has been recognized that RA may be associated with increased mortality. Life expectancy may be shortened by as much as 7 years in men and 3 years in women. Yet few have been able to attribute deaths directly to RA itself. Clinicians should therefore be constantly alerted to the development of other co-morbidities in RA patients, of which cardiovascular disease is the most important. Occurrence of cardiovascular disease has been reported in up to 42% of RA patients, and scrupulous management and correction of cardiovascular risk factors is of utmost importance to disease outlook. Although vasculitis, secondary amyloidosis and lymphoproliferative malignancies have been associated with the disease itself, these are rare, and renal, pulmonary, GI and infectious diseases are much more common. Furthermore, antirheumatic pharmacotherapy itself may compound these problems. The presence of co-morbidities is a known predictor for mortality in RA patients, and due attention must be given to its early identification.

Complimentary therapy

Although our discussion has focused on the pharmacotherapy of RA, it should be remembered that one of the main goals of management is restoration of function. In this respect, the roles of physiotherapy and occupational therapy and meticulous foot care cannot be overlooked. Advances in orthopaedic surgery have also benefited situations such as atlanto-axial subluxation, arthroplasties and tendon transfer and repair surgeries.

Further reading

Blom M, van Riel PL. Management of established rheumatoid arthritis with an emphasis on pharmacotherapy. *Best Practice & Research. Clinical Rheumatology* 2007; **21**: 43–57.

Chan ESL, Cronstein BN. Drugs that modulate the immune response. In: *Samter's Immunologic Diseases*, 6th edn. Lippincott Williams & Wilkins 2001: 1213–1223.

Fleischmann RM. Comparison of the efficacy of biologic therapy for rheumatoid arthritis: can the clinical trials be accurately compared? *Rheumatic Diseases Clinics of North America* 2006; **32** (Suppl. 1): 21–28.

Goldblatt F, Isenberg DA. New therapies for rheumatoid arthritis. *Clinical and Experimental Immunology* 2005; **140**: 195–204.

Lee SJ, Kavanaugh A. Pharmacological treatment of established rheumatoid arthritis. *Best Practice & Research. Clinical Rheumatology* 2003; **17**: 811–829.

CHAPTER 14

Spondyloarthritides

Andrew Keat[1] and Robert Inman[2]

[1]Northwick Park Hospital, Harrow, UK
[2]Toronto Hospital Western Division, Toronto, Canada

OVERVIEW

- Spondyloarthritides as a group occur with a similar prevalence to rheumatoid arthritis.
- The various spondyloarthritic syndromes share common clinical lesions, especially enthesitis, oligoarthritis, sacroiliitis, iritis, psoriasiform skin and mucosal lesions and overt or covert inflammatory bowel disease.
- Inheritance of HLA-B27 and other genes is common to all spondyloarthritides, the prevalence of these disorders varying with the local prevalence of HLA-B27.
- Diagnosis of ankylosing spondylitis is often long delayed; identification of inflammatory back pain is a key determinant in making the diagnosis early.
- Use of anti-tumour necrosis factor biologic drugs has revolutionized the treatment of severe ankylosing spondylitis.

Box 14.1 **The European Spondyloarthropathy Study Group Criteria for Spondyloarthropathy**

- Inflammatory spinal pain (defined as low back pain with morning stiffness, better on exercise, in patients <40 years old)

or

- Asymmetric or predominantly lower limb synovitis

plus

- Any one or more of the following: psoriasis, inflammatory bowel disease, alternating buttock pain, enthesopathy, sacroiliitis

The spondyloarthritides (SpA) comprise a group of syndromes that are distinct from rheumatoid arthritis and are characterized by inflammation of the spine in many, but not all, cases. Other key features include asymmetric oligoarthritis, enthesitis, psoriatic skin and mucous membrane lesions, and eye and bowel inflammation. Tests for rheumatoid factor, anti-cyclic citrullinated peptide antibody and other autoantibodies are negative, but there is a strong association with the human leukocyte antigen (HLA) B27. Spondyloarthritides occur in both adults and children, although spinal involvement is rare in children. A working definition has been provided by the European Spondyloarthritis Study Group (Box 14.1). A diagnosis of SpA requires one or two of the entry criteria plus one other. Skin, eye and bowel disease may become apparent only with the passage of time.

The classical forms of spondyloarthritis (also called "spondyloarthropathies") and the key physical features are listed in Table 14.1.

Together, spondylarthritides are roughly as common as rheumatoid arthritis in Europe and North America, although their prevalence varies in other areas, generally reflecting the prevalence of HLA-B27 in that population. Their prevalence and that of associated conditions is presented in Table 14.2.

Ankylosing spondylitis

Ankylosing spondylitis (AS) is an aseptic inflammatory condition of the joints and entheses of the spine. AS occurs in 0.2% of the general population, in 2% of the B27-positive population and in 20% of B27-positive individuals with an affected family member. Males predominate with a male:female ratio ranging from 2.5:1 to 5:1. AS typically begins in young adulthood, but symptoms may arise in adolescence or earlier. Up to 15% of children with juvenile idiopathic arthritis are classified as having juvenile-onset spondyloarthritis. Such children present with pauciarticular peripheral arthritis with a predilection for the tarsal joints; axial complaints, with the development of radiographic sacroiliitis, tend only to develop in late teenage years or later.

The first symptom of AS is usually inflammatory back pain—the insidious onset of low back pain and/or buttock pain that persists for more than 3 months, awakens the patient from sleep, is accompanied by early morning stiffness and is typically improved by exercise. Fatigue often accompanies inflammatory back pain, although it may also be present in fibromyalgia and other conditions. Inadequately controlled inflammation leads to persistent stiffness and progressive loss of spinal mobility.

ABC of Rheumatology, 4th edn. Edited by Ade Adebajo.
©2010 Blackwell Publishing Ltd. 9781405170680.

Table 14.1 Examples of spondyloarthropathies

Syndromes	Features
Ankylosing spondylitis	Sacroiilitis
	Enthesitis
	Spondylitis
Psoriatic arthritis	Oligoarthritis
	Dactylitis
	Skin and mucous membrane inflammation
	Psoriasis
Reactive arthritis (Reiter's syndrome)	Genito-urinary inflammation, iritis
Enteropathic arthritis	Small and large bowel inflammation
Undifferentiated spondyloarthritis	Possible infectious trigger
Childhood spondyloarthritis	Associated with HLA-B27

Table 14.2 Prevalence of spondyloarthropathies

	Prevalence (%) per 100,000	male:female
Ankylosing spondylitis	0.2	3.5
Psoriasis	2000	1.0
Psoriatic arthritis	20–100	1.3
Reactive arthritis	16	3.0
Crohn's disease	30–75	1.0
Ulcerative disease	50–100	0.8
Enteropathic arthritis	1–20% of inflammatory bowel disease	*

*Peripheral arthritis occurs more in women; sacroiliitis and spondylitis more often affect men

---

Box 14.2 **The modified New York criteria for ankylosing spondylitis (1984)**

A. Diagnosis
   1. Clinical criteria
      a. Low back pain and stiffness >3 months with improvement on exercise, not relieved by rest
      b. Limitation of spinal motion in both sagittal and frontal planes
      c. Limitation of chest expansion
   2. Radiologic criteria
      Sacroiliitis: Grade >2 bilaterally or Grade 3–4 unilaterally
B. Grading
   1. Definite ankylosing spondylitis if the radiologic criterion is associated with >1 clinical criterion
   2. Probable ankylosing spondylitis if:
      a. the three clinical criteria are present
      b. the radiologic criterion is present without any signs or symptoms satisfying the clinical criteria

Box 14.3 **Characteristics of inflammatory back pain (in patients <50 years old)**

- Morning stiffness >30 minutes duration
- Improvement in back pain with exercise but *not* with rest
- Awakening because of back pain during the second half of the night only
- Alternating buttock pain

If none of four parameters present post-test probability of AS 1.3%

If one of four parameters present post-test probability of AS 2.6%

If two of four parameters present post-test probability of AS 10.8%

If three or more parameters present post-test probability of AS 39.4%, with sensitivity of 33.6% and specificity of 97.3%

(See Rudwaleit *et al.*)

The diagnosis is based on the modified New York criteria (Box 14.2). Radiographic assessment is a key element of these criteria: classical changes in the sacroiliac joints include erosions in the joint line, pseudowidening, subchondral sclerosis and finally ankylosis, reflected as obliteration of the sacroiliac joint. Radiographs of the spine may reveal squaring and "shiny corners" of the vertebral bodies and, later, syndesmophytes and facet-joint fusion (Figure 14.1). As radiographic sacroiliitis often develops late, early diagnosis may be based on symptoms of inflammatory back pain (Box 14.3) combined with magnetic resonance imaging (MRI) evidence of sacroiliitis (Figure 14.2).

HLA-B27 is rarely the definitive factor for diagnosis, but when the clinical suspicion is high, the test has reasonably high sensitivity and specificity.

Up to 30% of patients with AS also develop peripheral arthritis. Typically this is asymmetrical oligoarthritis affecting leg joints, most commonly the knee. Involvement of the hip can occur at any point in the course of AS and may be highly destructive. Enthesitis—inflammation at attachments of tendon or ligament to bone—is also a characteristic feature of AS. Enthesitis at the calcaneal attachments of the Achilles tendon, usually accompanied by Achilles tendon bursitis (Figure 14.3) and plantar fascia, producing sometimes disabling heel pain, is highly characteristic of AS, although it also occurs in other SpAs. Dactylitis, usually affecting a toe ("sausage toe") (Figure 14.4), is also strongly suggestive of an SpA.

Ocular inflammation, usually acute anterior uveitis (iritis), occurs at some time in up to 40% of AS patients. Acute anterior uveitis typically causes pain, photophobia and, if untreated, impairment in visual acuity. Typically, it is unilateral and recurrent. Uncommon extra-articular manifestations of AS include aortic insufficiency, cardiac conduction defects and pulmonary fibrosis.

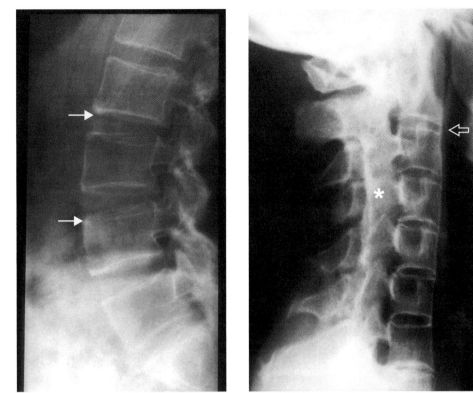

Figure 14.1 Radiographs of the spine showing early changes of "shiny corners" (→) late changes of syndesmophytes (⇨) and facet-joint fusion (*)

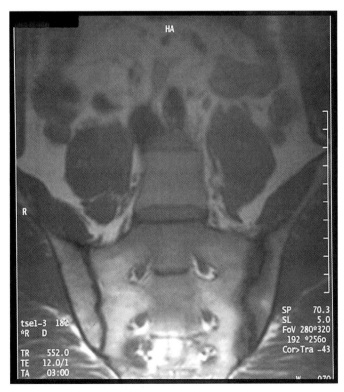

Figure 14.2 MRI scan showing right-sided sacroiliitis

Assessment of ankylosing spondylitis

In recent years several instruments have been devised for measuring disease activity, overall function, severity and progression of AS. Those most widely used are detailed below.

Disease Activity—Bath Ankylosing Spondylitis Disease Activity Index (BASDAI). A patient-completed set of six visual analogue scales assessing symptoms. The erythrocyte sedimentation rate and C-reactive protein are typically elevated, but levels do not usefully indicate inflammatory activity of spinal disease.

Overall patient function—Bath Ankylosing Spondylitis Functional Index (BASFI). A similar patient-completed set of 10 visual analogue scales assessing normal daily activities.

Spinal mobility—Bath Ankylosing Spondylitis Metrology Index (BASMI). A composite score derived from measurements of spinal mobility.

Radiologic progression—Modified Stoke AS Spinal Score (mSASSS). This uses lateral radiographs of the cervical and lumbosacral spine and can detect change over 2 years. It evaluates the anterior part of the lumbar spine and cervical spine and assesses chronic changes at each level with a score of 0 to 3 (0 = normal; 1 = erosion, sclerosis or squaring; 2 = syndesmophyte; 3 = bridging syndesmophyte).

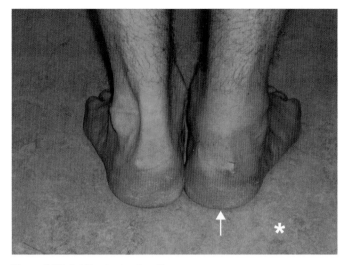

Figure 14.3 Achilles tendon bursitis

Box 14.4 **Patterns of psoriatic arthritis**

- Asymmetrical oligoarthritis (50%); involvement of one to five joints
- Predominantly distal interphalangeal joint disease (5–10%); distinctive but unusual form of psoriatic arthritis
- Rheumatoid pattern (25%); symmetrical small-joint arthritis particularly affecting metacarpophalangeal, wrist and proximal interphalangeal joints; may be indistinguishable from rheumatoid arthritis
- Arthritis mutilans (1–5%); osteolysis results in destruction of the small joints of the digits with shortening
- Spondyloarthritis (20%); may be isolated sacroiliitis, atypical or typical AS

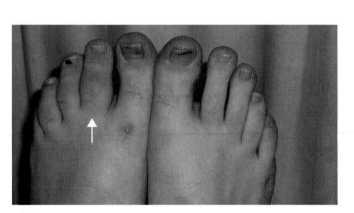

Figure 14.4 "Sausage toe"

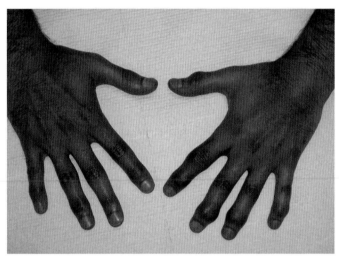

Figure 14.5 Distal interphalangeal joint involvement in psoriatic arthritis

The clinical course and disease severity of AS are highly variable. Inflammatory back pain and stiffness dominate the picture in the early stages, whereas chronic pain and deformity may develop over time. Osteoporosis tends to develop early in the disease, predisposing to spinal fractures later. One-third of AS sufferers give up work before retirement age because of their disease.

Psoriatic arthritis

Psoriatic arthritis is an inflammatory arthritis associated with psoriasis, usually with negative tests for rheumatoid factor. It is not a homogeneous clinical entity. In common with other spondyloarthritides, the key features are seronegative arthritis, enthesitis and, in a minority, sacroiliitis or spondylitis. It is the only SpA in which small joints of the hand are frequently affected. Five patterns of joint involvement are recognized (Box 14.4), although many patients have overlapping patterns of disease.

Psoriasis occurs in 5% of most white populations, and 5–15% of sufferers develop one or another form of associated arthritis. In a small minority of patients arthritis precedes the onset of psoriasis.

Typical psoriatic nail changes such as pitting, onycholysis and hyperkeratosis are seen in over 80% of patients with psoriatic arthritis, although skin lesions may be subtle and should be sought specifically in the scalp and natal cleft. Arthritis is characteristically oligoarticular and asymmetrical and may be associated with dactylitis of fingers or toes, often described as a "sausage digit" (Figure 14.4). Distal interphalangeal joint involvement at the fingers is uncommon but highly characteristic (Figure 14.5). Enthesitis plays a role in dactylitis but may also occur at more typical sites around the patella or around the heel at the Achilles tendon or plantar fascia insertion. Twenty per cent of patients with psoriatic arthritis develop low back pain with sacroiliitis and may develop typical or atypical spondylitis. Conjunctivitis and anterior uveitis may occur but less commonly than in AS.

Reactive arthritis

Reactive arthritis (ReA) is aseptic arthritis that occurs subsequent to an extra-articular infection, typically of the gastrointestinal (GI) or genito-urinary (GU) tract. The key GI pathogens are *Salmonella typhimurium*, *Yersinia enterocolitica*, *Shigella flexneri* and *Campylobacter jejuni*; the commonest GU pathogen is *Chlamydia trachomatis*. The true incidence and prevalence of ReA are not well defined. In epidemics involving *Salmonella* or *Yersinia*, ReA develops in up to 7% of infected individuals, but in as many as 20% of B27-positive individuals. In such epidemic studies, B27 confers risk not only for the onset of arthritis but also for axial involvement and chronicity. Typically, arthritis begins 1 to 3 weeks after the GI or GU infection.

As with other SpA syndromes, the pattern of joint involvement in ReA is one of asymmetrical oligoarthritis mainly affecting joints of the leg. As in AS, enthesitis may arise as Achilles tendonitis or plantar fasciitis, and dactylitis may occur at one or more toes. Sacroiliitis, with buttock pain, may occur in the acute phase, but radiographic changes are seen largely in the patients with a chronic course.

When ReA is accompanied by urethritis, conjunctivitis or muco-cutaneous lesions, the term "Reiter's syndrome" may be applied, but increasingly ReA is used to refer to this symptom complex. Urethritis may be manifest as dysuria or discharge and psoriasiform skin, and mucosal lesions include circinate balanitis and keratoderma blennorrhagicum (Figure 14.6), a painless papulosquamous

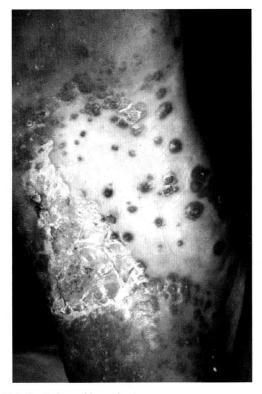

Figure 14.6 Keratoderma blennorhagicum

eruption on the palms or soles. Painless lingual or oral ulcers may also be seen. Conjunctivitis is usually bilateral and painful. Acute anterior uveitis is usually unilateral and may not be synchronous with the acute episode but may be clinically indistinguishable from conjunctivitis.

The most important differential diagnosis for ReA is septic arthritis, so appropriate culture of synovial fluid should precede the diagnosis of ReA whenever possible. The course of ReA is variable, and few prognostic markers are available for the clinician to predict the course in any individual case. The majority of patients have an initial episode lasting 2 to 3 months, but synovitis may persist for a year or longer. In patients with chronic disease a significant minority develop some degree of functional disability.

Enteropathic arthritis

Enteropathic arthritis is an inflammatory arthritis associated with inflammatory bowel disease (IBD), particularly ulcerative colitis and Crohn's disease. Two patterns of peripheral joint involvement are recognized, designated type 1 and type 2. Usually bowel and joint symptoms occur independently, and arthritis may wax and wane over many years. Non-specific arthralgia and myalgia without an inflammatory component, similar to that seen in fibromyalgia, is not uncommon in people with IBD.

Type 1 arthropathy affects approximately 5% of patients with IBD. Typically the peripheral arthritis is oligoarticular and principally affects the knees. It is usually self-limiting without leading to joint deformities. Joint symptoms can occur early in the course of bowel disease and may precede the onset of bowel symptoms. Enthesitis of the Achilles tendon and plantar fascia and dactylitis may also occur.

Type 2 arthropathy affects approximately 3% of patients with IBD. Arthritis is usually polyarticular, principally affecting the metacarpophalangeal joints, although the knees, ankles, elbows, shoulders, wrists, proximal interphalangeal joints and metatarsophalangeal joints may also be affected, sometimes in a migratory fashion.

Sacroiliitis and spondylitis occur in up to 20% of patients with either form of IBD. The course of spinal involvement is completely independent of the course of the IBD and may precede by years the first manifestations of bowel disease.

Undifferentiated spondyloarthritis

The development of inflammatory back pain or peripheral large joint arthritis, often in individuals who are positive for HLA-B27, with or without other features of the seronegative SpA but without fulfilling criteria for any particular subtype, is referred to as undifferentiated SpA. Most patients are young adults, although children may be affected; a proportion of cases will evolve over time to into a classifiable subset, particularly ankylosing spondylitis.

It is not unusual for the first feature of a spondyloarthritis to be an enthesitis, especially at the Achilles tendon or plantar fascia. These lesions may also occur independently of any arthritic conditions, especially in athletes. In spondyloarthritis, Achilles tendonitis typically affects the actual entheseal junction, often with marked bone oedema visible on MRI scanning and sometimes with Achilles tendon bursitis; in athletes pain and tendon swelling occur higher up in the tendon close to the muscle belly. Plantar fasciitis is not so easily differentiated, although it often occurs in overweight older adults.

There are no diagnostic criteria for undifferentiated SpA *per se*; however, the European Spondyloarthropathy Study Group (ESSG) has set out criteria, as in Box 14.1.

Treatment

The goals of treatment are to relieve symptoms, improve function and delay or prevent structural damage. To some extent treatment of spinal inflammation differs from that of peripheral joint synovitis and enthesitis, so treatment must be tailored to the actual problems in the individual patient at the time.

Sacroiliitis and spondylitis

First-line treatment—Regular physiotherapy and encouragement to exercise regularly; use of non-steroidal anti-inflammatory drugs (NSAIDS), such as naproxen or diclofenac, or COX-2 inhibitors such as etoricoxib or celecoxib.

Second-line treatment—Oral and intramuscular corticosteroids may control spinal symptoms, but long-term use should be avoided; local corticosteroid injections into one or both sacroiliac joints under radiographic imaging may be helpful.

Third-line treatment—Anti-tumour necrosis factor agents have been proven significantly to reduce spinal pain and stiffness and to increase spinal movement and patient function; reduction of spinal inflammation has been demonstrated by MRI scanning.

Adjunctive treatment—Bisphosphonates, calcium and vitamin D may improve bone density, although fracture reduction has not been demonstrated in AS; low-dose amitriptyline at night may improve sleep and reduce pain and fatigue.

Oligoarthritis and/or enthesitis

First-line treatment—Analgesics such as paracetamol/acetaminophen or codeine-based drugs may be helpful; intra-articular or intra-lesional corticosteroid injection can be useful for single peripheral joint involvement or enthesitis; injections into weight-bearing tendons should be avoided; NSAIDs may provide symptomatic relief (they must be used with caution in patients with IBD, as they may exacerbate the gut disease); orthotics, including heel pads, and carefully chosen footwear, including suitable trainer/running shoes, may provide the best symptomatic relief for arthritis or enthesitis affecting the feet; in patients with ReA, genital tract infection should be treated as in uncomplicated infection, with treatment of sexual contacts; antimicrobial treatment of gut infection is not usually indicated, and there is no clear evidence for long-term antimicrobial treatment of established arthritis.

Second-line therapy—Disease-modifying anti-rheumatoid drugs (DMARDs) may be effective for those patients with aggressive, erosive or polyarticular disease, as in the treatment of rheumatoid arthritis; methotrexate may be effective for both skin and joint disease, although the published evidence is scant; in individuals with enteropathic arthritis, sulphasalazine may be effective for both joint and bowel disease; rigorous monitoring of DMARD therapy, according to established practice guidelines, should be undertaken; oral or intramuscular corticosteroid treatment may be effective, especially in those with marked systemic features; in psoriatic arthritis, steroid therapy carries a risk of an exacerbation of skin disease on steroid withdrawal.

Third-line treatment—In those patients who have an inadequate response to conventional DMARDs and in whom the diagnosis is well established, anti-tumour necrosis factor therapy with etanercept, infliximab or adalimumab may be dramatically effective in the control of joint and skin disease; etanercept has not been shown to be effective for IBD.

Further reading

Carlin EM, Keat AC. European guidelines for the management of sexually acquired reactive arthritis. *International Journal of STD and AIDS* 2001; **12** (Suppl. 3) 94–102.

Hannu H, Inman RD, Granfors K, Leirisalo-Repo M. Reactive arthritis or postinfectious arthritis. *Best Practice and Research. Clinical Rheumatology* 2006; **20**: 419–433.

Holden W, Orchard T, Wordsworth P. Enteropathic arthritis. *Rheumatic Diseases Clinics of North America* 2003; **29**: 513–530.

Rudwaleit M, Metter A, Listing J, Sieper J, Braun J. Inflammatory back pain in ankylosing spondylitis: a reassessment of the clinical history for application as classification and diagnostic criteria. *Arthritis and Rheumatism* 2006; **54**; 569–578.

Zochling J, van der Heijde D, Burgos-Vargas R *et al.* ASAS/EULAR Recommendations for the management of ankylosing spondylitis. *Annals of the Rheumatic Diseases* 2006; **65**: 442–452.

CHAPTER 15

Juvenile Idiopathic Arthritis

Taunton R Southwood[1] and Ilona S Szer[2,3]

[1]University of Birmingham, and Birmingham Children's Hospital NHS Foundation Trust, Birmingham, UK
[2]UCSD School of Medicine, San Diego, CA, USA
[3]University of California, San Diego, CA, USA

OVERVIEW

- Juvenile idiopathic arthritis (JIA) is not the same disease as rheumatoid arthritis.
- JIA is an umbrella term that includes at least seven different conditions, each representing a unique form of childhood arthritis.
- JIA is characterized by persistent, non-recurrent, objective joint swelling.
- Joint pain and stiffness are presenting symptoms in most, but not all, children and young people with JIA.
- Early diagnosis is the key to optimal outcome.
- Effective treatment is available and positively affects long-term outcome.

Box 15.1 **Criteria for the diagnosis of juvenile idiopathic arthritis**

All three conditions must be met:

- Arthritis persisting for >6 weeks
- Onset before age 16 years
- Exclusion of other conditions associated with or mimicking arthritis

Introduction

The diagnosis of arthritis or other rheumatic conditions in children requires an awareness of the age-dependent manifestations of such conditions, skill in history taking, a meticulous approach to physical examination and judicious use of investigations. Such conditions may present with relatively common, non-specific, "constitutional" paediatric symptoms such as fever, rash, fatigue, weakness, anorexia and pain. Individually, or in combination, these are most likely to be features of common, insignificant, transient illnesses. Rheumatic diseases usually have additional clues, albeit subtle ones, that should alert the clinician to a possible rheumatic diagnosis. In arthritic disorders, joint swelling is the pivotal feature, but others include characteristic "rheumatic patterns" of fever, rash, weakness, diurnal variation or disease progression despite simple measures.

The key signs on physical examination may also be subtle, requiring experience and skill to discern and interpret them. A thorough physical examination (including detailed musculoskeletal assessment) of any child with potential rheumatic symptoms is essential. Joint swelling and pain with movement usually confirm the presence of arthritis (note that isolated joint pain/joint tender-ness without swelling are features of arthralgia). Investigations, especially during the first few weeks of illness, are aimed at ruling out the long list of conditions that comprise the differential diagnosis of childhood arthritis.

Juvenile idiopathic arthritis (JIA) is the most likely diagnosis in children with persistent symptoms and clinical features of arthritis for at least 6 weeks (Box 15.1), as most other illnesses either resolve or are treated and referred to other specialists during this time period. For the experienced paediatric rheumatologist, the child with arthritis or other chronic rheumatic illness presents with an almost instantly recognizable pattern of symptoms. The lack of timely detection of childhood inflammatory disease and delay in treatment may adversely affect the course and outcome of JIA. There are also dangers inherent in trying to make the diagnosis of JIA too precipitously, without ruling out other rare but important disorders, such as septic arthritis or malignancy. Diagnostic imaging and laboratory investigation must always be carefully considered, but there is no pathognomonic test for JIA. Disproportionate over-investigation may increase child and family anxiety without adding value to the diagnostic process. The overzealous investigator may even exacerbate the severity of some conditions, such as chronic idiopathic pain syndromes.

This chapter aims to give an overview of JIA, including clinical features, differential diagnosis, investigations, natural history and principles of treatment. No substitute exists, however, for actual clinical experience, and the reader is strongly recommended to practise the skills of paediatric musculoskeletal examination at every appropriate opportunity. An appreciation of the range of normality in children and young people is an absolute prerequisite to the detection of abnormality.

ABC of Rheumatology, 4th edn. Edited by Ade Adebajo.
©2010 Blackwell Publishing Ltd. 9781405170680.

Clinical features of JIA

JIA is one of the most common physically disabling conditions of childhood, with a prevalence of approximately one in a thousand children under the age of 16 years (surveys suggest that this may be higher, even as many as 4 in 1000 children; 10,000–40,000 affected children in the UK and up to 300,000 in the USA). The incidence of JIA is 1 in 10,000. In typical general practice, however, JIA is rare; one new case may be seen every 20 years. It is difficult to maintain a high index of suspicion for JIA in the face of this degree of rarity.

Most affected children are in their preschool or early school years, and often have difficulty describing their symptoms. Parents may notice joint swelling if one or more large peripheral joints are involved, such as the knee (the most common joint affected), ankle or wrist. It is rarer for children to present with isolated small joint (finger or toe) arthritis or axial joint involvement (such as the shoulder, hip, spine or temporomandibular joints), and parents are also less likely to notice swelling in these joints. Diurnal variation of symptoms, such as early morning joint stiffness or exacerbation after prolonged rest (joint "gelling") are characteristic. Stiffness improves with movement and may be helped by a warm bath or shower. Duration of morning stiffness may provide an index of improvement with treatment. Joint dysfunction may be manifest by limping, difficulty with writing or inability to carry out other activities of daily living (Table 15.1).

There is accumulating evidence that the natural history of JIA may not be as benign as first thought; between a third and a half of patients have persistent joint inflammation into their adult years. More aggressive treatment is being used in an attempt to induce early disease remission, an approach that has been complemented recently by a wider therapeutic armamentarium. Several targeted biologic drugs have been shown to be beneficial in JIA.

Physical findings in JIA

Peripheral joint arthritis in children is usually accompanied by joint swelling. In the knee, this may be demonstrated by balloting synovial fluid, palpating a fluid thrill on joint movement, eliciting a positive patella tap, or occasionally finding a Baker's cyst in the popliteal fossa. Swelling of the ankle may distort the contours of medial or lateral malleoli. When the ankle is dorsiflexed, the usually prominent anterior tendon surface markings may be obscured by arthritis, although this may be difficult to see in infants and overweight children. Other relevant observations include muscle wasting, particularly of the vastus medialis and gastrocnemius, and leg length discrepancy, which often indicates accelerated growth around affected joints.

Wrist arthritis may be best appreciated by asking the child to press the palms of their hands together in the "prayer" position; a dorsal bulge and reduced range of movement, especially if it is asymmetrical, are consistent features of synovitis. Swelling of the elbow can be palpated on either side of the olecranon and usually results in a flexion deformity of the elbow. Elbow swelling obscures the posterior dimple created when the elbow is fully extended.

The small joints of the hands and feet should be inspected and palpated individually; reliable signs of synovitis are the presence of joint margin tenderness, restricted movement, swelling and purplish discoloration, incomplete fist closure and diminished grip strength. Cervical spine involvement may be detected by inability to rotate the head laterally to place the chin on each shoulder and by reduced cervical extension. Temporomandibular synovitis is often missed; it may prevent full and symmetrical opening of the mouth. Involvement of sacroiliac joints and low back in patients with enthesitis-related arthritis (ERA) can be documented by a limited modified Schober test (less than 6 cm expansion of lumbar spine with forward bending) and documentation of tenderness of sacroiliac joints to direct palpation. Enthesopathy, a hallmark of ERA, is found at tendon insertions into bones, most frequently where the Achilles tendon inserts into the calcaneus. Careful observation of gait allows the examiner to evaluate the function of lower limb joints.

Children with JIA have a variety of extra-articular physical findings that help establish the diagnosis. For example, children with systemic arthritis may have little in the way of articular signs initially, but other characteristic features may be prominent, including a pink, macular, truncal rash (which may be pruritic and exhibit Koebner's phenomenon), lymphadenopathy, hepatosplenomegaly and myalgia. Children with oligoarthritis tend to appear very healthy and have few findings aside from arthritis (most frequently the knee). If asymptomatic chronic anterior uveitis has preceded the onset of arthritis, posterior synechiae and/or band keratopathy may be visible with a hand-held ophthalmoscope focused on the lens.

Once the presence of arthritis is confirmed objectively, it is vital to exclude conditions that may mimic JIA. Most serious among

Table 15.1 Typical symptoms of juvenile idiopathic arthritis

Present in all forms of JIA

Joint symptoms (pain, dysfunction, stiffness), particularly after sleep or prolonged sitting

Persistent joint swelling, particularly of the knee, ankle, wrist and small joints of the hand

Difficulty chewing, asymmetric mouth opening and micrognathia

Muscle atrophy

Flexion contracture deformity

Synovial hypertrophy

Constitutional symptoms (dramatic in children with systemic arthritis but mild in polyarthritis and ERA)

Fever (high and quotidian in systemic arthritis, low grade in polyarthritis, no pattern in ERA)

Rash (maculopapular, recurrent in systemic arthritis, nodules in polyarthritis, rheumatoid factor+, psoriasis and nail pitting in psoriatic arthritis)

Growth failure (almost always severe in systemic arthritis, mild in polyarthritis and localized to specific bones in oligoarthritis)

ERA = enthesitis-related arthritis

these are infection-related conditions (septic arthritis, osteomyelitis), trauma (including non-accidental injury), neoplasia (particularly acute lymphoblastic leukaemia and neuroblastoma), hidden inflammatory disorders (Crohn's disease and ulcerative colitis), acute inflammatory conditions (such as Kawasaki disease and Henoch–Schönlein purpura [HSP]), and other childhood rheumatic conditions such as reactive post-infectious arthritis, systemic lupus erythematosus (SLE) and its variants (mixed connective tissue disease [MCTD], SLE for antiphospholipid antibodies [APLA], subacute cutaneous lupus erythematosus [SCLE]), dermatomyositis (DMS), vasculitis syndromes and systemic sclerosis. Differentiating mechanical disorders and pain amplification syndromes from arthritis represents one of the greatest challenges in paediatric rheumatology.

An explanation of terms

"Juvenile idiopathic arthritis" is an umbrella term that has replaced previous nomenclatures, including juvenile rheumatoid arthritis (JRA) and juvenile chronic arthritis (JCA). The hallmark of JIA is persistent joint swelling in the absence of any defined cause in someone who is 16 years old or younger. Under the umbrella of JIA, children with at least seven unique types of arthritis can be classified both clinically and biologically, including the previously described onset subtypes of JRA/JCA (systemic-onset JRA/JCA, now called systemic arthritis; polyarticular-onset JRA/JCA, renamed polyarthritis; and pauciarticular-onset JRA/JCA, replaced by oligoarthritis), psoriatic arthritis (previously an illness separate from JRA) and enthesitis-related arthritis (ERA), which includes all of the conditions previously called (undifferentiated) spondyloarthropathy syndromes, seronegative arthritis and enthesopathy (SEA) syndrome and HLA-B27-related arthritis syndromes. In total, 95% of children and adolescents with JIA have a disease that is clinically and immunogenetically unique, and only 3–5% have features in common with rheumatoid arthritis (RA) of adulthood. The term adult-onset Still's disease is used when a patient older than 16 years of age develops systemic arthritis.

Differential diagnosis of JIA

Many common conditions of childhood present with musculoskeletal symptoms (Table 15.2; Box 15.2). The most frequent of these are mechanical disorders such as hypermobility and trauma, (including non-accidental trauma), followed by infectious and post-infectious illnesses, malignancies, acute and chronic inflammatory disorders and the idiopathic amplification pain syndromes. In young patients it is important to consider genetic disorders of inborn errors of metabolism, and in children with recurrent fevers the auto-inflammatory disorders need to be ruled out.

Mechanical disorders

Joint pain secondary to hypermobility is the most common non-inflammatory cause of pain in children newly referred to a paediatric rheumatologist (Box 15.3). In general, younger children are more flexible than older adolescents (babies and toddlers' joints are extremely mobile, and the finding of flat feet in children of this age is normal), girls are more flexible than boys, and black children are

Table 15.2 Differential diagnosis of juvenile idiopathic arthritis

Presenting with a single inflamed joint

Juvenile idiopathic arthritis: oligoarthritis, psoriatic arthritis or ERA

Septic arthritis: bacterial or tubercular: osteomyelitis

Lyme disease

Reactive arthritis: secondary to bacterial or viral infections

Haemarthrosis: secondary to trauma (including non-accidental) or bleeding disorder

Malignancy: leukaemia or neuroblastoma most common

Presenting with more than one inflamed joint

Juvenile idiopathic arthritis: polyarthritis (RF-positive or -negative), psoriatic, ERA or systemic arthritis

Other connective tissue diseases: SLE, juvenile dermatomyositis, sarcoidosis, Sjögren's syndrome, MCTD

Reactive arthritis: secondary to bacterial or viral infections

Lyme disease

Malignancy: leukaemia or neuroblastoma most common

Immunodeficiency state-associated arthritis

Inflammatory bowel disease-associated arthritis

Other: chronic recurrent multifocal osteomyelitis, CINCA (also known as NOMID) and auto-inflammatory disorders

Presenting with systemic features

Systemic arthritis

Other connective tissue diseases—SLE, MCTD, Kawasaki disease, chronic vasculitis syndromes

Infection: bacterial (streptococcal, including acute rheumatic fever, tuberculosis, Gonococcus, Lyme disease and Brucella), viral (Epstein–Barr virus and hepatitis B) or parasitic (malaria)

Inflammatory bowel disease

Auto-inflammatory disorders

CINCA (NOMID)

CINCA = chronic infantile neurological cutaneous and arthritis; ERA = enthesitis-related arthritis; MCTD = mixed connective tissue disease; NOMID = neonatal-onset multi-system inflammatory disease; RF = rheumatoid factor; SLE = systemic lupus erythematosus

more flexible than their white peers. These children may complain of pain after physical activity and in the evenings, unlike patients with JIA who feel worse in the mornings and with rest and better as the day progresses. The physical examination demonstrates an extra 10–15° degrees if motion in lax joints. Hypermobility may be localized or diffuse. Much of the musculoskeletal pain is confined to the lower limbs and low back. Lower limb findings may be improved by the use of custom-moulded semi-rigid insoles with shock-absorbing posts (as indeed may other postural abnormalities of the feet) that aim to support the longitudinal foot arch and stabilize the ankle. To be successful, such insoles need specialized source of infection should be undertaken before antibiotics are started. Arthrocentesis has the added advantage, particularly in the hip, of reducing intra-articular pressure and minimizing the risk of compromised blood supply to the epiphysis. Intravenous antibiotics are usually advocated until 48 hours after defervescence, with oral antibiotics continued until the erythrocyte sedimentation rate (ESR) has normalized and all clinical signs have resolved.

Osteomyelitis—Most children present with fever, bone pain and signs of toxicity. They cannot ambulate and have extreme pain at the site of infection. If the infection is located near a joint, it may cause a sterile (sympathetic) effusion that may be mistaken for arthritis. Radiographs may be normal initially or show periosteal reaction; a technetium bone scan helps establish bone infection and prevent chronic osteomyelitis.

Chronic rheumatic conditions

Systemic lupus erythematosus—SLE typically presents in an adolescent girl with malaise, fever and bone or joint pain. Multi-system inflammatory disease is characteristic, but clinical manifestations are protean. SLE is rare in prepubescent children. An erythematous, acneiform facial rash may be present, and the classic photosensitive malar rash is a frequent but not a uniform finding. Most children have hair loss, mouth sores, lymphadenopathy, organomegaly, other rashes and swollen joints. Elevated blood pressure suggests renal involvement. Tests for antinuclear antibodies (ANAs) are almost always positive, but auto-antibodies such as those to double-stranded DNA and Sm, are more specific for SLE and usually present along with complement consumption. Antibodies to SSA (Ro), SSB (La) and anti-cardiolipin are positive in less than 50% of paediatric patients but should be looked for because their presence is associated with particular complications (risk of neonatal lupus syndrome and risk of thrombosis, respectively). Lymphopenia, thrombocytopenia and Coombs' positive anaemia are regular findings. Simple urinalysis demonstrates the presence of proteinuria and casts, reflecting renal disease, the major cause of long-term morbidity that is more frequent in childhood than in adult-onset SLE. Adolescents presenting with Raynaud's phenomenon may have MCTD, whereas those whose cutaneous manifestations that overshadow major organ involvement may have SCLE, another variant of lupus. APLA represents the newest condition associated with thrombotic events and specific

assessment and fitting. Most mechanical causes of joint pain tend to be worse after exercise and as the day goes on, but early morning stiffness the day or two after exercise may also be a feature. A subset of patients with benign hypermobility complains of dizziness, poor tone and subjective weakness, and some children with significant laxity may indeed have more severe forms of Ehlers–Danlos syndrome. Diffuse pain syndromes have also been described in children with hypermobility.

Infection-related disorders

Reactive arthritis—This is the most common form of arthritis in childhood. It is characterized by self-limited, acute and painful joint swelling (usually lasting less than 6 weeks) that follows, or rarely accompanies, evidence of extra-articular infection (Box 15.4).

Septic arthritis—Almost exclusively monoarticular and associated with "pseudoparalysis" of the affected limb (extreme pain with the affected joint held rigidly in the position of maximum comfort). The child is usually systemically ill, with a high fever and signs of toxicity. It is important, however, to maintain a high index of suspicion of this condition in a child who is being, or has recently been, treated with antibiotics, because of the possibility of partially treated septic arthritis. Tuberculous septic arthritis may present more insidiously. Blood cultures and joint aspiration for bacterial autoimmune pattern (the presence of anti-cardiolipin antibodies, lupus anticoagulant and false-positive Venereal Disease Research Laboratory test).

Juvenile dermatomyositis—Children with juvenile DMS may present insidiously and are often labelled as malingerers before the true nature of the diagnosis is appreciated. Typical symptoms include malaise, progressive proximal muscle weakness and muscle pain or discomfort. Arthritis is found in 20% of the patients. Dermatological manifestations include heliotrope rash (purplish discoloration and oedema of the upper eyelids) (Figure 15.1) and malar rash travelling down the naso-labial folds (malar rash in SLE spares the naso-labial folds), Gottron's papules over the metacarpophalanges, elbows and knees (often mistaken for eczema) and cuticle hyperaemia (due to distended nailfold capillaries) (Figure 15.2). The diagnosis of juvenile DMS is usually made on the basis of typical rash and the finding of symmetrical proximal muscle weakness. Elevated serum muscle enzymes (CPK, aldolase, AST, ALT, LDH) confirm the presence of muscle inflammation. If the child has a typical rash but normal strength and enzyme levels, magnetic resonance imaging (MRI) of a large muscle demonstrates

otherwise subtle inflammation on T2 images. In very weak children, respiratory failure and aspiration pneumonia may be life-threatening.

Localized scleroderma syndromes—Most children with scleroderma have a localized disorder characterized by areas of oval (morphea) or linear lesions that traverse over joints, face (coup de sabre deformity) and trunk (Figure 15.3). Some children have frank arthritis and occasionally may develop extensive joint limitations that mimic polyarthritis but produce paucity of inflammatory signs, except morning stiffness.

Systemic vasculitis syndromes such Wegener's granulomatosis, polyarteritis nodosa or Churg–Strauss syndrome are extremely rare in childhood, and arthritis is not a common feature.

Acute inflammatory conditions

Henoch–Schönlein purpura—HSP is the most common vasculitis of childhood, manifested by purpuric rash over the lower legs and buttocks (Figure 15.4), often associated with cramping abdominal pain, bloody stools, haematuria and occasionally with arthritis of the ankles or knees. Haematuria is virtually always present, and proteinuria may be found, but significant renal disease is extremely rare.

Kawasaki disease—Arthritis is an uncommon feature at presentation in this illness of infants and toddlers; however, atypical cases of Kawasaki disease with fever, rash and elevated inflammatory markers, but without red eyes, raises the suspicion of systemic arthritis (Figure 15.5).

Malignancy

Acute lymphoblastic leukaemia—This may present with bone pain in children (sometimes primarily at night) and even frank arthritis, which can affect one, or sometimes more, joint(s). These children appear toxic and have pain over the affected bone(s). When these children present to the paediatric rheumatologist, their complete blood counts are normal, and a high level of suspicion is required. There is usually anaemia and elevated ESR. Bone-marrow biopsy confirms the presence of immature cells.

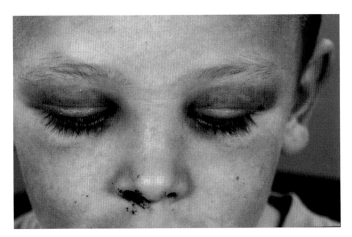

Figure 15.1 Heliotrope rash in a boy with dermatomyositis

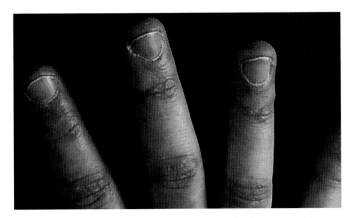

Figure 15.2 Gottron's papules in a boy with juvenile dermatomyositis

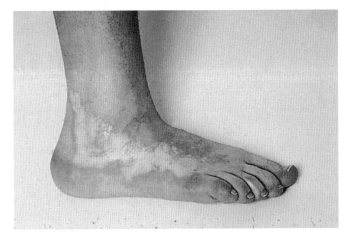

Figure 15.3 Localized scleroderma of the foot of an 11-year-old girl

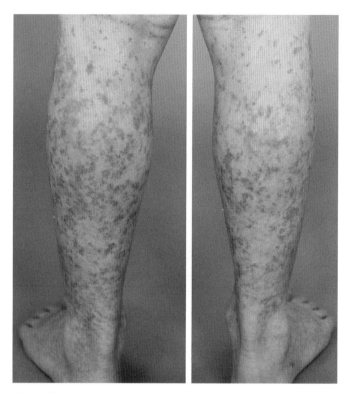

Figure 15.4 Leg purpura of Henoch–Schönlein purpura

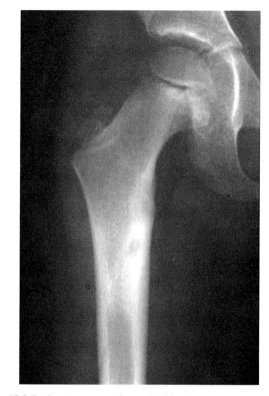

Figure 15.6 Benign tumours, such as osteoid osteoma, may present with night pain in the affected limb. These conditions should be considered in the assessment of a child with "growing pains"

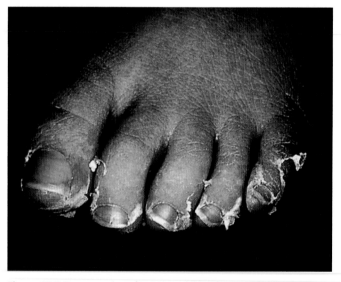

Figure 15.5 Desquamation of toes in a child with Kawasaki disease

Neuroblastoma—Neuroblastoma is a particularly concerning possibility in younger children who present with fever and joint pain. Early metastases to the bone cause pain that may be difficult for the doctor to localize.

Lymphoma—Lymphoma usually affects older children and may present with musculoskeletal symptoms.

Primary bone malignancies—These are rare and usually visible on plain X-ray radiographs (Figure 15.6).

Idiopathic pain syndromes

The most dramatic musculoskeletal pain in children is often found in the idiopathic pain syndromes. These may be localized (complex regional pain syndromes) or generalized (diffuse pain syndromes, also called fibromyalgia). Exogenous stress (including school pressures, bullying or other forms of abuse, and even parental pressure) is a common accompanying feature, although often unrecognized by the parents. These children and adolescents deserve meticulous physical examination and judicious investigation to rule out an underlying organic pathology. Too much investigation and vacillating doctor-to-patient communication, however, may perpetuate or exacerbate the clinical features of these disorders. Indeed, treatment should start while investigations are ongoing, because disability is common. Occasionally, an idiopathic pain syndrome may complicate a pre-existing condition, such as juvenile idiopathic arthritis. An individualized, intensive, multi-professional, rehabilitation regimen, either in the community or on an inpatient basis, is essential to restore function.

Complex regional pain syndromes—Previously called reflex sympathetic dystrophy, complex regional pain syndromes may begin after trauma (often minor) or without a clear precipitant. They are always associated with immobility, followed by increasing pain, hypersensitivity, cool skin and complete refusal to use the affected area (Box 15.5). Invariably, patients rate their pain as 9/10, whereas children with JIA typically rate their pain at 2–3/10. There is complete lack of correlation between physical findings and the patient's level of pain and disability. This condition seems to be increasing in frequency and affecting younger children.

Diffuse musculoskeletal pain syndromes—These poorly defined conditions are characterized by disturbed sleep patterns (initial insomnia, exhausted awakening and napping during the day), tenderness over soft-tissue "trigger" points (with facial grimacing and a sharp intake of breath), and the absence of other findings to suggest organic disease.

Investigations in children with arthritis

JIA is a label for children who fulfil classification criteria made on clinical features alone, as no diagnostic tests exist. Investigations are thus aimed at excluding a wide range of differential diagnoses. However, certain classic patterns emerge as features of history and physical examination combine with typical laboratory and imaging findings, allowing the clinician to arrive at the correct diagnosis.

Haematology

Complete blood count—To look for leucopenia, Coombs' positive anaemia and thrombocytopenia of SLE and MCTD, as well as the elevated white blood cell (WBC) count and anaemia of chronic inflammation of systemic arthritis. Malignancy may not be ruled out without bone-marrow biopsy.

Erythrocyte sedimentation rate—ESR is elevated in systemic arthritis and SLE but normal in up to half of patients with JIA and in most children with dermatomyositis.

Bone-marrow aspirate—To exclude malignancy, especially before instituting corticosteroid treatment.

Biochemistry

C-reactive protein—C-reactive protein (CRP) is elevated in systemic arthritis but normal in up to half of patients with JIA, as well as patients with SLE, MCTD and DMS.

Urinary catecholamines—To exclude neuroblastoma.

Liver function tests, creatinine kinase, aldolase, LDH—To rule out dermatomyositis.

Urinalysis—To rule out renal disease of SLE and HSP.

Immunology

Antinuclear antibodies—Positive in low titre in most children with JIA (especially oligoarthritis), and in up to 15% of the general paediatric population. High positive ANAs are seen in virtually all children with SLE and MCTD.

Rheumatoid factor—Negative in 95% of children with JIA but present in 25% of children with SLE.

Immunoglobulins—One in 500 children with JIA has a low level of immunoglobulin A (IgA). IgG is highly elevated in SLE.

Antistreptolysin "O" titre and viral serology—To help with acute rheumatic fever, post-streptococcal arthritis, viral and post-viral conditions.

Borrelia burgdorferi *serology*—To rule out Lyme disease if there is a history of travel in endemic areas.

Synovial fluid analysis—This is mandatory in suspected septic arthritis, but does not help in other differential diagnoses. Children do not get gout.

Radiology

Plain X-ray radiographs—To rule out fractures, avascular necrosis of bone, bone neoplasia, bone dysplasia and osteomyelitis.

Ultrasonography—To confirm the presence of joint effusion; to look for neuroblastoma.

Technetium-99 bone scan—To highlight bony inflammation secondary to infection, malignancy or benign tumours such as osteoid osteoma.

MRI of joints—To confirm the presence of early synovial inflammation and early erosions; to confirm the presence of myopathy; to rule structural abnormalities.

Classification of JIA

See Box 15.6 for a classification of JIA by the International League of Associations for Rheumatology.

Box 15.5 **Features of complex regional pain syndrome**

Characteristic
- Severe pain out of proportion to physical findings
- Hyperaesthesia
- Allodynia
- Immobility of affected limb, including adopting a bizarre posture or gait

Occasional
- Limb swelling
- Mottling of skin
- Cool pallor of skin

Box 15.6 **International League of Associations for Rheumatology classification of juvenile idiopathic arthritis**

- Systemic arthritis
- Oligoarthritis—persistent
- Oligoarthritis—extended
- Polyarthritis—rheumatoid-factor negative
- Polyarthritis—rheumatoid-factor positive
- Psoriatic arthritis
- Enthesitis-related arthritis
- Undifferentiated arthritis

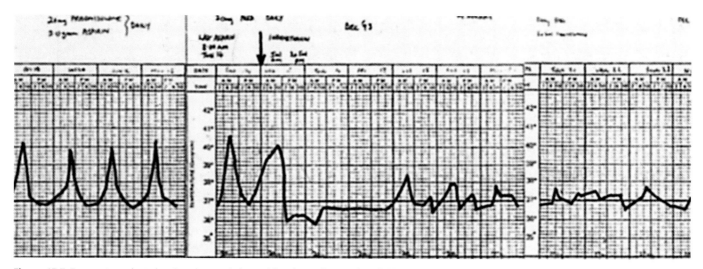

Figure 15.7 Temperature chart showing characteristic quotidian fever of systemic arthritis

Systemic arthritis

Systemic arthritis usually begins in early childhood (although it can occur at any age through to adulthood), with prominent extra-articular features of high quotidian fevers (Figure 15.7), rash (Figure 15.8), myalgia, arthralgia and irritability (Box 15.7). Laboratory studies show elevated WBC count, severe anaemia, thrombocytosis, high ESR, CRP, ferritin and positive d-dimers or fibrin split products. The systemic features usually resolve after a few months but may last indefinitely. The pattern of arthritis is variable, ranging from several swollen joints to a widespread pol-yarticular pattern that can be very difficult to control. These children have the worst prognosis of all, not only regarding erosions and loss of joint motion but also because of severe growth delay and sequalea of chronic corticosteroid use. Macrophage activation syndrome has been associated with systemic arthritis and carries a 10–15% mortality rate. Treatment with intravenous corticosteroids and cyclosporine is usually successful in reversing rapid deterioration and disseminated intravascular coagulation.

Oligoarthritis—persistent

The most common condition under the rubric of JIA, oligoarthritis accounts for over half of all cases of JIA. It mainly affects preschool girls, with a sex ratio of 5:1. The knee is the most frequently affected joint, followed by ankle and wrist (Figure 15.9). The hip is almost never affected. This group of otherwise healthy little girls is at the highest risk for the development of chronic asymptomatic anterior uveitis (20%). Chronic anterior uveitis is clinically silent and insidiously progressive; it produces visual loss and blindness if not detected by slit lamp examination and treated early (with recommended monitoring every 3 months). It is frequently associated with positive ANAs, but all other laboratory investigations are normal. Investigations have identified a complex genetic predisposition to both oligoarthritis and uveitis. Localized growth disturbances are common; the affected leg grows longer (presumably as a result of chronic hyperaemia and increased blood supply to the

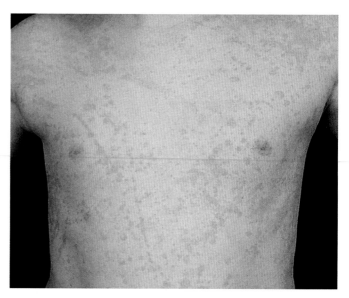

Figure 15.8 Typical erythematous and evanescent rash of systemic arthritis. Frequently, the rash is obvious only at the height of the fever and sometimes is confined to the axillary region, anterior chest wall and inside both thighs

Box 15.7 **Extra-articular features of systemic arthritis**

- Characteristic daily fever
- Evanescent erythematous maculopapular rash
- Hepatomegaly
- Splenomegaly
- Lymphadenopathy
- Serositis

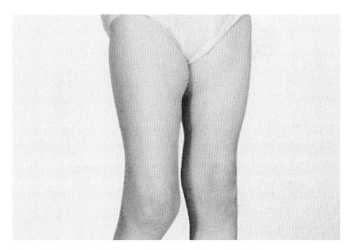

Figure 15.9 Oligoarthritis, persistent, in a 3-year-old girl

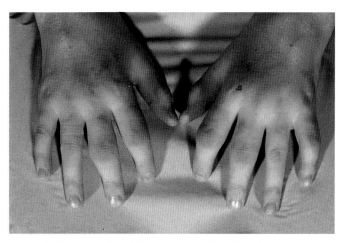

Figure 15.10 Symmetric arthritis in a young child with polyarthritis, negative for rheumatoid factor

inflamed area, resulting in leg length discrepancy) contributing to knee flexion contracture and atrophy of the muscle above the knee. The typical stance of a toddler with oligoarthritis is with the swollen knee bent and the other one straight.

Oligoarthritis—extended

One-third of children with oligoarthritis whose disease during the first 6 months affects less than four joints continue to develop arthritis in further joints thereafter; hence the nomenclature "extended." Many of these children have anterior uveitis. These patients have a different immunogenetic background than patients with persistent oligoarthritis and carry a prognosis similar to those with polyarthritis.

Polyarthritis—rheumatoid-factor negative

Polyarthritis accounts for 25–30% of children with JIA and usually affects preschool girls with a predominantly symmetrical arthritis of upper and lower limbs. Chronic anterior uveitis and growth disturbance are important but rare potential complications. This illness lasts most of childhood, and many children go into adulthood with active disease. These children have mild anaemia and usually positive ANAs. ESR and CRP may be mildly elevated.

Polyarthritis—rheumatoid-factor positive

This condition is similar in features and prognosis to adult RA and the only one deserving the name JRA. It affects girls primarily and usually presents in late childhood or adolescence. It affects less than 5% of patients with JIA and can be rapidly progressive and destructive. Rheumatoid nodules are common and failure to thrive more frequent than in seronegative polyarthritis. ANAs are usually positive (Figure 15.10).

Psoriatic arthritis

Arthritis may pre-date the onset of the classical skin findings of psoriasis by many years and is not required for the diagnosis in a

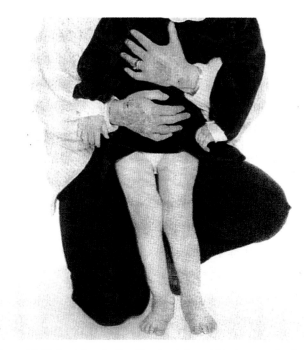

Figure 15.11 Psoriatic arthritis without rash in a child whose mother has psoriasis

child. The pattern of articular involvement in psoriatic arthritis is often asymmetrical, and tends to affects both small and large joints in a similar pattern to extended oligoarthritis, except for the presence of characteristic extra-articular features of psoriasis in a first-degree relative. Family history of a first-degree relative with psoriasis establishes the diagnosis. Asymptomatic uveitis with the same risk of blindness as in oligoarthritis affects many children, although the exact incidence is not known. These children should have a slit lamp evaluation every 3 months (Figure 15.11).

Enthesitis-related arthritis

ERA, or related conditions under the umbrella of JIA, typically begins after the age of 6 years and affects boys more often than girls. It is characterized initially by lower limb arthritis often complicated by enthesitis (inflammation of the point where tendon, ligament or fascia inserts into bone). The most common sites of enthesitis are at the insertions of plantar fascia (calcaneum, the base of the fifth metatarsal and the metatarsal heads), the insertion of the Achilles tendon into the calcaneum, and around and below the patella. Symptoms of sacroiliitis and spinal arthritis are uncommon at presentation. Although it may be a precursor illness to ankylosing spondylitis (AS), it is not known how many children with ERA progress to AS during their adult years. Uveitis affects these patients as well, but it tends to be symptomatic, presenting with red eyes, photophobia and pain. Some adolescent boys also complain of urethritis. A family history of similarly affected relatives is often positive, and HLA-B27 antigen may be found in 50% of patients, while ANA is usually negative.

Treatment

General principles

The aim of therapy is to maintain the child's or adolescent's quality of life while preserving joint function for as long as the disease is active. It helps to keep in mind that humans are living longer, and thus depending longer on the preservation of joint integrity. Second only to early recognition and referral, aggressive medical approach and timely physical interventions are of paramount importance. Whenever possible, the care of a child with JIA should be provided by an efficient, multidisciplinary team, a microsystem that prides itself on patient education and outreach (Boxes 15.8 and 15.9). The team should be led by a paediatric

---

Box 15.8 Members of the local community-based care team

- Primary care provider; the patient's general practitioner
- Rheumatologist
- Paediatrician
- Community rehabilitation and support staff
- School nurse
- Special education instructor
- Counsellor

Box 15.9 Members of the paediatric rheumatology care team

- Paediatric rheumatologist
- Paediatric nurse clinician
- Paediatric physiotherapist
- Paediatric occupational therapist
- Social worker
- Psychologist, parent liaison, nutritionist

---

rheumatologist working in tandem with a team of people who are expert in the specifics of paediatric rehabilitation, disease education, clinical and drug monitoring, the ethical conduct of clinical trials, school advocacy, nutrition, family and social support, and psychology. In addition, the need for ready access to other paediatric specialties, such as ophthalmology, orthopaedics, maxillofacial surgery, psychiatry, nephrology, infectious disease and dermatology, underscores the complexity of optimal management required for these children. Lastly, to fully maximize quality of care, the paediatric rheumatologist should be a member of one of the established networks of paediatric rheumatology professionals (clinicians including allied health professionals, scientists and all trainees), who collaborate in clinical trials augmented and enriched by translational research (such as the paediatric rheumatology international trials organization in Europe (PRINTO) and childhood arthritis and rheumatology research alliance (CARRA in the USA and Canada).

Hospital admission is often considered in European centres, intended for efficient initial investigation and team assessment of all patients with arthritis, particularly if they are significantly disabled or have prominent systemic features. In the USA, however, most children with arthritis, including JIA, are managed in outpatient settings, by paediatric rheumatologists heading up a painstakingly assembled multidisciplinary team. Most often, this team becomes a well-respected component of a clinical network employed within a tertiary referral structure (including children's hospitals and large academic, university-affiliated medical institutions), managing children with complex and chronic inflammatory diseases and evaluating youngsters with symptoms that prove too challenging for their primary care physicians. Ideally, this tertiary team communicates well with the local team led by the primary care provider, or school nurse, or physio- and occupational therapists, working in a variety of community settings. Computerized systems of care will ease communication among different providers.

Drug treatment of JIA usually starts with oral non-steroidal anti-inflammatory drugs (NSAIDs). However, most patients need better control than can be accomplished with NSAIDs alone. Within 4–12 weeks, slow-acting antirheumatic drugs such as methotrexate or sulfasalazine, can be considered if signs of inflammation persist even without disability (Table 15.3). Seventy per cent of children with polyarthritis improve (much fewer with systemic arthritis do so), but many continue to have radiologic progression and risk a lifetime of disability and decreased productivity. The addition of one of the new biologic agents, such as anti-tumour necrosis factor alpha (TNF-α) receptors and monoclonal antibodies, is considered quite early in the USA, especially in children threatened with long-term disability from both chronicity and aggressiveness of their inflammatory synovitis (as documented in children with polyarthritis, systemic arthritis and psoriatic arthritis). The use of these agents has revolutionized the approach to potentially disabling arthritis in both adults and children, and the resulting outcomes have dramatically altered natural history and stopped progression of disease in thousands of patients. No longer are children with JIA kept in strollers or wheelchairs. If the experience of the last 10 years holds, prognosis is now excellent for

Table 15.3 Drug treatment

Non-steroidal anti-inflammatory drugs

Ibuprofen 10 mg/kg/dose four times a day
Piroxicam 0.2–0.3 mg/kg/dose once a day
Naproxen 10 mg/kg/dose twice a day

Intra-articular corticosteroids

Triamcinolone hexacetonide

1 mg/kg/joint for large joints
0.5 mg/kg/joint for medium joints
1–2.5 mg/joint for digits

Triamcinolone acetonide

2 mg/kg/joint for large joints
1 mg/kg/joint for medium joints
2–4 mg/joint for digits

Methotrexate*

0.3–1 mg/kg/dose once weekly orally or subcutaneously

Sulfasalazine*

25 mg/kg/dose twice daily

Etanercept*

0.4 mg/kg/dose twice weekly or 0.8 mg/kg once weekly, both subcutaneously

Parenteral corticosteroids

Methylprednisolone 10–30 mg/kg/dose daily over 1–3 days
Prednisolone 0.2–2 mg/kg/dose once a day

*Need regular monitoring with blood counts, chemistry and metabolic tests and urinalysis

children with arthritis who have access to the latest therapies. Repeat intra-articular therapy and periods of intensive rehabilitation may still be needed for truly recalcitrant arthritis, but most children, particularly in the USA, where access to these new and expensive biologics is not restricted, face an increasingly positive future.

Whereas in the past ongoing physiotherapy services were required components of high-quality management, viewed as important as medical treatment, this is no longer the case. Children diagnosed and treated during the biologic era avoid ravages of chronic inflammation because biologic agents rapidly resolve stiffness and pain, allowing uninterrupted joint motion and muscle strength, thus preventing scarring, atrophy, asymmetric growth and subsequent reliance on assistive devices. The role of physiotherapists now is to keep children with arthritis strong

and flexible, engaged in regular exercise and open to a healthy lifestyle.

As with all chronic treatment, the issue of non-compliance is of particular importance in children and adolescents. Drugs that need to be given more than twice daily or taste badly should be avoided, if possible. School absence (and associated loss of work by parents) ought to be minimized and physical education classes adjusted to the student's physical tolerance. Great care should be given to minimizing pain associated with repeated injections. Meticulous attention to detail and routine utilization of health-related quality-of-life measures work synergistically to manage complications and prevent progression, resulting in high quality of care and improved outcomes.

Non-steroidal anti-inflammatory drugs

Treatment of children with arthritis usually begins with NSAIDs. These are used in higher doses, relative to body weight, than in adults because children have increased rates of metabolism and renal excretion. An individual NSAID, if free of significant adverse effects, could be continued for 4–8 weeks before a judgement about efficacy is made and the treatment is escalated. Adverse effects include abdominal pain (usually minimized by taking the NSAID with food and treated successfully with ranitidine, omeprazole or misoprostol), change in mood (usually transient) and rarely, bronchospasm (mild asthma is not a contraindication to the use of NSAIDs in children). Naproxen has the additional side effect of inducing pseudo-porphyria, particularly in children with reddish-blonde hair and fair complexions.

Selective COX-2 inhibitors were tested in paediatric trials and found as effective and safe as the widely used traditional NSAIDs. However, only one, celecoxib, is labelled for use in children with arthritis, owing to increased incidence of myocardial infarction in adults. Cessation of NSAIDs may be considered if the patient has been free of active disease for at least 6 months. The majority of patients with early JIA do not respond completely to NSAIDs and need more aggressive treatment. In children with single joint involvement, an intra-articular corticosteroid with a long half-life is often recommended after 6 weeks.

Corticosteroids

Intra-articular preparations are the most frequently used form of corticosteroids in JIA. Triamcinolone hexacetonide has the highest efficacy and longest duration of action, although drug supplies are unreliable and at times limited within the UK and the USA. In children with oligoarthritis, intra-articular injections have largely replaced other interventions, including NSAIDs. A single injection usually resolves all signs of inflammation for several months. In the UK, intra-articular medication in children is usually given under general anaesthesia and multiple injections are common, whereas in the USA, where usually no more than one or two joints are injected, local anaesthetic is acceptable for most children.

Systemic steroids must be avoided if possible, because of a nearly unacceptable range of adverse effects, including growth and immune suppression, cataract formation, diabetes, avascular necrosis of bone, vertebral collapse and the horrible and predictable physical changes of Cushing's stigmata, in virtually all patients. In some situations, however, large pulses of intravenous methylprednisolone help gain control of active and devastating features of systemic arthritis and may be lifesaving in the face of significant pericarditis with tamponade or rapidly progressive macrophage activation syndrome.

The use of oral prednisolone is limited to low-dose, preferably alternate-day administration, for children with severe polyarthritis or systemic arthritis who are unable to function in school or the community despite having taken all available steroid-sparing medications. "Steroid-sparing agents" refers to aggressive interventions, including chemotherapy, biologics and stem-cell replacement, which should only be tried by experts in childhood rheumatic diseases.

Short stature, a common and severe sequel of poorly controlled systemic arthritis, may be treated with daily injections of growth hormone. Most children, as reported in several studies, have a statistically improved rate of growth while receiving growth hormone and seem to achieve higher ultimate height. Similarly, and often in addition to the above, short stature associated with chronic corticosteroid use also improves after the addition of growth hormone and appears well tolerated.

Slow-acting antirheumatic drugs

Methotrexate—Methotrexate is effective in approximately 70% of children with polyarthritis but much less in systemic arthritis. It should be considered for any child whose arthritis is not well controlled with a trail of NSAIDs and intra-articular steroids, alone, after 4–12 weeks. Initial doses of 0.3–0.5 mg/kg of methotrexate are usually given by mouth once a week (recommended 1 hour before food to improve absorption). For recalcitrant disease, subcutaneous methotrexate provides serum levels up to 40% higher than the oral route. Once methotrexate is started, efficacy may be determined after 1–3 months.

The most common adverse events associated with methotrexate are nausea, followed by mouth sores. Subcutaneous administration may be less of a problem in this regard than oral administration. Oral folate supplements or ondansetron may be helpful, and leucovorin rescue is often used if symptoms persist after 24 hours. Other side effects include abdominal pain; elevated liver enzymes; and rarely, hair loss and bone-marrow suppression. Patients taking methotrexate must have blood monitoring on a monthly basis to screen for abnormal liver function and bone-marrow suppression. Adolescents must refrain from drinking alcohol.

Recent trials with leflunomide have shown the same efficacy and less toxicity in children taking leflunomide than methotrexate. While very similar to methotrexate in mode of action, leflunomide seems better tolerated, particularly by patients who develop some of the more recalcitrant side effects (such as nausea before the drug is even administered) (Silverman *et al.*, 2005).

Sulfasalazine—Sulfasalazine has been shown to be efficacious in oligoarthritis and polyarthritis, but seems particularly effective in ERA. It is usually well tolerated, but an erythematous rash may be an adverse event. There are rare reports of aplastic anaemia. The usual doses of 2–4 g per day are divided into two doses. It is not of value in systemic arthritis, with a poor clinical response and an increased incidence of side effects such as macrophage activation syndrome.

Biologic agents

Currently three TNF antagonists exist, and two have been studied well in children: etanercept and infliximab. Adalimumab, a fully humanized monoclonal antibody to TNF, is also available. There remain significant long-term concerns relating to the unknown effects of these agents, particularly in young children. Many years of practice are needed to identify potential disruption of immune surveillance in children; however, to date with over 10 years and millions of prescriptions worldwide, experience has been overwhelmingly positive.

Etanercept—Therapy with this anti-TNF-α receptor is approved for the treatment of children with JIA whose disease is not adequately controlled with methotrexate or who are intolerant of it. Large multicentre trials showed that children with severe, methotrexate-resistant polyarthritis demonstrated sustained clinical improvement with more than 2 years of continuous etanercept treatment. Etanercept was generally well tolerated, and there were no increases in the rates of adverse events over time (Lovell *et al.*, 2003). Etanercept may be initiated if methotrexate fails to control signs of inflammation or if there are unacceptable adverse drug reactions. Regular (1–2 month) monitoring of blood counts and chemistry studies is recommended. Etanercept should be discontinued in the event of fever or other signs of significant infection. Methotrexate is often discontinued when etanercept is started, but may be continued indefinitely after initiation of etanercept if it is well tolerated. Combinations of medical interventions appear to have the best long-term outcome.

Infliximab—Infliximab is a biologic agent developed for the treatment of RA in adults and is a chimeric monoclonal antibody against TNF-α. It is highly effective but not yet labelled for use in JIA. It is approved for use in childhood Crohn's disease and being increasingly used for children with JIA who fail etanercept or have associated uveitis. In adults, infliximab is now approved for treatment of seronegative spondyloarthropathies. It is used in combination with methotrexate to minimize the risk of immune reactions. A dose of 5 mg/kg/dose is usually associated with improvement in the majority of children. Reactions are common and infusions should be done in paediatric settings where staff is experienced in handling intravenous infusions.

Other drugs

Hydroxychloroquine—Hydroxychloroquine is a relatively safe antimalarial drug that has been used widely in adults with RA, mostly as adjunctive therapy. Studies in children do not support its use in JIA, and the availability of successful interventions has largely superseded its use. It does show efficacy in RA and thus is still advocated for adolescents with RF-positive polyarthritis.

Cyclosporin A—Cyclosporin A is a Il-2 inhibitor that targets T-cells and is used (with falling frequency and in combination with methotrexate) to control features of systemic arthritis. It is initially well tolerated but only anecdotally successful. It has also been combined with methotrexate to treat uveitis. Side effects include gingival hyperplasia and hirsuitism. Over time, cyclosporin A contributes to hypertension and progressive renal disease. It is still used routinely to treat macrophage activation syndrome associated with systemic arthritis either solo or in combination with high-dose methylprednisolone.

Cyclophosphamide—Borrowing from oncology, high doses of chemotherapy are sometimes advocated for patients unresponsive to all other available therapies, particularly children with severe recalcitrant systemic arthritis whose quality of life is poor and for whom even the newest biologic therapies are not working.

Autologous stem-cell transplantation

A number of children with truly recalcitrant systemic arthritis have been successfully transplanted in Europe, and the procedure is being investigated in the USA for JIA unresponsive to all other therapies. It is a high-risk procedure but seems to offer a reasonable chance of inducing disease remission.

Natural history

JIA is a diverse group of conditions, each unique but all associated with persistent arthritis. The spectrum of JIA varies from: mild to severe; smouldering to rapidly progressive; uniphasic and polyphasic to chronic and continuous; affecting one to affecting most joints; associated with no extra-articular symptoms to such severe extra-articular manifestations as to overshadow the presence of arthritis. Accordingly, few children may remit spontaneously (predictive factors for this are unknown), while another small fraction will have devastating disease, recalcitrant to all, including experimental, treatments. For the remaining majority of children with JIA, however, long-term follow-up studies highlight a much poorer prognosis than previously believed (Foster *et al.*, 2003). These studies show a profound impact on later productivity and on quality of life of adults diagnosed at a time when biologic therapies had not yet been found. It follows then that early diagnosis and rapid referral to an experienced paediatric rheumatology team would be associated with improved outcome and that the longer duration of inflammation, the higher the impact on quality of life, in particular on independence in activities of daily living.

Studies of large numbers of children with JIA followed longitudinally show that as many as 30% continue to have active arthritis into their adult years. These studies include children with persistent oligoarthritis whose natural history of illness has been well described and tends to be limited to an average of 2 years of monoarthritis. That leaves children with polyarthritis and systemic arthritis, in addition to 20% with extended oligoarthritis, comprising the group who continues to have disease into adulthood. Today, many of these young adults are left with the chronic sequelae of short stature, restricted joint movement, asymmetrical growth and extra-articular abnormalities. An appreciation of the true natural history of JIA and the availability of successful treatments have imparted great urgency to prompt referral, initiation of aggressive treatment regimens, improved access to clinical trials and renewed hope for children with arthritis. Over the next decade, new treatments will be developed and tested in children, while concomitant translational research, including studies in pharmacogenetics, will all result in custom-designed individualized and uniquely targeted therapies.

References

Foster HE, Marshall N, Myers A, Dunkley P, Griffiths ID. Outcome of adults with juvenile idiopathic arthritis; quality of life study. *Arthritis and Rheumatism* 2003; **48**: 767–775.

Lovell DJ, Giannini EH, Reiff A *et al.* for the Pediatric Rheumatology Collaborative Study Group. Long-term efficacy and safety of etanercept in children with polyarticular course juvenile rheumatoid arthritis. *Arthritis and Rheumatism* 2003; **48**: 218–226.

Silverman E, Mouy R, Spiegel L *et al.* Leflunomide or methotrexate for juvenile rheumatoid arthritis. *New England Journal of Medicine* 2005; **352**: 1655–1666.

Further reading

Brooks CD. Sulfasalazine for the management of juvenile rheumatoid arthritis. *Journal of Rheumatology* 2001; **28**: 845–853.

Jung JH, Jun JB, Yoo DH, Kim TH, Jung SS, Lee IH *et al.* High toxicity of sulfasalazine in adult-onset Still's disease. *Clinical and Experimental Rheumatology* 2000; **18**: 245–248.

Ruperto N, Lovell DJ, Cuttica R *et al.* for the Pediatric Rheumatology International Trials Organisation and the Pediatric Collaborative Study Group. A randomised placebo controlled trial of infliximab plus methotrexate for the treatment of polyarticular-course juvenile rheumatoid arthritis. *Arthritis and Rheumatism* 2007; **56**: 2815–2816.

Szer IS, Kimura Y, Malleson PN, Southwood TR, eds. *Arthritis in Children and Adolescents: juvenile idiopathic arthritis*. Oxford University Press, Oxford, 2006.

CHAPTER 16

Musculoskeletal Disorders in Children and Adolescents

Helen Foster[1] *and Lori Tucker*[2]

[1]Newcastle University, Newcastle upon Tyne, UK
[2]British Columbia's Children's Hospital, Vancouver, Canada

OVERVIEW

- Musculoskelelal complaints in children are common, often benign and self-limiting, but can be presenting features of significant, severe and potentially life-threatening conditions.

- Making a diagnosis rests on competent clinical skills, knowledge of normal variants, knowledge of common clinical scenarios, "red flags" to suggest severe conditions and judicious use and interpretation of investigations.

- Common clinical scenarios include the limping child, "growing pains", back pain and knee pain.

- Knowledge of "red flags" to suggest infection, malignancy, multi-system disease and inflammatory joint disorders are important.

- The management of musculoskeletal conditions involves a multidisciplinary approach.

- Many chronic conditions that begin in childhood continue into adult life, and the process of transitional care to adult services starts in early adolescence.

Introduction

Musculoskeletal (MSK) presentations in childhood are common, with a spectrum of causes (Box 16.1), the majority of which are benign and self-limiting. It must be remembered, however, that severe, potentially life-threatening conditions such as malignancy, sepsis, vasculitis and non-accidental injury may also present with MSK complaints. Furthermore, MSK features are common in association with chronic conditions other than rheumatic disorders, such as inflammatory bowel disease and cystic fibrosis. Diagnosis relies on competent MSK clinical skills, with the minimum of a screening MSK examination (Foster *et al.*, 2006), appropriate knowledge of normal variants (Box 16.2), "red flags" to raise suspicion of malignancy or sepsis and clinical scenarios at different

ABC of Rheumatology, 4th edn. Edited by Ade Adebajo.
©2010 Blackwell Publishing Ltd. 9781405170680.

Box 16.1 **Differential diagnosis of musculoskeletal pain**

Life-threatening conditions
- Malignancy (leukaemia, lymphoma, bone tumour)
- Sepsis (septic arthritis, osteomyelitis)
- Non-accidental injury

Joint pain with no swelling
- Hypermobility syndromes
- Idiopathic pain syndromes (reflex sympathetic dystrophy, fibromyalgia)
- Orthopaedic syndromes (e.g. Osgood–Schlatter disease, Perthes disease)
- Metabolic (e.g. hypothyroidism, lysosomal storage diseases)

Joint pain with swelling
- Trauma
- Infection
  - Septic arthritis and osteomyelitis (viral, bacterial, mycobacterial)
  - Reactive arthritis (post-enteric, sexually acquired)
  - Infection related (rheumatic fever, post-vaccination)
- Juvenile idiopathic arthritis
- Arthritis related Inflammatory bowel disease
- Connective tissue diseases (SLE, scleroderma, dermatomyositis, vasculitis)
- Sarcoidosis
- Metabolic (e.g. osteomalacia, cystic fibrosis)
- Haematological (*e.g.* haemophilia, haemoglobinopathy)
- Tumour (benign and malignant)
- Chromosomal (e.g. Downs related arthritis)
- Auto-inflammatory syndromes *e.g.* CINCA, (Figure 16.1) periodic syndromes, CRMO)
- Developmental/congenital (e.g. spondylo-epiphyseal dysplasia)

---

ages (Box 16.3). The approach to MSK assessment in children is different to that of adults; as young children may have difficulty in localizing or describing symptoms, the history is often given by the parent/carer, and complaints may be non-specific, such as "my child is limping". Clinical assessment usually distinguishes between mechanical and inflammatory problems and an approach to assess-

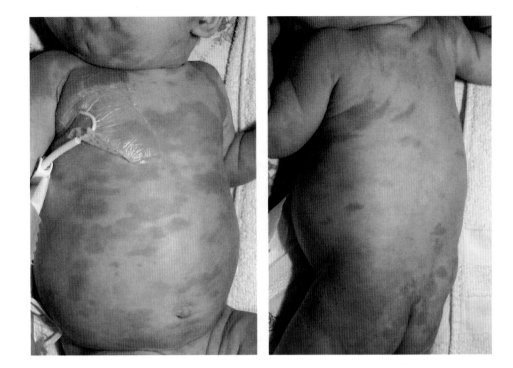

Figure 16.1 Chronic infantile neurological cutaneous arthritis (CINCA) syndrome: widespread rash

Box 16.2 **Normal variants in gait patterns and stance**

- Intoeing can be due to:
  - Hip—persistent femoral anteversion—commonly between ages of 3–8 years
  - Lower leg—(internal tibial torsion)—commonly from onset of walking to 3 years
  - Feet—metatarsus adductus—most resolve by the age of 6 years
- Bow legs (varus)—birth to early toddler—most resolve by 3 years
- Knock knees (valgus)—most resolve by age of 7 years
- Flat feet—most resolve by 6 years, and normal arches are evident on tiptoeing
- Crooked toes—most resolve with weight bearing

Indicators to cause concern

- Persistent changes that fail to resolve by the expected age
- Progressive changes
- Lack of symmetry
- Associated pain or functional disability
- Systemic upset
- Dysmorphic features/short stature

Table 16.1 A strategy for characterizing musculoskeletal pain in children

Localized pain		Diffuse pain	
"Well" child	"Unwell"** child	"Well" Child	"Unwell" Child
Strains and sprains	Septic arthritis	Hypermobility	Leukaemia
Bone tumours	Osteomyelitis	Diffuse idiopathic pain syndromes	Neuroblastoma
JIA (oligoarticular subtype)			JIA (systemic and polyarticular onset subtypes)
Localized idiopathic pain syndromes			SLE
"Growing pains"			Juvenile dermatomyositis
			Vasculitis

**associated with one or more "red flags", such as fever, anorexia, weight loss, malaise and raised inflammatory markers
JIA = juvenile idiopathic arthritis; SLE = systemic lupus erythematosus
This table is adapted from Malleson and Beauchamp, 2001

Box 16.3 **"Red flags" to warrant concern in children presenting with musculoskeletal symptoms**

- Systemic upset (fever, malaise, anorexia, weight loss or raised inflammatory markers)
- Bone pain and/or night pain
- Regression of motor milestones
- Functional disability

ment (Table 16.1) incorporates potential diagnoses according to whether pain is localized or diffuse, whether the child is "well" or not and the presence or absence of "red flags". The presence of multi-system features broadens the differential to include connective tissue diseases.

The "limping child"

This is a common presentation, with a spectrum of age-related

Table 16.2 Common/significant causes of limping according to age

Toddler/preschool

Infection (septic arthritis, osteomyelitis—hip, spine)
Mechanical (trauma and non-accidental injury)
Congenital/developmental problems (e.g. hip dysplasia, talipes)
Neurological disease (e.g. cerebral palsy, hereditary syndromes)
Inflammatory arthritis (JIA)
Malignant disease (e.g. leukaemia, neuroblastoma)

5–10 years

Mechanical (trauma, overuse injuries, sport injuries)
Reactive arthritis/transient synovitis—"irritable hip"
Perthes' disease
Inflammatory arthritis (JIA)
Tarsal coalition
Idiopathic pain syndromes
Malignant disease

10–17 years

Mechanical (trauma, overuse injuries, sport injuries)
Slipped capital femoral epiphysis
Inflammatory arthritis (JIA)
Idiopathic pain syndromes
Osteochondritis dissecans
Tarsal coalition
Malignant disease (leukaemia, lymphoma, primary bone tumour)

JIA = juvenile idiopathic arthritis
Reproduced by kind permission of the Arthritis Research Campaign (www.arc.org.UK)

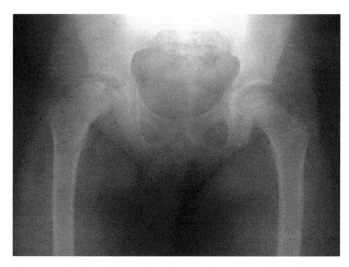

Figure 16.2 Perthes' disease, showing avascular necrosis of the right hip

Box 16.4 **The "rules" of growing pains**

- Pains are *never* present at the start of the day after waking
- The child does not limp
- Physical activities are not limited by symptoms
- Pains are symmetrical in the lower limbs
- Physical examination is normal (evidence of joint hypermobility is common)
- The child is systemically well
- Gross motor milestones are normal
- Age range 3–11 years

causes (Table 16.2), and the site of the problem may be broad (from a foreign body in the sole of the foot to a tumour in the spine). Orthopaedic conditions at the hip are common and often present acutely, with a well (albeit limping) child, with possible diagnoses including slipped upper femoral epiphysis (usually the older, often overweight, child) and Perthes' disease (Figure 16.2) (which may follow a transient synovitis or "irritable hip" in the younger child). The hip joint is unusual as a monoarthritis in juvenile idiopathic arthritis (JIA), and in isolation, sepsis (including mycobacterial infection) needs to be considered. The concept of referred pain from the hip or thigh, for example, must be sought in situations where the child has knee pain but there is no evidence of localized disease at the knee.

Back pain

Back pain is a common complaint, and is frequently mechanical with contributory factors such as poor posture, physical inactivity or abnormal loading (such as carrying heavy school bags on one shoulder). Certain sporting activities such as cricket, bowling or gymnastics pose increased risk of back pain, with possible consequences such as spondylolysis and spondylolisthesis. "Red flags" for referral for a child with back pain include a painful scoliosis,

neurological symptoms suggestive of nerve-root entrapment or cord compression and systemic findings to suggest malignancy or sepsis. Inflammatory back pain may be a late feature of enthesitis-related arthritis (a subtype of JIA), often presenting in late adolescence and with a strong association with expression of HLA-B27.

Mechanical pain

Osteochondritis of the knee (Osgood–Schlatter disease) is common, especially in adolescent boys who are physically active (particularly those who play football or basketball). Sever's disease (osteochondritis of the calcaneum) may present with a painful heel. Flat feet (Figure 16.3) are common, and standing on tiptoe should create a normal medial longitudinal arch; inability to do so or painful fixed flat feet warrant further investigation to exclude tarsal coalition. High fixed arches, or pes cavus, may suggest neurological disease. Non-specific mechanical MSK pain in children is often labelled as "growing pains". Making a diagnosis of "growing pains" requires careful assessment, and Box 16.4 suggests when alternative diagnoses need to be sought. Many children and adolescents with non-

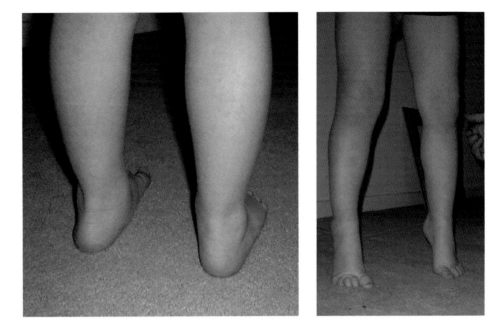

Figure 16.3 Normal variant: mobile flat feet are common

specific aches and pains, including growing pains, are found to have joint hypermobility, which is suggested by symmetrical hyper-extension at the fingers, elbows and knees (genu recurvatum), and flat pronated feet. It is important, however, to consider and exclude "non-benign" causes of hypermobility (e.g. Marfan's, Stickler's and Ehlers–Danlos syndromes), which are rare but important, as these children are at risk of retinal and cardiac complications. Non-specific aches and pains are also a feature of idiopathic pain syndromes, which are mostly seen in older female children/adolescents; such patients are often markedly debilitated by their pain and fatigue—the pain can be incapacitating—but the child/adolescent is otherwise well, and physical examination is usually normal. Localized idiopathic pain syndromes most commonly affect the foot or hand, may be triggered by trauma (often mild) and are likened to reflex sympathetic dystrophy.

Neoplasia

It is important to differentiate joint pain from bone pain. Bone pain is a "red flag" and is a common feature of leukaemia, meta-static neuroblastoma and primary bone tumours (Figure 16.4). It is important to note that these malignancies may also present with frank arthritis. Osteoid osteomas (the most common benign bone tumour) are usually located in the femoral neck or posterior ele-ments of the spine, and typically cause night pain that can be relieved by salicylates.

Arthritis and infection

Children with septic arthritis are usually febrile, appear unwell and have severe pain with joint movement. Septic arthritis usually occurs in large joints. Reactive arthritis is usually monoarticular or

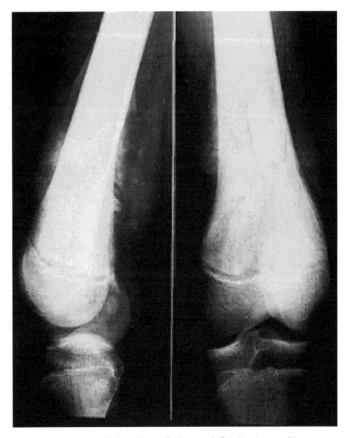

Figure 16.4 Periosteal elevation: soft-tissue calcification in a malignant tumour of the distal femur

oligoarticular and follows bacterial infection in the gut (*Salmonella, Shigella, Campylobacter, Yersinia*), although in the older child and adolescent it is important to consider sexually acquired infection (*Chlamydia,* gonorrhoea*)*. Rheumatic fever (a form of reactive arthritis that follows pharyngeal streptococcal infection) is uncommon in the UK, but common in developing countries. Lyme disease following tick-transmitted infection with *Borrelia burgdorferi* is suggested by the presence of an oligoarthritis, erythema chronicum migrans, and a travel history to an endemic area.

Chronic arthritis (JIA)

In the absence of sepsis or trauma, JIA is the most likely cause of a single swollen joint in a child and is covered in more detail in Chapter 15.

Connective tissue diseases

Systemic lupus erythematosus

Systemic lupus erythematosus (SLE) may be confused with chronic arthritis, because some patients present with arthritis as the primary clinical finding. SLE is rare but is more common in non-white individuals, with a predominance of girls affected in the adolescent group and more boys affected in young children. The arthritis of SLE is usually polyarticular, non-deforming and non-erosive. Extra-articular features are variable, and a diagnosis is made with a combination of clinical and laboratory features (Table 16.3). It is worth considering drug-induced SLE, which can develop from the use of anti-convulsants, oral contraceptives or minocycline. The medical management of SLE is complex and requires specialist supervision, and many patients require corticosteroid and immunosuppressive medication. In addition, patients often require anti-hypertensives, anticoagulation (related to antiphospholipid syndrome), and medications to control dyslipidaemias and avoid osteoporosis.

Juvenile dermatomyositis

Juvenile dermatomyositis (JDM) may present at any age, with characteristic skin involvement (Figure 16.5), and proximal muscle weakness which can present acutely or indolently. JDM has a broad range of severity; contrary to adult-onset DM, there is no association with malignancy. Patients with JDM may develop calcinosis as a late complication of poorly controlled disease (Figure 16.6). Severe complications at the time of active disease include risk of aspiration pneumonia and interstitial lung disease. Diagnosis usually rests on clinical assessment, and elevated serum muscle enzymes; most children do not require electromyography or a muscle biopsy in the absence of atypical features. Magnetic resonance imaging of the muscles is very useful to demonstrate muscle involvement and monitor disease activity. Treatment of JDM requires rapid initiation of high-dose corticosteroids, frequently accompanied by methotrexate, although other medication such as intravenous immunoglobulin, cyclophosphamide or anti-cytokine agents are used in severe or refractory disease. Physical therapy input is essential to optimize outcome.

Table 16.3 SLE in children and adolescents

Common presenting symptoms

Malar rash
Arthritis
Fatigue
Fever
Weight loss
Oral ulcers
Alopecia
Pleuritis/pericarditis
Central nervous system findings
Photosensitivity
Raynaud's phenomenon
Lymphadenopathy
Hepatosplenomegaly

Laboratory findings

Anaemia (may be haemolytic with positive red cell autoantibodies)
Leukopaenia, lymphopaenia
Thrombocytopaenia
Elevated liver enzymes
Elevated kidney function tests (blood urea nitrogen, creatinine)
Decreased complement components C3 and C4
Positive antinuclear antibody
High titre positive anti-double-stranded DNA antibody
Positive autoantibodies to extractable antigens (anti-Ro (SSA); anti-La (SSB); anti-Sm; anti-RNP)
Positive antiphospholipid antibodies (anti-cardiolipin, lupus anticoagulant)

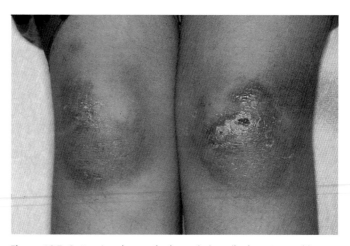

Figure 16.5 Gottron's rash over the knees in juvenile dermatomyositis

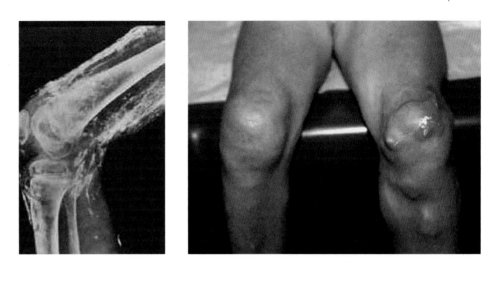

Figure 16.6 Calcinosis in juvenile dermatomyositis

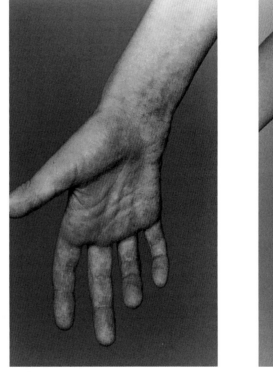

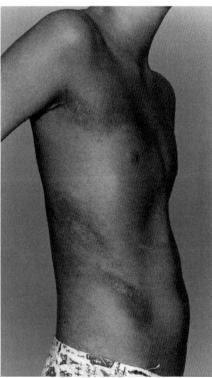

Figure 16.7 Localized scleroderma with morphoea skin lesions and underlying muscle wasting of the right hand

Sclerodermas

Scleroderma in childhood is rare and heterogeneous, and subtypes are determined by the type and number of lesions, the area of involvement and serological abnormalities. Localized scleroderma (Figure 16.7) is the most common and can present at any age, with the appearance of a patch of abnormal skin, which when untreated, generally follows a course of active expanding disease, fibrosis and eventual softening with some "remission". The functional and cosmetic impact can be profound, as the lesions may interfere with growth of a limb and subcutaneous tissues (of the face or a limb). Current practice advocates aggressive treatment regimes (corticosteroid and methotrexate) to control disease and limit severe disfigurement and disability. Systemic scleroderma is very rare in children and includes progressive diffuse fibrous changes of the skin and fibrous changes involving internal organs—most commonly lungs, gastrointestinal tract, heart and kidneys—with a significant mortality. Systemic scleroderma is slowly progressive, has a guarded prognosis and requires potent immunosuppression, although clinical trials are lacking to guide practice.

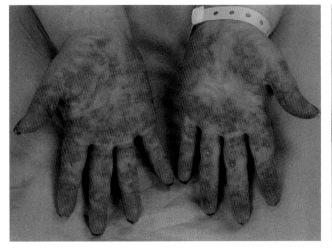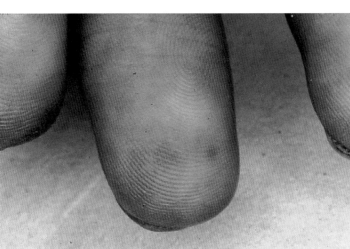

Figure 16.8 Vasculitis of the hands

Box 16.5 **Features of Kawasaki disease**

Fever for more than 5 days plus at least four of the following signs:

- Bilateral conjunctival injection
- Changes in the oropharyngeal membranes (swollen fissured lips, strawberry tongue, injected pharynx)
- Changes in peripheral extremities (erythema and swelling of hands and feet followed by desquamation of the skin)
- Polymorphous rash
- Cervical lymphadenopathy (at least one node >1.5 cm)

Vasculitis

Vasculitis (Figure 16.8) is a heterogeneous group of disorders, most commonly classified by the size of involved blood vessels. A diagnosis may be suggested by multi-system clinical involvement and laboratory features (Table 16.4). The common childhood vasculitides Henoch–Schönlein purpura (HSP) and Kawasaki (KD) disease (Box 16.5) often have transient arthritis affecting large joints. HSP is characterized by palpable purpura (Figure 16.9) over the legs and buttocks, abdominal pain, haematuria and arthritis. In general, HSP resolves completely within 4 weeks of onset; however, some patients have recurrences of rash and gastrointestinal symptoms, and a small percentage of children who develop renal disease with HSP go on to renal failure. KD is an acute systemic vasculitis, predominantly in young children (less than 5 years); it is usually self-limiting but has the potential for causing severe long-term complications due to the involvement of coronary and other blood vessels with aneurysms. Prompt recognition of KD is essential in providing early treatment with intravenous immunoglobulin, which decreases the risk of developing coronary aneurysms significantly.

Table 16.4 Vasculitides in childhood

Type according to size of vessel

Large-vessel vasculitis

Takayasu's arteritis
[Giant cell (temporal) arteritis—rarely seen in adolescents/children]

Medium-vessel vasculitis

Polyarteritis nodosa
Kawasaki disease

Small-vessel vasculitis

Wegener's granulomatosis
Churg–Strauss syndrome
Microscopic polyangiitis
Henoch–Schönlein purpura
Cutaneous leukocytoclastic vasculitis
[Cryoglobulinaemic vasculitis—rarely seen in adolescents/children]

Features suggesting a vasculitis in adolescents and children

Clinical
Fever, weight loss, persistent fatigue
Skin rash: palpable purpura, vasculitic urticaria, nodules, ulcers
Neurologic signs: headache, mononeuritis multiplex, focal CNS lesions
Arthritis or arthralgia, myalgia or myositis
Hypertension
Pulmonary infiltrates or haemorrhage

Laboratory
Increased acute-phase reactants (ESR, CRP)
Anaemia, leukocytosis
Eosinophilia
Antineutrophil cytoplasmic antibodies (ANCA)*
Elevated factor VIII-related antigen (von Willebrand factor)
Haematuria

*ANCA: cytoplasmic (c-ANCA) associates specifically with Wegener's granulomatosis and perinuclear (p-ANCA) associates with microscopic polyangiitis and a variety of other vasculitides
CRP = C-reactive protein; ESR = erythrocyte sedimentation rate
Reproduced by kind permission of the Arthritis Research Campaign (www.arc.org.UK)

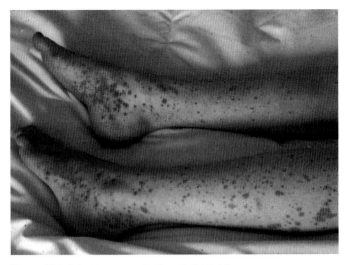

Figure 16.9 Palpable purpura in Henoch–Schönlein purpura

Box 16.6 Inherited periodic fever syndromes

- Familial Mediterranean fever
- Hyerimmunoglobulinaemia D—also known as mevalonic kinase deficiency
- Tumor necrosis factor receptor-associated periodic syndrome
- The cryopyrinopathies:
  - Familial cold auto-inflammatory syndrome
  - Muckle–Wells syndrome
  - Chronic infantile neurologic cutaneous and articular syndrome—also known as neonatal-onset multi-system inflammatory disease
- Periodic fever with aphthous stomatitis, pharyngitis and adenitis
- Cyclic neutropenia

Rare inflammatory syndromes

Inherited auto-inflammatory syndromes

These syndromes (Box 16.6) are rare, and children may present with repeated unexplained bouts of fever with a variety of clinical findings associated with the fevers, which may include rash (Figure 16.1), MSK complaints, abdominal pain and ocular and neurologic complaints. There is often a broad range of severity among patients with the same genetic disorder, making diagnosis on clinical grounds often challenging. New treatment options have become available for some patients with periodic fever syndromes, and patients require specialist supervision.

Chronic recurrent multifocal osteomyelitis

Chronic recurrent multifocal osteomyelitis (CRMO) is a condition that presents similarly to bacterial osteomyelitis, but no organism can be isolated and there are often multiple involved sites with recurring episodes. Children or adolescents present with bone pain, sometimes accompanied by swelling; most common affected areas are long bones (tibia), but ribs, clavicle, vertebrae or

Table 16.5 Health-care transition planning in the paediatric rheumatology clinic

Planning for transition

Begin to discuss eventual transition from pediatrics with child and parent at an early stage (by puberty)

Engage the child in health-care visits directly at their developmental level

Begin to encourage the child/youth to spend time alone with health-care providers during visits

Transition tasks

Education about disease, prognosis, treatments and roles of health-care providers specifically directed at youth

Education about generic youth health issues (diet, dental care, sleep, exercise, smoking, alcohol, sexual health, recreational drugs)

Address adherence to medical plan at every visit

Career and vocational planning

Promote youth self-management, advocacy and independence in health-care decision-making

Assist with separation from parents with respect to medical issues

Acknowledge and be respectful of broader adolescent transitional tasks

Ultimately transfer them to adult rheumatologist and health-care providers (who are ideally youth-friendly) and forward adequate health records

Reproduced by kind permission of the Arthritis Research Campaign (www.arc.org.UK)

mandible can be involved. Radiographs show osteolytic changes similar to osteomyelitis, and a bone scan may show lesions that are asymptomatic. Antibiotics are not effective, and many children with CRMO have good symptomatic relief with non-steroidal anti-inflammatory drugs. For those with persistent disease, bisphosphonates are often effective.

The role of the multidisciplinary team

The paediatric rheumatology multidisciplinary team (MDT) is highly skilled in the provision and coordination of comprehensive and often complex management regimes for the child and family, providing education and support, with other specialist services as well as community services, schools and health-care providers within shared care clinical networks. Many children with rheumatic diseases have continuing disease activity or relapses in adulthood, or sequelae from previous disease activity, which require ongoing medical treatment. Health-care transition, for youths with childhood-onset rheumatic diseases describes the movement of patients from child- and family-centred paediatric care to adult-oriented health-care systems. The MDT coordinate transitional care, addressing generic and disease-specific health issues (Table 16.5), and ultimately transfer to adult rheumatology services. Education and support are paramount, particularly with complex treatment regimes and the impact on adolescent behaviours, such as avoidance of pregnancy and excess alcohol in those taking methotrexate.

References

Foster HE, Kay LJ, Friswell M, Coady DA, Myers A. pGALS—a paediatric musculoskeletal screening examination for school aged children based on the adult GALS screen. *Arthritis Care Research* 2006; **55**: 709–716. A web-streamed demonstration of pGALS, supplementary materials and DVD are available online, at: http://www.arc.org.uk/arthinfo/emedia.asp

Malleson PN, Beauchamp P. Diagnosing musculoskeletal pain in children. *Canadian Medical Association Journal* 2001; **165**: 183–188.

Further reading

Cassidy JT, Petty RE. *Textbook of Pediatric Rheumatology*, 5th edn. WB Saunders, Philadelphia, PA, 2005.

Compeyrot-Lacassagne S, Feldman B. Inflammatory myopathies in children. *Pediatric Clinics of North America* 2005; **52**: 493–520.

Foster HE, Cabral DA. Is musculoskeletal history and examination so different in paediatrics? *Best Practice & Research. Clinical Rheumatology* 2006; **20**: 241–262.

Klein-Gitelman, M, Reiff A, Silverman ED. Systemic lupus erythematosus in childhood. *Rheumatic Disease Clinics of North America*. 2002; **28**: 561–577.

McDonagh JE. Transition of care from adult to paediatric rheumatology. *Archives of Disease in Childhood* 2007; **97**: 802–807.

Murray KJ, Laxer RM. Scleroderma in children and adolescents. *Rheumatic Disease Clinics of North America* 2002; **28**: 603–624.

Ozen, S. The spectrum of vasculitis in children. *Best Practice & Research Clinical Rheumatology* 2002; **16**: 411–425.

CHAPTER 17

Polymyalgia Rheumatica and Giant Cell Arteritis

Eric L Matteson[1] and Howard A Bird[2]

[1]Mayo Clinic, Rochester, USA
[2]Chapel Allerton Hospital, Leeds, UK

OVERVIEW

- Patients with polymyalgia rheumatica are over 50 years of age, and on average over 70 years old.
- Hallmark symptoms of the disease are shoulder and hip girdle pain with marked stiffness.
- Giant cell arteritis may be present in at least 30% of patients.
- Treatment is with glucocorticosteroids, initially 15–20 mg a day of prednisone equivalent. Treatment is often required for several years.

Polymyalgia rheumatica (PMR) is a clinical syndrome that affects older patients and comprises proximal muscle group stiffness, particularly in the shoulder, and systemic features such as fatigue and weight loss. It is associated with an increased erythrocyte sedimentation rate (ESR) and responds dramatically to relatively small doses of steroids.

Giant cell arteritis (GCA) is a systemic vasculitis that affects large- and medium-sized arteries. Although it may involve any artery, it has a propensity to affect the branches of the external carotid artery, particularly the posterior ciliary arteries that supply the optic nerve and the superficial temporal artery; hence its alternative (often interchangeable) name "temporal arteritis" (Figure 17.1).

There are clinical and pathogenetic links between temporal arteritis, GCA and PMR, which has led to the concept that they are manifestations of a disease spectrum that affects the same disease population (Box 17.1). The two entities may occur in the same patient simultaneously, at different time points, or independently. PMR has been observed in 40–60% of cases of GCA, and 30–80% of patients with PMR have GCA.

Causes

The cause of GCA or PMR is likely to be polygenic, with both genetic and environmental factors contributing to disease susceptibility and severity.

Environmental

Acute-onset prodromal events and synchronous variations in incidence of PMR and GCA suggest a possible environmental infectious trigger. Several studies have shown concurrence in the incidence of PMR and GCA with epidemics of *Mycoplasma pneumoniae*, *Chlamydia pneumoniae*, parvovirus B19, respiratory syncytial virus and adenovirus. Despite this, no definite causative infectious agent has been identified.

Genetics

Racial differences in incidence and familial aggregation suggest a common genetic susceptibility factor. PMR and GCA are linked with human leukocyte antigen DR4 (HLA-DR4). Patients who are positive for HLA-DR4 and those who are negative for HLA-DR4 do not present differently. A conserved sequence within the second hypervariable region located in the antigen-binding groove of the HLA-DR molecule has been identified. Differential expression of genes responsible for inflammatory cytokine expression are likely to account for the variable disease manifestations.

Clinical features

In the absence of a specific diagnostic test, apart from biopsy of the temporal artery when GCA is also present, the diagnosis of PMR is based on clinical features (Table 17.1) and made by exclusion

---

Box 17.1 **Epidemiology of polymyalgia rheumatica and giant cell arteritis**

- Giant cell arteritis is the most common of the vasculitides, and polymyalgia rheumatica is more common than giant cell arteritis
- Pre-eminently affect Northern European people; can occur in any ethnic group
- Rare under the age of 50 years
- Woman:man ratio = 3:1
- Annual incidence approximately 18 per 100,000 for giant cell arteritis and 100 per 100,000 for polymyalgia rheumatica in people aged >50 years
- Possible cyclic pattern in incidence
- Siblings at increased risk

ABC of Rheumatology, 4th edn. Edited by Ade Adebajo.
©2010 Blackwell Publishing Ltd. 9781405170680.

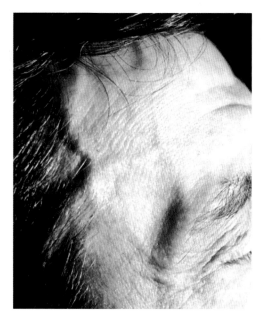

Figure 17.1 Markedly dilated temporal arteries in a 74-year-old man with giant cell arteritis. The arteries are visibly thickened and inflamed; palpation of the vessel is painful. Courtesy of Dr Lester Mertz, Mayo Clinic, Rochester, MN, USA

Table 17.1 Clinical features

Polymyalgia rheumatica	Giant cell arteritis
Bilateral shoulder pain, stiffness	Age >50 years
Duration onset <2 weeks	New headache
Initial ESR >40 mm/hour	Temporal artery abnormal
Stiffness >1 hour	to palpation
Age >50 years, typically >65 years	Elevated ESR
Depression or weight loss, or both	Abnormal findings on
Bilateral upper arm tenderness	temporal artery biopsy
Probable PMR: 3 or more <3 with clinical abnormality of temporal artery	
Definite PMR: probable PMR responding to corticosteroids	

ESR = erythrocyte sedimentation rate; PMR = polymyalgia rheumatica

(Boxes 17.2 and 17.3). Several diagnostic criteria sets have been suggested.

In PMR, the onset is relatively rapid, over a matter of days to several weeks. The shoulder pain and stiffness are invariably bilateral and can be profound. Acute-phase reactants such as ESR and C-reactive protein (CRP) are usually (>95%) elevated (Box 17.4). Systemic features may include low-grade fever, fatigue, weight loss and depression. Sometimes, the muscles of the upper arms and thighs are tender on direct palpation, although muscle strength is usually unimpaired. Patients may have difficulty turning over in bed, particularly early in the morning. It may be hard to lift heavy objects, painful to walk up stairs, or tender to sit on the toilet. Patients comment on their "overwhelming illness". Unusual upper-arm tenderness when blood pressure is taken should raise suspicion of the disease, especially in patients with other constitutional symptoms.

Box 17.2 Polymyalgia: rarer mimics

- Polyarteritis nodosa
- Parkinson's disease
- Thyrotoxic myopathy and hypothyroidism
- Carcinomatous myopathy
- Systemic lupus erythematosus
- Calcium pyrophosphate deposition
- Multiple myeloma
- Paget's disease
- Osteomalacia
- Polymyositis
- Subacute bacterial endocarditis
- Malignancy

Box 17.3 Polymyalgia rheumatica: differential diagnoses

- Polymyalgia
- Osteoarthritis
- Cervical spondylosis
- Frozen shoulder
- Rheumatoid arthritis
- Giant cell arteritis
- Cluster headache
- Non-inflammatory ophthalmic ischemia
- Systemic amyloidosis
- Other forms of vasculitis, including polyarteritis nodosa
- Occipital myalgia
- TMJ syndromes

Box 17.4 Markers of disease activity

Although there are numerous non-specific acute-phase reactants such as heptoglobin and cytokines such as interleukin-6 and vascular endothelial growth factor, as well as plasma viscosity, which may be elevated in polymyalgia rheumatica/giant cell arteritis, only two have routine clinical utility:
- Erythrocyte sedimentation rate
- C-reactive protein
- Other common laboratory abnormalities include a non-specific normochromic, normocytic anaemia and elevation of alkaline phosphatase (bone and/or liver fraction)

GCA usually may be viewed as inflammation of the aorta and its major branches. Its clinical features are related to the affected arteries. The scalp is tender to the touch, and it may even hurt to wear spectacles. Jaw claudication may occur while chewing. Clinical signs (Table 17.1) vary according to the duration of the disease. In the early stages, the pulse is full and bounding, and the arteries tender. Later, fibrosis and repair may predominate, the artery may have a nodular indurated feel to it, and the pulse is almost absent. Diplopia, partial or complete loss of vision, and cranial nerve palsy

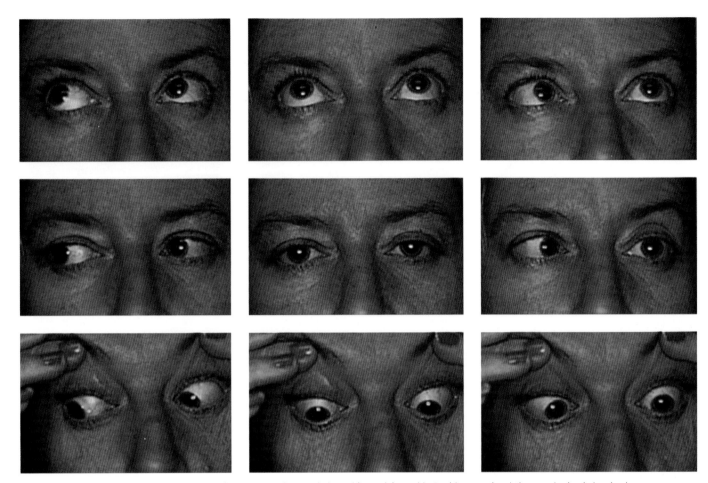

Figure 17.2 Temporary or permanent nerve palsy can occur in association with cranial arteritis. In this case, the sixth nerve is clearly involved

Box 17.5 **Biopsy for giant cell arteritis**

- Biopsy is most useful just before or within 24 hours of treatment initiation with steroids, but treatment should not be delayed for the sake of obtaining a biopsy
- Skip lesions occur, so a negative result does not exclude giant cell arteritis
- A positive result may resolve later doubt about diagnosis, particularly if the response to treatment is not rapid and classical
- It may not be possible to biopsy all patients; the decision depends on local resources
- One week after starting steroid treatment, the chance of obtaining positive biopsy falls to 10%, although the biopsy may still reveal evidence of inflammation >1 year after initiation of treatment

(Figure 17.2) may all occur if the condition remains untreated. Late complications of large-vessel involvement, including aortic aneurysm and stenosis, may complicate the disease course. Patients should be followed long term for aortic disease with computed tomography and aortic magnetic resonance imaging (MRI) and complemented by ultrasonography of the aortic root and abdominal aorta by clinical and imaging assessment, as aneurysmal rupture is a cause of premature mortality in these patients. The value of biopsy for GCA is discussed in Box 17.5.

Histopathology

Giant cell arteritis—The inflammatory features of GCA are typically described as illustrating the "skip" phenomenon due to the patchy or segmental involvement of the arteries. GCA is principally a disease driven by T-cells that is limited to vessels with an internal elastic component. Histologically, the lesions are characterized by a mainly lymphocytic and macrophage infiltrate with the presence of giant and epithelioid cells (Figure 17.3). The CD3+ and T-cell population comprises CD4+ or CD8+ subsets, of which CD4+ T-cells predominate. The initial immunological event—probably the induction of CD4+ T-cell proliferation by an unknown antigen—occurs in the outer vessel layer: the adventitia. These CD4 cells produce interferon-©, which attracts macrophages to the arterial wall, where they fuse to form multinucleated giant cells in the intima-media junction (Figure 17.4). The giant cells produce express adhesion molecules, nitric oxide and collagenases to result in, for example, tissue injury and in situ thrombosis.

Polymyalgia rheumatica—The histopathological features of PMR are defined less clearly than for GCA. Biopsy of synovium, especially of shoulder-joint structures, have confirmed synovitis in about one-third of patients, which is nonerosive and self-limiting arthritis.

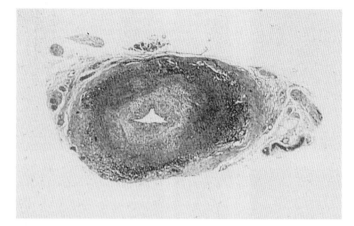

Figure 17.3 Histology of temporal arteritis. The elastic tissue appears black, while various types of collagen stain yellow. Remnants of the internal elastic lamina are indicated by an arrow. An inflammatory infiltrate is found in the media and intimal fibrosis. Multinucleated giant cells and macrophages are attacking the elastic tissue and ingesting it. There is extensive intimal proliferation and fibrosis. Luminal narrowing has occurred almost completely. Involvement of other arteries may occur, including the ophthalmic artery, which results in loss of vision

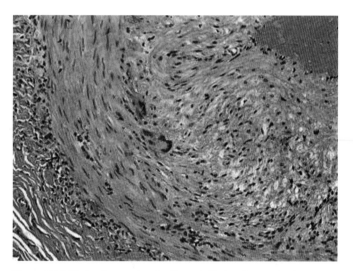

Figure 17.4 Photomicrographs of active arteritis in a temporal artery biopsy. High-power view showing proliferation of intimal fibroblasts and transmural inflammation with multinucleated giant cells present at the media-intima junction (Hematoxylin-Eosin, 200×)

Inflammation of the temporal artery may also be demonstrated even in patients without overt GCA. The characteristics of synovitis on biopsy confirm a predominance of CD4+ T-cells and macrophages. Similar to features described in GCA, the vascular infiltrate reveals CD4+ interferon-©-positive cells in the adventitia; macrophages that produce interleukin-1®, interleukin-6 (IL-6), endothelial cell adhesion molecules with matrix metalloproteinases, and inducible nitric oxide are seen in the media intima.

Increasingly used in clinical evaluation, ultrasonography of the shoulders (Figure 17.5) and hips may reveal synovitis of the joints or bursa. MRI studies also give evidence of an inflammatory process affecting distal articular or extra-articular (tenosynovial) structures, or both (Figure 17.6). Although skeletal muscle is not

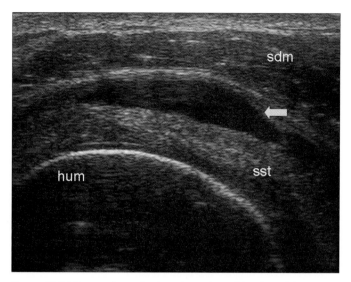

Figure 17.5 Ultrasound examination of a patient with polymyalgia rheumatica and subdeltoid bursitis. Anterior transverse ultrasound image of the right shoulder with maximum internal rotation of the arm: the dark area (arrow) between the subdeltoid muscle and supraspinatus tendon represents subdeltoid bursitis. hum = humerus; sdm = subdeltoid muscle; sst = supraspinatus tendon. Courtesy of Dr Wolfgang Schmidt, Humboldt University, Berlin, Germany

considered to be a site of pathology, focal changes in muscle ultrastructure and mitochondria abnormalities have been noted, but their significance remains unclear. Muscle enzymes and biopsies are normal.

Investigations

ESR and/or CRP are the most accepted and easily available markers of active inflammation in PMR (Figure 17.7). They are initially elevated in over 90% of patients, although PMR and even blindness from GCA can occur in the presence of a normal ESR. The ESR and CRP fall with effective treatment; the CRP falls faster. With treatment, the normocytic normochromic anaemia corrects, and the slight increase in hepatic alkaline phosphatase sometimes noted in active disease is reduced.

In parallel, to these basic laboratory studies, additional investigations should be arranged to exclude conditions that cause diagnostic confusion, including thyroid function studies and age- and symptom-appropriate malignancy screening. Additionally, an evaluation should be performed in all patients to screen and follow common conditions of elderly patients, which may be induced or exacerbated by protracted corticosteroid use, including diabetes, osteoporosis and cardiovascular disease.

Vascular assessment with ultrasound, computed tomography/ MRI, or conventional angiography may be required to assess the activity and extent of vascular involvement (Figure 17.8). Ultrasound and MRI may reveal a characteristic "halo" around inflamed vessels, even of the caliber of the temporal arteries. Positron emission tomography may occasionally be useful in defining disease activity, but remains experimental.

The basic investigations described above are summarized in Box 17.6.

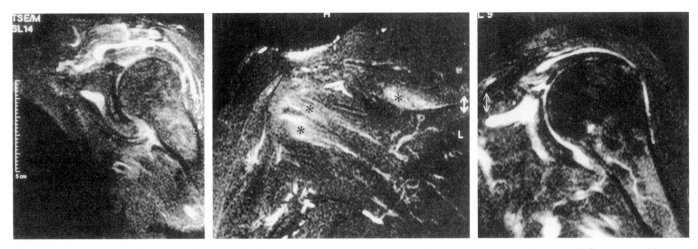

Figure 17.6 MRI of shoulder in polymyalgia rheumatica (T2 fat suppressed corona). Oblique MRI sequences shows modest synovial inflammation with substantial fluid in the subacromial bursa associated with diffuse capsular edema extending into the adjacent tendons and muscle bellies. Courtesy of Dr D. McGonagle and Dr H. Marzo-Ortega, Academic Unit of Musculoskeletal Disease, Leeds General Infirmary, Leeds, UK

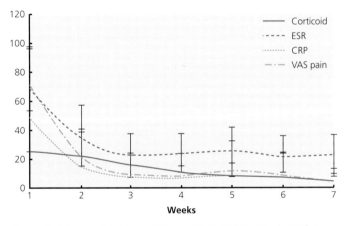

Figure 17.7 Improvement in erythrocyte sedimentation rate, C-reactive protein, and the patient's perception of pain (measured on a visual analogue scale) in response to corticosteroid therapy in a group of 76 patients with polymyalgia rheumatica. Courtesy of Dr Burkhard Leeb, Lower Austria Centre for Rheumatology, Stockerau, Austria

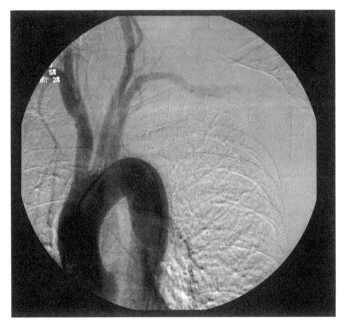

Figure 17.8 Arterial thrombosis complicating polymyalgia rheumatica, supporting a generalized vasculitic aetiology of this condition. Courtesy of Dr C. Pease, Academic Unit of Musculoskeletal Disease, Leeds General Infirmary, Leeds, UK

Box 17.6 **Basic investigations**

- Complete blood count with differential
- Alkaline phosphatase
- Blood glucose
- Acute-phase reactants (erythrocyte sedimentation rate and/or C-reactive protein)
- Creatinine
- Blood lipids
- Thyroid function studies
- Creatine phosphokinase
- Bone mineral density
- Tuberculosis testing (PPD skin test; QuantiFERON gold)

Polymyalgia rheumatica
- Ultrasonography of hip and shoulder (where available and appropriate)

Giant cell arteritis
- Temporal artery biopsy
- Large-vessel evaluation with echocardiography, ultrasound, computed tomography, magnetic resonance imaging of the vessel wall, and magnetic resonance or computed tomographic angiography, as appropriate to the vessels of interest
- Position emission tomography

Box 17.7 **Treatment of polymyalgia rheumatica**

- "Treat the patient, not the sedimentation rate"
- Initial dose of corticosteroid should be adjusted to patient's size and weight
- Typically start prednisone, equivalent of 10–20 mg daily for 1 month
- After 1 month, aim to reduce the dose by 2.5 mg every 2–4 weeks, titrating against clinical response and level of acute-phase reactants, with the aim of reducing to 10 mg daily
- After 6 months, try a further cautious reduction in increments of 1 mg daily every month, in the hope of reducing to 5 mg daily, as long as symptoms do not recur; in general, symptoms are a better guide to the need for continued treatment than persistent modest elevation in the acute-phase reactants
- Most patients require treatment for 3 years, but withdrawal over a period of some 6 months can be attempted at 1–2 years, if the response has been good; the duration of treatment may range from about 9 months to over 9 years
- Relapsing symptoms with reduction of the corticosteroid dose is common; the need for protracted treatment is associated with increased risk of corticosteroid-related side effects, prompting interest in the use of corticosteroid-sparing agents

Treatment

The only known effective treatment for PMR is with corticosteroids. Data from the pre-steroid era suggest that untreated PMR and GCA burn themselves out after a mean of 2 years (range 6 months to 10 years), although long-term vascular complications in GCA are more common than realized (2 to 3-fold increased risk of aneurysm and increased risk of death from aneurysm rupture).

The treatment of PMR and GCA is summarized in Boxes 17.7 and 17.8, respectively.

Appropriate doses of corticosteroids depend on the condition and symptom activity. Once a patient has been weaned off corticosteroids at 2–3 years, it should be remembered that about 10% of patients will relapse within a 10-year period. Often, the symptoms of relapse are more pronounced than the increase in acute-phase reactants. In the case of relapse, the original dose of prednisolone should be reinstated.

For long-term therapy, the correct dose of corticosteroids remains the lowest that keeps symptoms in complete remission, but if any doubt exists, a higher dose of corticosteroids should be prescribed. Related adverse events are common, even in patients with PMR, and include increased rates of cataracts, osteoporosis and insufficiency fractures, hypertension, avascular necrosis, infections, diabetes and steroid myopathy. Management of co-morbidities including prophylaxis for osteoporosis is necessary, particularly if treatment is of long duration and the patient is not rendered mobile, or if other risk factors are present (see Chapter 1).

Box 17.8 **Treatment of giant cell arteritis**

- Doses of prednisone/prednisolone should be higher than for polymyalgia rheumatica and the period of treatment longer; the incentive to reduce is much less than with polymyalgia rheumatica because of the possibility of vascular compromise
- For headaches alone, the starting dose of prednisolone should be in the range of 20–40 mg daily; with clinical signs of vasculitis or visual symptoms, the dose should be in the range of 40–60 mg daily; for impending or recent blindness, 80 mg daily should be given, possibly with the addition of intravenous hydrocortisone
- Dosage reduction can then be at a rate of about 5 mg every 3 or 4 weeks until a maintenance level of 10 or 15 mg daily is achieved, depending on response
- At 1 year, an effort should be made to reduce the dose to 5 mg daily in 1-mg steps
- Maintenance therapy at this low dose is likely to last up to 5 years
- As with polymyalgia rheumatica, relapses are common, and extended treatment may be needed; persistently elevated acute-phase reactants in the face of clinically quiescent disease should alert the clinician to the possibility of subclinical disease; physicians should be vigilant for the development of large vascular disease and assess appropriately
- Addition of low-dose aspirin as 81–325 mg daily has potential ancillary benefit in control of inflammation as well as cardiovascular protective value

Response criteria

The European Collaborating Polymyalgia Rheumatica Group recently proposed response criteria (Box 17.9) that aim to compli-

Box 17.9 **European Collaborating Polymyalgia Rheumatica Group's response criteria**

Clinical improvement in pain (on visual analogue scale) and three out of four from:

- Reduction in C-reactive protein or erythrocyte sedimentation rate, or both
- Improvement in morning stiffness
- Ability to raise shoulders
- Improvement of physicians' global assessment on visual analogue scale

ment existing diagnostic criteria, as corticosteroid response remains so important in diagnosis.

Corticosteroid-sparing agents

There is no proven benefit of any corticosteroid-sparing agent for GCA, and a paucity of evidence for the efficacy of methotrexate and anti-tumour necrosis alpha (TNF-α) agents in the treatment of PMR. A small placebo-controlled study recently suggested that initial treatment of GCA with "pulse" methylprednisolone at 1 g daily for 3 days followed by standard oral prednisone therapy may result in more rapid, durable treatment response and lower long-term corticosteroid therapy burden. Theoretical reasons lead to a suspicion that modification of interleukins might be helpful. This might be achieved by using drugs to block TNF-α drugs yet to be marketed to block IL-6. The use of such drugs remains experimental at present.

Further reading

Gabriel SE, Sunku J, Salvarani C, O'Fallon WM, Hunder GG. Adverse outcomes of and inflammatory therapy among patients with polymyalgia rheumatica. *Arthritis and Rheumatism* 1997; **40**: 1873–1878.

Hunder GG. Clinical features of GCA/PMR. *Clinical and Experimental Rheumatology* 2000; **18**: 56–58.

Levine SM, Hellmann DB. Giant cell arteritis. *Current Opinion in Rheumatology* 2002; **14**: 3–10.

Salvarani C, Cantini F, Boiardi L, Hunder GG. Polymyalgia rheumatica and giant cell arteritis. *New England Journal of Medicine* 2002; **347**: 261–271.

Weyand CM, Goronzy JJ. Giant cell arteritis and polymyalgia rheumatica. *Annals of Internal Medicine* 2003; **139**: 505–515.

CHAPTER 18

Systemic Lupus Erythematosus and Lupus-like Syndromes

Caroline Gordon[1] and Rosalind Ramsey-Goldman[2]

[1]University of Birmingham, Birmingham, UK
[2]Northwestern University Feinberg School of Medicine, Chicago, USA

OVERVIEW

- Systemic lupus erythematosus (SLE) is a multi-system autoimmune disease associated with genetic and environmental risk factors.
- SLE is most common in women and those from non-white ethnic backgrounds.
- Lupus nephritis occurs in up to 50% of SLE patients.
- SLE patients should receive pre-pregnancy counselling to ensure optimal disease control and drug therapy before conception.
- Premature cardiovascular disease is an increasing cause of death in SLE patients.

Box 18.1 **Genetic factors involved in predisposition to SLE**

- Major histocompatibility complex genes, e.g. HLA-DR2 and HLA-DR3
- Complement genes, e.g. C1q, C4 and C2
- Fc gamma receptor genes, e.g. FCγRIIA, FcγRIIIA, FcγRIIB
- Cytotoxic T-lymphocyte antigen-4 (CTLA-4, a negative regulator of T-cells)
- Programmed cell death-1 (PDCD-1, an immunoreceptor of the CD28 family)
- Cytokine genes, e.g. interferon-α and TNF-α

Box 18.2 **Environmental factors involved in susceptibility to, or triggering of, SLE**

- Drugs, e.g. hydralazine, procainamide, minocycline
- Ultraviolet light (UV-A and UV-B)
- Viral infections, e.g. EBV, CMV, retroviruses, parvovirus B19
- Hormones, e.g. oestrogens, prolactin
- Chemicals and heavy metals, e.g. silica and mercury
- Diet, e.g. L-canavanine in alfalfa (but still debatable)

Systemic lupus erythematosus (SLE) is a multi-systemic autoimmune disease of unknown cause (Mok and Lau, 2003) with a wide variety of manifestations that is usually characterized by remissions and relapses. SLE is part of a spectrum of autoimmune diseases that also includes discoid lupus, drug-induced lupus, neonatal lupus, Sjögren's syndrome, antiphospholipid antibody syndrome, dermatomyositis/polymyositis and overlap syndromes. Antiphospholipid antibody may occur as a primary disorder or secondary to SLE or another autoimmune condition, such as autoimmune hypothyroidism or chronic active hepatitis. As no cure exists for these conditions, life-long follow-up is needed, so it is important that the primary care physician, patient and hospital specialists are involved closely in the management of these diseases (Bertsias *et al.*, 2008).

Causes

SLE is a multifactorial disease caused by a complex interplay of genetic and environmental factors that vary between individuals and are still not well understood (Mok and Lau, 2003) (Boxes 18.1 and 18.2). SLE is characterized by multiple immune abnormalities, including dendritic, B- and T-cell dysfunction resulting in the development of autoantibodies and autoreactive T-cells. Defective clearance of apoptotic cells and of immune complexes contributes to pathogenesis with the activation of complement playing a major role in tissue damage. There is increasing evidence that the cytokine interferon-alpha (IFN-α) plays a role in activating genes involved in the disease, and that interleukin-6 (IL-6) and Il-10 levels are increased in active disease. Antiphospholipid antibodies are a specific family of autoantibodies directed against anionic phospholipids located in cell membranes. The pathogenic mechanisms in antiphospholipid syndrome relate to the prothrombotic effects of these antibodies in vivo.

ABC of Rheumatology, 4th edn. Edited by Ade Adebajo.
©2010 Blackwell Publishing Ltd. 9781405170680.

Table 18.1 Prevalence and incidence of systemic lupus erythematosus worldwide

Country	Prevalence (per 100,000)	Incidence (per 100,000)
United Kingdom (Nottingham, Birmingham)		
• Adults	27.7	3.8
• Women	49.6	6.8
• White	36.3	2.5–3.4
• Afro-Caribbean	197.2	11.9–31.9
• Asian	96.5	4.1–15.2
Iceland	35.9	3.3
Spain	34.1	2.2
Sweden	38.9	4.8
USA		
• Adults	4.8–78.5	0.7–7.2
• Women	7.7–131.5	1.1–11.4
• White	4.8–9.9	0.7–2.2
• African-Americans	9.3–29.6	1.7–7.2
• Puerto Rican (NY, NY only)	18.0	2.3
Canada	20.6–42.3	0.9–7.4
Australia (Aborigine)	11.0	13.4–89.3
Japan	3.7–19.3	0.9–2.9
Martinique	64.2	4.7

Table 18.2 Cumulative percentage incidence of clinical features of systemic lupus erythematosus

Feature	(%)
Arthritis	72–94
Alopecia	52–80
Skin rash	74–90
Photosensitivity	10–62
Malar rash	37–90
Oral ulcers	30–61
Fever	74–91
Neuropsychiatric	19–63
Renal	35–73
Cardiac	10–29
Pleuropulmonary	9–54

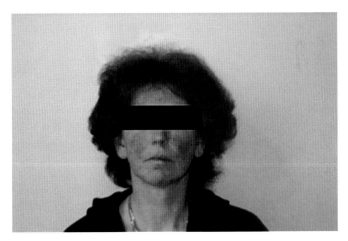

Figure 18.1 Malar rash in systemic lupus erythematosus

Epidemiology

There are significant disparities in the incidence and prevalence rates of SLE disease worldwide (Danchenko *et al.*, 2006) (Table 18.1) and in the cumulative incidence of clinical features (Table 18.2). This variability may be due to true population differences or to dissimilar methods of case ascertainment. Nevertheless, the consistent trend reflects that the burden of disease is highest in women and higher among non-white ethnic groups.

Clinical presentations

Systemic lupus erythematosus

The American Rheumatology Association's 1982 classification criteria (Tan *et al.*, 1982) for SLE (Box 18.3) were revised in 1997 (Hochberg, 1997). These criteria were designed not for diagnosis but for classifying patients into studies and clinical trials. The diagnosis of SLE should be considered if a patient has characteristic features of lupus (Table 18.2), even if they do not fulfil four of the eleven criteria. For example, a 25-year-old woman with malar rash (Figure 18.1), positive antinuclear antibody and histologically proven glomerulonephritis obviously has SLE, despite fulfilling only three of the criteria (Box 18.3).

> Box 18.3 **The American Rheumatology Association's revised classification criteria for systemic lupus erythematosus (taken from Tan *et al.*, 1982)**
>
> • Malar rash
> • Discoid rash
> • Photosensitivity
> • Mucosal ulcers
> • Arthritis
> • Serositis
> • Neurological disorder (psychosis, seizures)
> • Renal disorder
> • Haematological disorder
> • Immunological disorder
> • Positive antinuclear antibodies

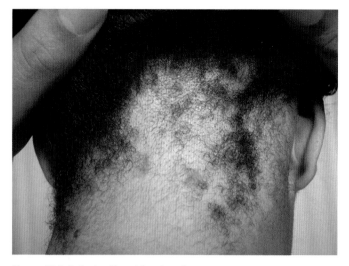

Figure 18.2 Patient with patchy alopecia

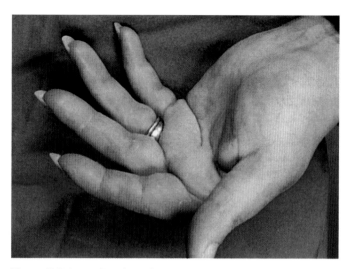

Figure 18.3 Jaccoud's arthropathy

General features

Fatigue is common, troublesome and difficult to evaluate. It may be associated with depression or fibromyalgia secondary to SLE, hypothyroidism (often autoimmune in nature), anaemia and pulmonary or cardiovascular problems. Other constitutional symptoms of active disease include fever, malaise, anorexia, lymphadenopathy and weight loss.

Mucocutaneous manifestations

The most common mucocutaneous features are painful or painless mouth ulcers, diffuse alopecia (Figure 18.2), butterfly or malar rash, and photosensitivity. Nasal or vaginal ulcers may also occur. Mucocutaneous features are more prominent in Asian and white people. Subacute cutaneous lupus erythematosus is a non-scarring rash that is found in areas of the body exposed to sunlight. Discoid lesions are chronic scarring lesions that heal with hypo- or hyperpigmentation. Non-scarring alopecia may be patchy or diffuse. Rapid, spontaneous hair loss indicates active disease. Raynaud's phenomenon is usually milder than in scleroderma.

Musculoskeletal manifestations

Generalized arthralgia with early morning stiffness and no swelling is very common. A non-erosive arthritis with joint tenderness and swelling may develop. Deformities are unusual but may occur due to ligamentous laxity (Jaccoud's arthropathy; Figure 18.3), compared with rheumatoid arthritis, in which the deformities are due to joint erosions. Myalgia is common, but inflammatory myositis occurs in only 5% of patients. Indeed, secondary causes of myopathy are more common and can be caused by corticosteroids, antimalarials and lipid-lowering agents. Avascular necrosis and infection should be suspected if the patient complains of sudden-onset severe pain in only one joint. In addition, the risk of osteoporosis and subsequent fracture due to minimal or no trauma can be increased in patients with SLE.

Haematological manifestations

Leucopaenia may be an early clue to the diagnosis of SLE. Lymphopaenia is the most common manifestation of SLE other than positive antinuclear antibodies and, in untreated patients, is caused by lymphocytotoxic antibodies. Mild neutropenia is relatively common in black people even without SLE, but values $<1.5 \times 10^9$/l are usually related to disease or drugs. Anaemia is the second most common haematological abnormality seen in lupus patients and may be multifactorial. The differential diagnosis of anaemia is shown in Box 18.4. Thrombocytopenia may occur as an immune-mediated condition associated with a risk of bleeding, as in idiopathic thrombocytopenic purpura, or as a milder abnormality with platelet counts $>80 \times 10^9$/l associated with a risk of thrombosis in antiphospholipid syndrome (see below).

Renal manifestations

Renal disease is an important determinant of the outcome of SLE. Renal disease can occur in up to 50% of white patients and 75% of black patients. Studies have shown that renal disease is also more severe in non-white patients. Early nephritis is often asymptomatic, so regular urinalysis for protein, blood and casts is essential. Some patients present with nephrotic syndrome and a few with devastating accelerated hypertension and renal shutdown. Renal biopsy is helpful for assessing the severity, nature, extent and reversibility of the involvement and is an important guide to treatment and prognosis. For example, those with mesangial nephritis (class I) rarely progress to renal failure, in contrast to those with diffuse proliferative glomerulonephritis (class IV), who are at risk for end-stage renal disease.

Nervous system manifestations

SLE may affect the central and peripheral nervous systems. Definitions for these manifestations have been proposed by a consensus group (American College of Rheumatology, 1999) (Boxes 18.5 and 18.6). The most common manifestations are headache, seizures, aseptic meningitis and cerebrovascular accidents. Antiphospholipid antibodies (including anticardiolipin antibodies) have been implicated in cerebrovascular accidents and chorea. It often is hard to determine whether the depression and headaches are due to lupus itself; in many cases, they are related to psychosocial issues. Other possible causes such as sepsis, drugs, uraemia, severe hypertension and other metabolic causes must be sought and treated. Steroids are often blamed for inducing psychosis, but if any doubt exists, patients should be given more, not less, steroid while under medical supervision, particularly if active lupus is evident in other systems.

> **Box 18.5 Central nervous system manifestations of systemic lupus erythematosus**
>
> - Aseptic meningitis
> - Cerebrovascular disease
> - Demyelinating syndrome
> - Headache (including migraine and benign intracranial hypertension)
> - Movement disorders (including chorea)
> - Myelopathy
> - Seizure disorders
> - Acute confusional state
> - Anxiety disorder
> - Cognitive dysfunction
> - Mood disorder
> - Psychosis

> **Box 18.6 Peripheral nervous system manifestations of systemic lupus erythematosus**
>
> - Acute inflammatory demyelinating polyradiculoneuropathy (Guillain–Barré syndrome)
> - Autonomic disorder
> - Mononeuropathy (single or multiplex)
> - Myasthenia gravis
> - Neuropathy, cranial
> - Plexopathy
> - Polyneuropathy

> **Box 18.7 Risk of atherosclerosis in lupus**
>
> Survival and disease control have improved in patients with SLE, but complications of premature vascular disease are recognized increasingly: the relative risk for myocardial infarction in women aged 35–44 years with SLE is 52.3 times the risk for women without lupus

Pulmonary and cardiovascular manifestations

Pleurisy, often without physical signs, is common in SLE. Less common manifestations are lupus pneumonitis, pulmonary haemorrhage, pulmonary embolism and pulmonary hypertension. Pulmonary haemorrhage can be sudden and acute and has high mortality. Pulmonary hypertension is associated with a poor prognosis, especially in pregnancy. Pericarditis is common but often asymptomatic. Other cardiac manifestations are myocarditis, endocarditis and rarely pericardial tamponade. Coronary artery disease is occasionally caused by vasculitis, but more often results from premature atherosclerosis (Box 18.7).

Gastrointestinal manifestations

Abdominal pain, nausea, vomiting and diarrhoea occur in up to 50% of SLE patients at some stage of the disease. Although the presentation of greatest importance is mesenteric vasculitis, in which the patient presents with an acute abdomen and is at high risk of death, there have been recent reports of patients with subacute abdominal pain or aseptic peritonitis. This is usually associated with other serological signs of active disease and generally improves with steroid therapy. Other abdominal manifestations include subacute bowel obstruction, hepatitis, sclerosing cholangitis, protein-losing enteropathy, pancreatitis and ascites. Exclusion or treatment of infection is essential in patients with these conditions.

Pregnancy and SLE

No evidence suggests that SLE reduces fertility, but active disease and the presence of antiphospholipid antibody syndrome (see below) may increase the risk of intrauterine growth retardation, premature delivery, miscarriages and stillbirth (Gayed and Gordon, 2007). Doses of prednisolone >10 mg/day predispose to preeclampsia, isolated hypertension in pregnancy, premature rupture of membranes and maternal infection. No evidence shows that prednisolone crosses the placenta and causes fetal abnormalities in humans. Increasing evidence shows that azathioprine (<2 mg/kg/day) and hydroxychloroquine (200 mg daily) can be continued in pregnancy (Ostensen et al., 2006). If patients are on an angiotensin-converting enzyme (ACE) inhibitor or mycophenolate mofetil for renal disease, then medications must be discontinued due to their association with congenital malformations in exposed fetuses (Ostensen et al., 2006). Other anti-hypertensive medications such as methyldopa, labetalol and nifedipine are the most widely used to control blood pressure, and steroids and azathioprine can be added for lupus manifestations needing ongoing treatment.

> **Box 18.8 Management of pregnancy**
>
> Pregnant women with lupus need close monitoring for optimal fetal and maternal outcome and are best managed in specialist units

> **Box 18.9 Management of congenital heart block**
>
> Most babies born with congenital heart block need a pacemaker during the first year of life

> **Box 18.10 Sjögren's syndrome**
>
> Sjögren's syndrome is often misdiagnosed as rheumatoid arthritis or systemic lupus erythematosus

Pulmonary hypertension is associated with a 50% risk of mortality, particularly in the first 72 hours after delivery. This is usually a contraindication to planned pregnancy and needs specialist multidisciplinary care if diagnosed in pregnancy (Gayed and Gordon, 2007) (Box 18.8).

Neonatal lupus syndrome

This is a syndrome that occurs in about 10% of babies born to mothers with anti-Ro or anti-La antibodies. The most common manifestation is a rash induced by ultraviolet light a few days after birth. It resolves spontaneously if the babies are removed from sunlight or ultraviolet light. A more serious, but much rarer, manifestation of this syndrome is congenital heart block (CHB). This is usually detected in utero about 16–28 weeks into the pregnancy and may need treatment before or after delivery (Box 18.9).

Sjögren's syndrome

This clinical syndrome is characterized by sicca symptoms: dry eyes and dry mouth due to failure of salivary and mucosal glands, often preceded by salivary gland swelling, and is associated with autoantibody formation as described below. It may occur as a secondary disorder in patients with SLE or other conditions, including rheumatoid arthritis, systemic sclerosis and primary biliary cirrhosis, or as a primary disorder with features that resemble a mild form of SLE (mild symmetrical arthritis, photosensitivity, fatigue and diffuse alopecia) (Box 18.10). The primary syndrome is associated with hypergammaglobulinaemia with very high total immunoglobulin G levels and definitely positive antinuclear antibody, rheumatoid factor, and anti-Ro and anti-La antibody tests. Patients with these immunological abnormalities may benefit from special-

ist advice, as they are at risk of systemic complications. Hydroxychloroquine and pilocarpine with other local symptomatic measures, such as artificial tears, are used to treat the condition.

Overlap syndromes and other lupus-like conditions

Up to 25% of patients with connective tissue disorders do not fit into classical descriptions and present with overlapping clinical features. Some may evolve into well-defined connective tissue disorders, while others have manifestations of more than one definite connective tissue disorder—e.g. systemic sclerosis combined with SLE and inflammatory myositis (see Chapter 21). Raynaud's phenomenon is often present and may occur in isolation as the first manifestation of a connective tissue disorder. Patients with mild undifferentiated connective tissue disorders may have inflammatory arthritis, oedema of hands and acrosclerosis. Generally prognosis is good as long as patients do not develop pulmonary hypertension.

Polymyositis and dermatomyositis

Proximal muscle weakness, elevated muscle enzymes, myopathic changes on electromyography and inflammatory changes on muscle biopsy are diagnostic criteria for polymyositis. The presence of a characteristic rash in the presence of the above features defines dermatomyositis. These diagnoses are made by fulfilling these criteria in combination and excluding other potential aetiologies for these test abnormalities.

Antiphospholipid syndrome

Antiphospholipid syndrome (Box 18.11) is an important cause of recurrent arterial and venous thrombosis and miscarriages that are associated with antiphospholipid antibodies (Box 18.12).

Thrombosis

The most common presentation of antiphospholipid syndrome is venous thrombosis in the arms or legs, which is often recurrent, multiple and bilateral, with a propensity for pulmonary embolism. Arterial thrombosis is less common but most frequently manifested by features of ischaemia or infarction. The severity of presentation depends on the acuteness and extent of the occlusion. The brain is the most common site, where thrombosis presents as stroke and transient ischaemic attacks. Other sites for arterial occlusion are the coronary arteries, and subclavian, renal, retinal and pedal arteries.

Obstetric syndromes

Recurrent pregnancy losses in the second or third trimester are typical (Box 18.11). Patients should be monitored for intrauterine growth restriction due to placental insufficiency and pre-eclampsia in a specialist unit. Planned early delivery is often required. (See below for treatment during pregnancy in the setting of antiphospholipid antibody syndrome.)

Other manifestations

Other prominent features include thrombocytopenia (up to 50% of patients), haemolytic anaemia, livedo reticularis (Figure 18.4), chronic ulcers, typically near the medial malleolus, and cutaneous vasculitis.

Catastrophic antiphospholipid syndrome

This is an acute and devastating syndrome characterized by multiple simultaneous vascular occlusions throughout the body, which are often fatal. The kidney is affected most often, followed by the lungs, central nervous system, heart and skin.

Outcome of SLE and antiphospholipid syndrome

Although survival has improved substantially over the last 50 years (90% of patients survive at least 5 years and over 80% at least 10

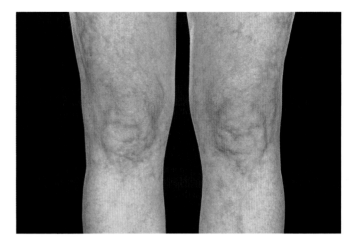

Figure 18.4 Livedo reticularis

years), awareness is increasing that these patients succumb to late complications of the disease or its therapy. In particular, hyperlipidaemia, hypertension, premature ischaemic heart disease, diabetes mellitus and osteoporotic fractures may develop. Compliance with medications, clinic visits and lifestyle modifications is essential to prevent or reduce the risk of these associated problems, which may be iatrogenic or disease-related in origin (Bertsias *et al.*, 2008). The long-term prognosis of antiphospholipid syndrome is poor, with organ damage in about one-third and functional impairment in up to one-fifth of patients at the end of 10 years.

Investigations

Investigations in SLE

A full blood count with differential white count, urinalysis and serum creatinine should be done for diagnosis and monitoring of the activity of SLE. Creatinine clearance or other assessment of glomerular filtration rate is more reliable for detecting early impairment of renal function. Patients with proteinuria or haematuria, or both, on dipstick must have microscopy done to look for casts if infection, stones and menstrual blood loss have been excluded.

For diagnosis, antinuclear antibody and anti-extractable nuclear antigen tests (see Chapter 24) should be done. No value is gained by repeating these tests, unless a change in clinical features is noted. Anti-ribonucleoprotein is associated with mixed connective tissue disease. Anti-dsDNA antibodies are useful for predicting patients at risk of developing renal disease and for monitoring disease activity. Although levels usually rise before a disease flare, they may fall at the time of flare. Levels of C3 and C4 fall with disease activity because of complement consumption, particularly in patients with renal disease. Levels also relate to the rate of synthesis in the liver and may rise in infections and pregnancy. Measurement of complement degradation products (for example, C3d, C4d) is less widely available but is more reliable for monitoring disease activity, as these reflect complement consumption alone. In women who are planning pregnancy, it is important to check for anti-Ro and anti-La antibodies and for antiphospholipid antibodies.

Table 18.3 Management of systemic lupus erythematosus

Risk factor advice	Further management
Avoid sun and other ultraviolet light	Wear sun block
Avoid infection	Treat bacterial infections early with antibiotics
Avoid unplanned pregnancy	Advise appropriate contraception
Use non-steroidal anti-inflammatory drugs with care	Use other analgesics as needed
Use oral steroids with care	Consider local and intramuscular or intravenous steroids and cytotoxic agents
Monitor for active disease	Urinalysis, full blood count, creatinine, anti-dsDNA antibodies, C3, C4
Screen for hypertension	Treat with calcium-channel blockers or angiotensin-converting enzyme inhibitors
Screen for diabetes and lipids	Advise on diet and give drugs if needed
Assess osteoporosis risk	Give postmenopausal women bisphosphonates

Table 18.4 Steroid-sparing and cytotoxic drugs used in systemic lupus erythematosus

Drug	Range
Hydroxychloroquine	≤6.5
Azathioprine	1–2.5
Methotrexate	7.5–25 mg per week
Cyclosporin A	1–2.5
Lefluonamide	10–20 mg daily
Cyclophosphamide	Intravenous pulses or ≤2 mg/kg/day orally
Mycophenolate mofetil	1–3 g/day

Investigations in antiphospholipid syndrome

Overall, 80–90% of patients with antiphospholipid syndrome are positive for antibodies to a complex of anticardiolipin antibodies and β_2-glycoprotein I. Lupus anticoagulant is only found in 20% of patients with antiphospholipid syndrome but is associated with a high risk of thrombosis. Low levels of antiphospholipid antibodies of no clinical consequence may develop transiently after infections (Boxes 18.12 and 18.13).

Management

General measures

Patients must be educated about the nature of their disease and the need for therapy. Leaflets from patient support organizations and references to reliable internet websites are useful. More than just drug therapy is required (Table 18.3; Box 18.14). Patients with sun-induced rashes should use sunblock regularly for about 6 months over the summer. Other patients with SLE should be aware that sun exposure may precipitate a disease flare.

Infections should be avoided and treated promptly if appropriate, as they can precipitate flares. Similarly, contraceptive pills that contain oestrogen may exacerbate lupus disease or thrombosis and should be used with caution. In general, barrier methods or progesterone-only contraception are preferred. Pregnancy should be planned, as the outcome is better, with fewer complications in both mother and fetus, if the mother has inactive disease at the time of conception. Drug therapy should be reviewed before conception.

Overlap and lupus-like conditions are managed in much the same way as mild SLE (Table 18.3; Box 18.14). Dry eyes should be managed by the frequent use of artificial tears. Dry mouth is best managed by taking sips of plain water, sucking ice cubes, or eating sugar free sweets. Artificial saliva preparations are disappointing.

Drug therapy in SLE

Milder cases with intermittent rashes, arthritis and other mucocutaneous features can usually be treated with steroid creams, short courses of non-steroidal anti-inflammatory drugs (NSAIDs) and hydroxychloroquine (<6.5 mg/kg/day). These drugs are also widely used in overlap syndromes, with the exception of NSAIDs, which are contraindicated in patients with features of systemic sclerosis or renal disease. More severe cases of SLE usually require oral corticosteroids. Patients who need 10 mg/day of prednisolone or more despite hydroxychloroquine, or those who present with more severe manifestations (such as nephritis, gastrointestinal vasculits or central nervous system disease) that need higher initial doses of prednisolone (0.5–1 mg/kg/day) are likely to need azathioprine, methotrexate or cyclophosphamide as steroid-sparing immunosuppressive agents (Table 18.4; Box 18.15). Mycophenolate mofetil

Box 18.15 **Cyclophosphamide therapy in severe lupus**

Cyclophosphamide is often given as intermittent intravenous "pulse therapy" and is used predominantly for proliferative glomerulonephritis and systemic vasculitis

Box 18.16 **Management of Raynaud's phenomenon**

Raynaud's phenomenon is best treated with calcium-channel blockers, local nitrate creams if mild to moderate, and intravenous prostacyclin infusions in severe cases. Angiotensin-converting enzyme inhibitors may be tried if calcium-channel blockers are not tolerated.

Box 18.17 **Goals of treatment in antiphospholipid syndrome**

- Prophylaxis
- Treatment of acute thromboses
- Prevention of further thrombotic events
- Management of pregnancy in antiphospholipid syndrome

is a promising alternative drug for the treatment of severe lupus; it has been best studied for lupus nephritis as an alternative to cyclophosphamide, but it is not licensed for SLE yet. Cyclosporin A, tacrolimus and lefluonamide are sometimes used for patients intolerant or resistant to other immunosuppressive agents (Table 18.4). Steroids should always be reduced slowly.

In pregnancy, patients may be given prednisolone, hydroxychloroquine and/or azathioprine, as the advantages are now considered to outweigh the risks. During lactation, prednisolone and hydroxychloroquine are acceptable, and azathioprine rarely causes problems at low doses. Methotrexate, mycophenolate, lefluonamide and cyclophosphamide are contraindicated in pregnancy and while breastfeeding. Cyclosporin A has been used in pregnancy in patients who have undergone transplants, but is not usually recommended during lactation.

Meticulous screening and treatment of blood pressure, diabetes, hyperlipidaemia and osteoporosis are essential. In general, calcium-channel blockers, ACE inhibitors and angiotensin receptor blockers are the preferred anti-hypertensive agents, as they are helpful in the management of Raynaud's phenomenon and renal disease, and because β-blockers aggravate Raynaud's phenomenon (Box 18.16). Bisphosphonates are often required in postmenopausal women, but they should be used with great care in women who may want to become pregnant in the future. Bisphosphonates, statins, ACE inhibitors and angiotensin-receptor blockers should be stopped before a planned pregnancy. Calcium and vitamin D can be used in all age groups. Treatment with anticoagulation and anti-epileptic, antidepressant, or antipsychotic drugs should be considered early in the management of patients with neuropsychiatric disease.

Oestrogen-containing contraceptives and hormone replacement therapy should be used with care in women with stable mild/moderate lupus and should be avoided in women with antiphospholipid antibodies, especially those with a history of thrombosis or pregnancy loss. Progesterone-only contraception is acceptable but is associated with a theoretical increased osteoporotic risk. Intrauterine devices can be used in women in stable relationships with a low risk of infection.

Therapy in antiphospholipid antibody syndrome

There is no evidence for prophylactic treatment of patients serologically positive for antiphospholipid antibody syndrome but without a history of thrombosis, although aspirin is often given in practice. Oestrogen-containing contraceptives and hormone replacement therapy are best avoided in patients with antiphospholipid syndrome and in patients with antiphospholipid antibodies without thrombosis or fetal loss. Treatment for thrombosis is usually initiated with intravenous or subcutaneous heparin and is soon changed to oral anticoagulation with warfarin. Most doctors recommend maintaining the international normalized ratio (INR) at 2–3 to prevent venous thrombosis and between 3 and 4 to prevent arterial thrombosis, as studies suggesting that INR in the range 2–3 was sufficient for patients after arterial thrombosis were flawed. Anticoagulation is usually life-long unless a contraindication, such as poorly controlled hypertension, is present (Box 18.17).

Pregnancy—A combination of low-molecular-weight heparin and low-dose aspirin is preferred. Pregnant women need close monitoring by the obstetrician, haematologist and rheumatologist, preferably in combined clinics at specialist units. Heparin dosage will depend on the clinical circumstances (Derksen *et al.*, 2004).

Conclusion

SLE is more common than many people realize. The presentations are diverse, and it may take a few years to realize that a variety of symptoms and signs can all be attributed to SLE, Sjögren's syndrome or an overlap syndrome. Antiphospholipid antibody syndrome should be sought actively in patients with a history of recurrent fetal loss or thrombosis, or both, because of the risk of future thrombotic complications. These diagnoses should not be made without appropriate clinical and serological features, as there are many social consequences of these diagnoses, such as implications for obtaining insurance and mortgages. With appropriate treatment, the outcome of these conditions is good, but the risk of late complications, particularly those of atherosclerosis, is important. In future, the management of patients with these conditions should seek to reduce these risks as well as control active disease.

References

American College of Rheumatology. American College of Rheumatology nomenclature and case definitions for neuropsychiatric lupus syndromes. *Arthritis and Rheumatism* 1999; **42**: 599–608.

Bertsias GK, Ioannidis JP, Boletis J *et al.* EULAR recommendations for the management of systemic lupus erytematosus (SLE): report of a task force of the European Standing Committee for International Clinical Studies Including Therapeutics. *Annals of the Rheumatic Diseases* 2008; **67**: 195–205.

Danchenko N, Satia JA, Anthony MS. Epidemiology of systemic lupus erythematosus: a comparison of worldwide disease burden. *Lupus* 2006; **15**: 308–318.

Derksen RH, Khamashta MA, Branch DW. Management of the obstetric antiphospholipid syndrome. *Arthritis and Rheumatism* 2004; **50**: 1028–1039.

Gayed M, Gordon C. Pregnancy and rheumatic diseases. *Rheumatology (Oxford)* 2007; **46**: 1634–1640.

Hochberg MC. Updating the American College of Rheumatology revised criteria for the classification of systemic lupus erythematosus. *Arthritis and Rheumatism* 1997; **40**: 1725.

Miyakis S, Lockshin MD, Atsumi T *et al.* International consensus statement on an update of the classification criteria for definite antiphospholipid syndrome (APS). *Journal of Thrombosis and Haemostasis* 2006; **4**: 295–306.

Mok CC, Lau CS. Pathogenesis of systemic lupus erythematosus. *Journal of Clinical Pathology* 2003; **56**: 481–490.

Ostensen M, Khamashta M, Lockshin M *et al.* Anti-inflammatory and immunosuppressive drugs and reproduction. *Arthritis Research and Therapy* 2006; **8**: 209.

Tan EM, Cohen AS, Fries JF *et al.* The 1982 revised criteria for the classification of systemic lupus erythematosus. *Arthritis and Rheumatism* 1982; **25**: 1271–1277.

CHAPTER 19

Raynaud's Phenomenon and Scleroderma

Christopher P Denton and Carol M Black

Royal Free Hospital, London, UK

OVERVIEW

- Survival from systemic sclerosis (SSc) is much better than in the past, owing to better and more effective treatment of organ-based complications, including scleroderma renal crisis and pulmonary arterial hypertension.

- Lung fibrosis is present in approximately one-third of systemic sclerosis patients but may be trivial and not progress. Progressive disease is currently treated with intravenous cyclophosphamide.

- Internal organ manifestations of systemic sclerosis occur in both of the major subsets (limed cutaneous SSc and diffuse cutaneous SSc). Association of anti-topoisomerase 1 with lung fibrosis and anti-RNA polymerase III autoantibodies with renal crisis is seen in both subsets.

- In most cases of dcSSc, peak severity of skin sclerosis is within the first 18 months of disease and the skin often plateaus or improves.

- Approximately 10% of patients with isolated Raynaud's phenomenon that have positive antinuclear antibodies and abnormal digital nailfold capillaroscopy will later develop clinical features of connective tissue disease.

The scleroderma spectrum

Scleroderma, meaning "hard skin", is a generic term used to describe a number of related connective tissue disorders. There is a spectrum from localized dermal sclerosis, through systemic conditions featuring cutaneous and internal organ fibrosis together with vascular dysfunction, to purely vascular disorders of Raynaud's phenomenon (Table 19.1). These conditions overlap clinically and pathologically, and in approximately 20% of cases there are additional features of other connective tissue diseases such as lupus, myositis or inflammatory arthritis (overlap systemic sclerosis). Although there are other causes for skin sclerosis, including scleroedema/scleromyxoedema, amyloidosis and nephrogenic systemic fibrosis, most of the differential diagnoses lie within the scleroderma spectrum. Distinguishing localized forms of the

disease from those in which internal organ complications may develop is central to management. Absence of antinuclear antibodies, altered nailfold capillaroscopy and Raynaud's phenomenon all point towards localized scleroderma (see below).

Raynaud's phenomenon

Episodic cold-induced vasospasm (Figure 19.1), triggered by cold or emotional stress, affects around 5% of the adult population, especially young females. In Primary Raynaud's (90%) there are no other clinical or investigational abnormalities. Secondary Raynaud's (10%) implies there are other features, usually an underlying autoimmune rheumatic disease. Investigation of Raynaud's symptoms includes the identification of secondary causes (Box 19.1). Such causes of Raynaud's, or acrocyanosis, include vibrating machine tools, thoracic-outlet obstruction, drugs such as β-blockers, and haematological abnormalities such as cryoglobulinaemia. Macrovascular arterial disease, embolization and systemic vasculitis, including Berger's disease, are important but rare differential diagnoses. Some patients with isolated Raynaud's

---

Box 19.1 **Points to consider when looking for underlying cause of Raynaud's phenomenon**

- Occupation—working outdoors, fishing industry, using vibrating tools, exposure to chemicals such as vinyl chloride
- Examination of peripheral and central vascular system for proximal vascular occlusion
- Drugs—such as β-blockers, oral contraceptives, bleomycin, migraine therapy
- Symptoms of other autoimmune rheumatic disorders:
  - Arthralgia or arthritis
  - Cerebral symptoms
  - Mouth ulcers
  - Alopecia
  - Photosensitivity
  - Muscle weakness
  - Skin rashes
  - Dry eyes or mouth
  - Respiratory or cardiac problems

ABC of Rheumatology, 4th edn. Edited by Ade Adebajo.
©2010 Blackwell Publishing Ltd. 9781405170680.

Table 19.1 The spectrum of scleroderma and scleroderma-like disorders

Localized scleroderma	Dermal inflammation and fibrosis. No visceral disease, few vascular symptoms
Plaque morphoea	Fewer than four localized areas of involvement
Generalized morphoea	More than four areas or widespread lesions
Linear scleroderma	Skin sclerosis follows dermatomal Distribution; commonest form of childhood-onset scleroderma
En coup de sabre	Scalp and facial linear lesion often with underlying bone changes
Systemic sclerosis	
Diffuse cutaneous systemic sclerosis	Skin involvement proximal to elbows or knees, short history of Raynaud's phenomenon; associated with anti-scl70 or anti-RNA polymerase antibodies
Limited cutaneous systemic sclerosis	Skin tightening affects extremities only, long history of Raynaud's phenomenon, associated with anti-centromere autoantibodies
Overlap syndromes	Clinical features of systemic sclerosis associated with those of another autoimmune rheumatic disease (SLE, myositis, arthritis)
Systemic sclerosis *sine* scleroderma	Serological, vascular and visceral features of SSc without detectable skin sclerosis
Isolated Raynaud's phenomenon	
Primary	Common, onset in adolescence, female predominance, normal nailfold capillaroscopy and negative autoantibody profile
Secondary	Raynaud's with abnormal nailfold capillaries and/or positive autoantibody testing

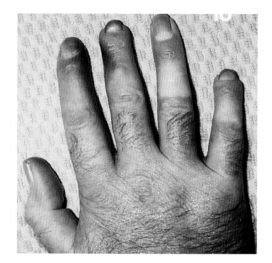

Figure 19.1 Well-defined blanching of skin, characteristic of Raynaud's phenomenon

Raynaud's phenomenon and connective tissue diseases

Many patients with a defined connective tissue disease have Raynaud's phenomenon. For SSc this approaches 95% and emphasizes a likely central role for vascular abnormalities. In lupus or dermato/polymyositis the frequency of Raynaud's is around 50%. It is less common in other rheumatic diseases, including Sjögren's syndrome and rheumatoid arthritis. There are many patients with overlap syndromes who have Raynaud's and also features such as arthralgia, malaise or photosensitivity but who do not fulfil classification criteria for a defined disease. These are best termed "undifferentiated connective tissue disease" cases, which may later evolve into more significant diseases (see also Chapters 18 and 21).

Systemic sclerosis

The most important disease within the scleroderma spectrum is SSc. This has high mortality, and approximately 60% of patients diagnosed with SSc will ultimately die from the disease. Most often this is due to cardio-respiratory complications. Nevertheless, there has been significant improvement in survival recently due to better treatment of organ-based complications, and the overall 5-year survival now approaches 80%. Cardinal features of SSc are the association of skin sclerosis with Raynaud's phenomenon, which is almost always present, and with internal organ involvement, which varies in extent between patients.

The majority of cases fall into one of two major subsets (Table 19.1). The diffuse cutaneous subset (dcSSc) is determined by involvement of skin proximal to the knees and elbows and may actually be confused with an inflammatory arthropathy in its early stages. Most of the important complications develop within the first 3 years of dcSSc, and skin sclerosis tends to be maximal at

phenomenon have positive antinuclear antibodies and abnormal nailfold capillaroscopy. These cases are at increased risk of developing a defined connective tissue disease, with approximately 15% of such cases progressing within 10 years. The significance of a hallmark scleroderma-associated antibody is less clear, but it has been suggested that some cases could be labelled "limited" systemic sclerosis (SSc) as they are at high risk of evolving to limited cutaneous SSc (lcSSc). These cases should not be confused with patients who have Raynaud's phenomenon, positive serology and overt visceral complications of SSc (lung fibrosis, renal crisis or severe gut disease). These are termed "systemic sclerosis sine scleroderma" and comprise around 1% of cases of SSc (see below). The negative predictive value of normal nailfold capillaroscopy and negative autoantibody screening is powerful, allowing robust reassurance. Benign primary Raynaud's must be distinguished from a more serious condition, which may have actuarial implications for life insurance and mortgage protection, for example.

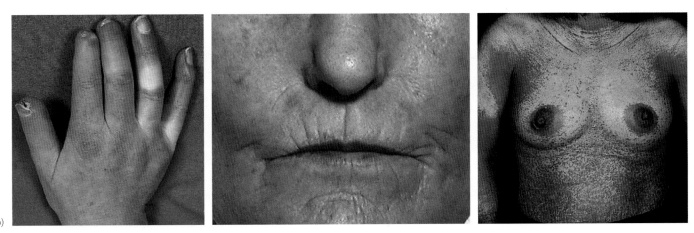

(a), (b)   (c)

Figure 19.2 Characteristic features of limited cutaneous scleroderma. (a) Puffy fingers, tight skin, Raynaud's phenomenon, loss of distal digits and ulceration of tips of digits. (b) Microstomia and telangiectasia. (c) Hypopigmentation caused by diffuse cutaneous scleroderma.

Box 19.2 Characteristic findings and suggested treatment for limited cutaneous scleroderma

Early stage (≤5 years after onset)
- Constitutional symptoms—fatigue common
- Skin thickening—no or minimal progression
- Organs affected—Raynaud's phenomenon, ulcers of digital tips, oesophageal symptoms
- Treatment—vascular treatment (oral or intravenous) with or without digital sympathectomy, removal of calcinosis, treat oesophageal problems

Late stage (>10 years after onset)
- Constitutional symptoms—fatigue common and aggravated by effects of vasculopathy and gut disease
- Skin thickening—stable or slow progression
- Organs affected—Raynaud's phenomenon, ulcers of digital tips, calcinosis, oesophageal stricture, small bowel malabsorption, pulmonary arterial hypertension, lung fibrosis
- Treatment—vascular treatment (oral or intravenous) with or without digital sympathectomy, removal of calcinosis, treat oesophageal and midgut problems

Box 19.3 Characteristic findings and suggested treatment for diffuse cutaneous scleroderma

Early stage (≤5 years after onset)
- Constitutional symptoms—fatigue, weight loss, pruritis
- Skin thickening—rapid progression with peak involvement by 2 years typical
- Organs affected—risk of renal, cardiac, pulmonary fibrosis, gastrointestinal, articular and muscular damage
- Treatment—vascular therapy, physiotherapy and occupational therapy as appropriate; immunosuppression for lung fibrosis and severe or progressive skin involvement; low-dose corticosteroids

Late stage (>5 years after onset)
- Constitutional symptoms—generally diminished
- Skin thickening—stable or regression
- Organs affected—musculoskeletal deformities, progression of existing visceral diseases but reduced risk of new complications
- Treatment—treat complications, gradual withdrawal of immunosuppression

around 18–30 months. Thereafter skin involvement tends to stabilize or improve. Despite stabilization or improvement in skin sclerosis, internal organ complications may develop at a later stage, and so long-term follow-up is mandatory. The characteristics of patients with each subset at different times in their disease are summarized in Boxes 19.2 and 19.3. Raynaud's generally develops concurrently with the skin disease or shortly afterwards. The limited cutaneous subset of SSc (Figure 19.2) accounts for around 60% of cases in most North American or European series. Skin involvement is much less extensive and may be confined to the fingers (sclerodactyly), face or neck. Raynaud's phenomenon is very prominent and may precede development of SSc by several years. The designation "CREST syndrome" is popular in the USA, referring to a subgroup of lcSSc in whom calcinosis, Raynaud's

phenomenon, oesophageal dysmotility, sclerodactyly and telangiectasia occur. It is probably better not to distinguish such cases, as these manifestations are not universal and under-emphasize the life-threatening complications that develop in a significant proportion of lcSSc patients. These include pulmonary arterial hypertension, severe midgut disease and interstitial pulmonary fibrosis. Other SSc cases include overlap syndromes with features of polyarthritis, myositis or systemic lupus erythematosus, and the small group of SSc sine scleroderma who have major visceral involvement, Raynaud's phenomenon and a hallmark autoantibody— typically anti-topoisomerase 1. The term "MCTD" is probably best avoided, as most of the patients with this designation evolve into a defined overlap syndrome, often with prominent features of SSc or lupus.

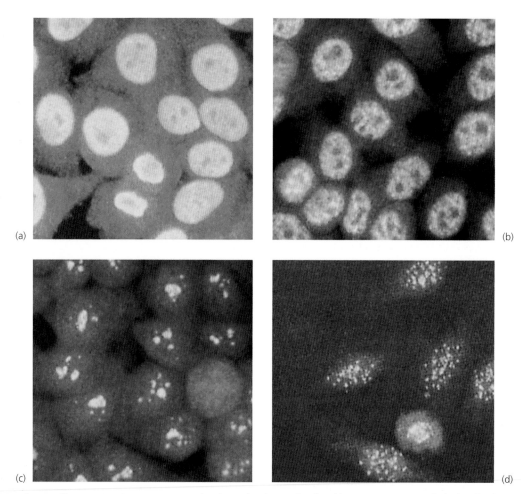

Figure 19.3 Common immunofluorescent patterns seen on testing for antinuclear antibodies. (a) Homogeneous—typical of antibodies to DNA, with or without histones. (b) Speckled—typical of antibodies to Ro, La, Sm and ribonucleotide protein. (c) Nucleolar—typical of scleroderma. (d) Centromere—mainly found with limited cutaneous scleroderma

Autoantibody profiles

The major hallmark autoantibodies associated with SSc are mutually exclusive (Figure 19.3). Thus, if a patient has anti-centromere antibodies they will almost never have anti-topoisomerase 1 or another reactivity associated with SSc. This appears to reflect the immunogenetic background of these individuals and may explain the clinical differences between patients with hallmark reactivity. The SSc-associated patterns of autoantibody reactivity are summarized in Table 19.2.

Risk stratification in SSc

The clinical heterogeneity of SSc and differences in natural history between the two major subsets and the life-threatening nature of some of the SSc-associated complications have led to attempts to risk-stratify patients at diagnosis and initial assessment. Abnormalities reflecting systemic inflammation (elevated erythrocyte sedimentation rate), pulmonary disease (impaired diffusion capacity, DLCO) or renal involvement (proteinuria) identifies patients with a poor 5-year survival. In addition, the clinical association of antibody profiles allows patients at increased risk of

Table 19.2 Autoimmune serology in SSc

Antibody	Prevalence	Comments
ACA	60% lcSSc	Associated with typical CREST
Scl-70	40% dcSSc, 15% lcSSc	Predictive of interstitial lung involvement, especially in lSSc
RNApol	20% SSc	Anti-RNApol I or III associated with diffuse subset and renal disease
U1-RNP	10% SSc	Associated with overlap features
U3-RNP	5% SSc	Poor outcome and isolated PHT in dcSSc
PM-Scl	3% SSc	Myositis overlap
Th/To	5% SSc	Lung fibrosis in lcSSc
anti-M2	5–10% SSc	Especially in lcSSc with PBC

See also chapters 18 and 20

pulmonary or renal complications to be identified. In the future, such information is likely to direct management and screening. Antibodies can predict particular complications such as anti-topoisomerase and lung fibrosis, anti-RNA polymerase and renal crisis or anti-Th/To and respiratory involvement in lcSSc. At present the strongest genetic associations relate to SSc-specific autoantibodies, but other genetic factors that determine the disease profile are being sought. Recently a genetic variant in connective tissue growth factor (CTGF) was associated with SSc (Fonseca *et al.*, 2007).

Management of SSc

The principles of effective management of SSc are summarized in Box 19.4. Unfortunately at present there are no disease-modifying treatments of proven efficacy. Most patients benefit from vascular therapy, and a number of agents that suggest the potential for vascular remodelling have been used in trials (Table 19.3). Immunosuppressive treatment is generally reserved for patients with early and aggressive dcSSc or with a major organ-based complication such as interstitial lung disease or myositis. Cyclophosphamide has been demonstrated to have modest benefit in prospective clinical trials (Hoyles *et al.*, 2006; Tashkin *et al.*, 2007). A number of approaches are being evaluated in clinical trials. High-dose immunosuppression with autologous peripheral stem-cell rescue is currently being evaluated in clinical trials. There are currently no effective antifibrotic agents for established SSc, but a number are under development. They include biological therapies that neutralize key potential cytokines driving SSc, including transforming growth factor beta 1 (TGFβ1) and CTGF.

Organ-based complications

The outcome of SSc is largely determined by the extent and severity of organ-based complications. Some of these are almost universal, such as oesophageal reflux, while many of the severe complications occur in around 10–15% of cases overall.

Pulmonary hypertension—Pulmonary hypertension is the single largest cause of death directly attributable to SSc. The frequency of the complication is likely to be around 10% overall, although published prevalence studies have varied largely owing to differences in diagnostic methods and variation in study cohorts. It occurs in both limited and diffuse cutaneous subsets, although as an isolated

Table 19.3 Drugs to treat Raynaud's phenomenon

Pharmaco-nutrients

Antioxidant vitamins: vitamins C and E at high dose may reduce oxidant stress in Raynaud's and SSc
Fish oils: maxepa, cod liver oil supplements may favour endothelial production of vasodilatory prostanoids
Gamolenic acid: mechanism uncertain
Seredrin: *Gingko biloba*, vasodilator giving symptomatic benefit in Raynaud's

Vasodilators

Calcium channel blockers: nifedipine and others may be effective; primary Raynaud's responds better than secondary; different agents may demonstrate varied effectiveness and side effects; side effects are frequent and often dose-limiting, including headache, ankle swelling and postural hypotension
Angiotensin receptor blockers: effective for SSc-associated hypertension; may also help Raynaud's symptoms and have potential beneficial effect on vascular remodelling
Nitroglycerin: topical glyceryl trinitrate ointment or patches may benefit ischaemic digits, but limited by side effects; new microemulsions under evaluation with better tolerability

Other agents

5HT reuptake inhibitors: give well-tolerated and effective symptom relief in many Raynaud's patients; mechanism of action probably involves depletion of platelet serotonin
Surgical options include lumbar sympathectomy for lower limb symptoms and digital sympathectomy (adventectomy) for severely affected digits; cervical sympathectomy disappointing and only temporarily helpful
Lifestyle adjustments (especially cold avoidance and cessation of smoking), silk-lined gloves and chemical hand-warmers often provide substantial benefit

complication it is most often seen in established lcSSc. Diagnosis can only be made robustly using right-heart catheterization and is determined by a mean pulmonary arterial pressure in excess of 25 mm Hg at rest, without elevated pulmonary capillary wedge pressure, but with increased pulmonary vascular resistance.

Distinction should be made between pulmonary arterial hypertension (PAH) and pulmonary hypertension secondary to severe interstitial lung fibrosis. The latter is uncommon in SSc, although some degree of lung fibrosis in association with PAH is frequent and may impact on survival. Historically the outcome in SSc-associated PAH was dismal, with a 2-year survival of 47%. With the advent of modern advanced therapies, including endothelin receptor antagonists (e.g. bosentan, sitaxentan) and selective phosphodiesterase inhibitors that promote nitric-oxide-induced vasodilatation (e.g. sildenafil) given in the context of a multidisciplinary pulmonary hypertension service, outcome for confirmed PAH has improved and currently survival of greater that 69% at 2 years has been demonstrated. Nevertheless, this is much inferior to outcome in idiopathic (previously primary) PAH using the same therapies, and so there is much scope for improvement.

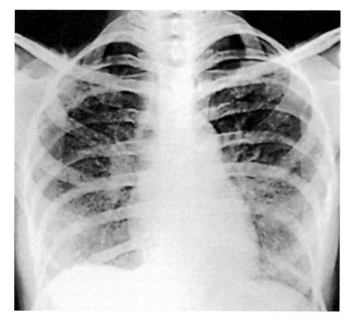

Figure 19.4 Chest radiograph of diffuse interstitial lung disease in a patient with scleroderma

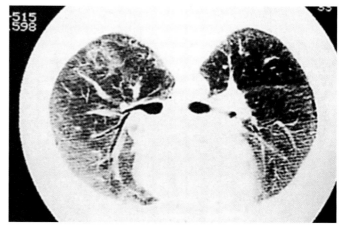

Figure 19.5 High-resolution computed tomography scan showing evidence of early interstitial lung disease

In SSc there is the potential for earlier diagnosis through screening, and currently it is recommended that all cases of SSc have annual assessment by echo-Doppler and lung function tests. Elevation of estimated right ventricular systolic pressure based on tricuspid regurgitant jet velocity (above 35 mm Hg) or fall in carbon monoxide transfer factor (DLCO) below 55% predicted with preserved lung volumes should prompt consideration for right-heart catheter study. Less invasive tests are being developed, including plasma N-terminal pro-BNP, which has been shown to predict outcome and associate with haemodynamic variables in PAH. In the future is likely that earlier detection and intervention, possibly using combination therapy including ERA, PDE5 inhibition and prostacyclin analogues, will further improve outcome in this difficult problem.

Lung fibrosis—Interstitial lung fibrosis is a common internal organ manifestation of SSc (Figures 19.4 and 19.5). It is present in more than 30% of cases but may not be inexorably progressive. The anti-scl70 autoantibody provides a useful clinical marker and is generally associated with lung fibrosis in both SSc subsets. High-resolution computed tomography (HRCT) imaging is currently the gold-standard test to detect and determine the pattern and extent of disease. Bronchoalveolar lavage is favoured in some centres and certainly correlates with the extent of disease, but not always with activity. Lung biopsy is not routinely indicated, but histologically most cases of SSc-associated lung fibrosis are classified as non-specific interstitial pneumonia, rather than the usual interstitial pneumonia pattern of idiopathic lung fibrosis. This may explain the better outcome for most patients with SSc compared with idiopathic pulmonary fibrosis. Immunosuppressive treatment with cyclophosphamide has recently been shown to be superior to placebo in a large controlled clinical trial, but the effect was modest.

Therefore new and better treatments are needed. It has been suggested that alveolar epithelial damage may be more important than inflammation in driving the fibrosis, and research data confirm that markers of epithelial injury or permeability such as serum KL-6 or DTPA clearance may provide predictive information about future decline in lung function. At present having determined the presence of fibrosis by HRCT, the cornerstone of management is serial pulmonary function testing. Progressive deterioration, even if gradual, is a clinical indicator for active treatment. At present immunosuppressive strategies are used. In severe advanced disease without major co-morbidity, single lung transplantation has been shown to be beneficial.

Scleroderma renal crisis (SRC)—There have been major advances in management of renal disease in SSc. The major problem is one of recognition, and education of both patients and physicians is important. SRC often presents non-specifically with headaches and visual disturbances before encephalopathy, cardiac failure or acute oliguric renal failure develop. Treatment with angiotensin-converting enzyme inhibition is mandatory. Patients should be admitted for blood pressure control and monitoring of renal function. Fifty per cent of cases require dialysis, which is temporary in many individuals. There may be significant recovery in renal function for up to 2 years after a renal crisis, and decisions regarding transplantation should be delayed until that time. There is no evidence that prophylactic administration of ACE inhibitors is helpful in preventing renal crisis or improving outcome, and the cornerstone of management is patient education, vigilant blood pressure monitoring, and avoidance of nephrotoxic drugs or high-dose corticosteroids with prompt initiation or appropriate therapy early in the course of the SRC.

Gut disease—The gastrointestinal tract is the most frequently affected organ in SSc. Up to 90% of patients demonstrate oesophageal dysmotility with reflux, and the proton pump inhibitors have dramatically improved symptomatic disease. Strictures are now relatively rare, although vigilance for Barrett's metaplasia is required. Midgut disease with bacterial overgrowth may respond to broad-spectrum antibiotics, although maintenance treatment may be required. Paradoxically, colonic involvement may lead to severe constipation, and anorectal incontinence is prevalent. It is important that acute abdominal complications of SSc are managed conservatively as far as possible, because major abdominal surgery is poorly tolerated owing to SSc-related co-morbidity, prolonged post-operative ileus and poor healing.

Patient Support organizations are listed in Box 19.5.

References

Fonseca C, Lindahl GE, Ponticos M *et al.* A polymorphism in the CTGF promoter region associated with systemic sclerosis. *New England Journal of Medicine* 2007; **357**: 1210–1220.

Hoyles RK, Ellis RW, Wellsbury J *et al.* A multicenter, prospective, randomized, double-blind, placebo-controlled trial of corticosteroids and intravenous cyclophosphamide followed by oral azathioprine for the treatment of pulmonary fibrosis in scleroderma. *Arthritis and Rheumatism* 2006; **54**: 3962–3970.

Tashkin DP, Elashoff R, Clements PJ; Scleroderma Lung Study Research Group. Effects of 1-year treatment with cyclophosphamide on outcomes at 2 years in scleroderma lung disease. *American Journal of Respiratory and Critical Care Medicine* 2007; **176**: 1026–1034.

Further reading

Akram MR, Handler CE, Williams M *et al.* Angiographically proven coronary artery disease in scleroderma. *Rheumatology (Oxford)* 2006; **45**: 1395–1398.

Bouros D, Wells AU, Nicholson AG *et al.* Histopathologic subsets of fibrosing alveolitis in patients with systemic sclerosis and their relationship to outcome. *American Journal of Respiratory and Critical Care Medicine* 2002; **165**: 1581–1586.

Coghlan JG, Mukerjee D. The heart and pulmonary vasculature in scleroderma: clinical features and pathobiology. *Current Opinion in Rheumatology* 2001; **13**: 495–499.

Denton CP, Black CM. Scleroderma and related disorders: therapeutic aspects. *Bailliere's Best Practice & Research. Clinical Rheumatology* 2000; **14**: 17–35.

LeRoy EC, Medsger TA Jr. Criteria for the classification of early systemic sclerosis. *Journal of Rheumatology* 2001; **28**: 1573–1576.

Silver RM. Clinical aspects of systemic sclerosis (scleroderma). *Annals of the Rheumatic Diseases* 1991; **50** (Suppl. 4): 854–861.

Steen VD, Medsger TA Jr. Severe organ involvement in systemic sclerosis with diffuse scleroderma. *Arthritis and Rheumatism* 2000; **43**: 2437–2444.

Williams MH, Das C, Handler CE *et al.* Systemic sclerosis associated pulmonary hypertension: improved survival in the current era. *Heart* 2006; **92**: 926–932.

Williams MH, Handler CE, Akram R *et al.* Role of N-terminal brain natriuretic peptide (N-TproBNP) in scleroderma-associated pulmonary arterial hypertension. *European Heart Journal* 2006; **27**: 1485–1494.

CHAPTER 20

Reflex Sympathetic Dystrophy

Chris Deighton[1] and Paul Davis[2]

[1]Derbyshire Royal Infirmary, Derby, UK
[2]University of Alberta, Edmonton, Canada

OVERVIEW

- Reflex sympathetic dystrophy (RSD) is a descriptive term for a condition mainly affecting the limbs, with severe pain, a preceding event that might be relatively trivial in traumatic terms, and abnormal blood flow and sweating in the affected area.

- Eventual structural changes to superficial and deep structures lead to atrophic, shiny skin, contractures and patchy osteoporosis around joints on X-rays.

- The cause is not clearly understood, but probably a variety of central and peripheral voluntary and involuntary neurological pathways play a part.

- The diagnosis is usually clinical, although X-rays and bone scans may show a characteristic appearance.

- Treatment is empirical, but relies on pain reduction, early mobilization and restoration of function. Further randomized controlled trials are needed to improve the therapeutics of this difficult condition.

Introduction

Reflex sympathetic (osteo)dystrophy (RSD) is a descriptive term for a poorly understood clinical condition of unknown aetiology. It has also been variously termed shoulder-hand syndrome, Sudeck's atrophy and algodystrophy. It has often been confused and compared with causalgia, a different condition with similar clinical symptoms. Generally speaking, the more words used in the description of a condition, the less we understand that condition. In 1993, it was suggested that reflex sympathetic dystrophy be renamed "complex regional pain syndrome (CRPS) type I". This change in nomenclature has done little to reassure the non-specialist that our understanding of the condition has substantially improved. The change in terminology has also failed to catch on, so that many specialists still refer to RSD, even though it is clear that the reflexes are not necessarily involved, and the sympathetic nervous system cannot be implicated in many patients (for example, sympathetic ganglia blockade only relieves the pain in some patients).

To have the "full house" clinically, the following should be present: (a) severe pain, usually starting peripherally, and working more proximally over time in a non-dermatomal fashion (allodynia)—the pain is disproportionate to the triggering event and clinical findings (hyperpathia); (b) usually a preceding event that might be relatively trivial in traumatic terms; (c) abnormal blood flow to the affected area (usually a limb), with colour changes (blues, whites and reds) and oedema; (d) abnormal sweating in the area; (e) changes in the motor system, with weakness and sometimes tremor; (f) eventual structural changes to superficial and deep structures leading to atrophic, shiny skin, contractures and patchy osteoporosis around joints on X-rays.

Although diagnostic criteria have been proposed, these have not been validated and are complicated by the fact that not all features may be present at the same time and may vary in their intensity. The condition tends to affect upper limbs more commonly than lower limbs. Usually one limb is affected, but it can become bilateral, or affect another limb. It is usually most evident distally (hand and wrist, or foot and ankle), but a whole limb can be affected, such as in "shoulder-hand syndrome".

This chapter explores the following areas: What causes RSD? How is RSD diagnosed? What is the treatment of RSD?

What causes RSD?

The cause of RSD is far from understood, but it appears to involve an exaggeration of normal physiological responses and involves changes at multiple levels in the central and peripheral nervous systems. Some epidemiological features of RSD are shown in Table 20.1. Taking total knee arthroplasty as an example, a prevalence of between 0.8 and 1.2% of persistent RSD has been quoted. However, a recent prospective study suggested that 21% of patients fulfilled diagnostic criteria 1 month after operation, falling to 12.7% at 6 months, suggesting that symptoms and signs of RSD are not

ABC of Rheumatology, 4th edn. Edited by Ade Adebajo.
©2010 Blackwell Publishing Ltd. 9781405170680.

Table 20.1 Some epidemiological factors in reflex sympathetic dystrophy

Triggers	Usually some noxious event such as:
	Wrist and tibial fractures (about 30% may demonstrate mild features, but only a minority go on to severe disease)
	Trauma: mild or moderate
	Rotator cuff tendonitis or subacromial bursitis
	Surgery: carpal tunnel decompression, arthroscopy, arthroplasty, lumbar spine surgery
	Central nervous system disorders: head injury, hemiplegia, spinal cord injury, neuropathy
	Myocardial infarction
	Immobilization: in any of the above may be an important factor
Sex	More common in women than men, with a ratio of 3:1 quoted
Age	Any age, although the mean in some studies is quoted as 52 years; now well recognized in children
Genetics	Some evidence to support a familial predisposition
Personality traits	No convincing evidence to support an association
Psychological factors	Some patients can have motor weakness and movement disorders relieved by placebo, nerve blocks or infusions

uncommon after operation, but persistent full-blown disease is mercifully unusual. Figures of up to 35% and 5% have been reported for Colles' fracture and peripheral nerve injury, respectively. The pathology of RSD is bedevilled by the lack of tissue studies, either pre- or post-mortem. Limited histological investigations have suggested that microangiopathy or other vascular abnormalities may be a key driver. A crucial question that has not been satisfactorily answered is: Why do the majority of patients who suffer the potential triggers listed in Table 20.1 make a full and uneventful recovery, but a minority go onto develop RSD? A number of theories have been propounded, but revolve around peripheral mechanisms, central mechanisms and neurogenic inflammation with microvascular dysfunction. These interrelate in a series of vicious circles that result in the characteristic features of RSD, which are summarized below.

Peripheral mechanisms

Trauma to C fibres and A™ afferents is likely to be an initiating event. Many patients have sympathetically maintained pain, which may activate both mechanoreceptors and nociceptors. Some patients experience benefit from alpha blockade, supporting a role for ⟨-adrenoceptors in the pathogenesis of RSD. These receptors become expressed on nociceptors in some cases of soft-tissue and nerve injury. Some patients demonstrate supersensitivity to catecholamines, consistent with increased ⟨-adrenoceptor responsiveness.

Central mechanisms

In RSD an initial activation of nociceptors may lead to alteration of central information processes, resulting in central sensitization. Patients exhibit normal thresholds for the detection of cold and heat, but reduced thresholds for cold-pain and heat-pain, suggest-

ing a central nervous disturbance. Activation of low-threshold mechanoreceptors is interpreted as noxious, and results in normal sensations being interpreted as painful ("allodynia"). There is a close similarity between the autonomic features of RSD, and those of autonomic failure after stroke. The latter occur in the absence of pain, suggesting an uncoupling of the mechanisms that underpin the pain and sensory symptoms from the autonomic features. Tests on normal volunteers that create conflict between motorsensory central nervous processing can lead to pain and sensory disturbances, such as using mirrors during congruent and incongruent limb movements. It has been proposed that central processing of persistent sensorymotor conflict may lead to chronic pain in some vulnerable individuals.

Neurogenic inflammation

Release of vasoactive peptides, including substance P and calcitonin gene-related peptide, from afferent nerve fibres cause vasodilatation, with increased vascular permeability and protein leakage. Neuropetides may also be released in response to impaired blood flow, oxygen deficiency and an increase in protons and skin lactate levels. This might explain why some of the early clinical features of RSD appear to be inflammatory.

Microvascular dysfunction

A number of investigators have confirmed microvascular dysfunction in RSD, although it remains unknown whether these changes, reflected by colour and temperature changes, drive the disease process or are secondary to it.

Bringing these factors together, it has been suggested that RSD is initiated by trauma to C fibres and A™ afferents in soft tissue or nerves, resulting in neurogenic inflammation. Signs of inflammation predominate in early disease, with redness, increased skin temperature due to inhibition of cutaneous vasoconstrictor neurons, with subsequent loss of function and pain. Early in the disease, the sympathetic nervous system plays a role, but when central sensitization takes over, with changes at the dorsal root ganglion level, the pain becomes independent of sympathetic nerves. There is a competition between the continued inhibition of vasoconstriction and supersensitivity of the peripheral vessels to circulating adrenaline. Late intractable disease can be characterized by a cold, painful limb with poor or no function, with disuse leading to immobility and contractures.

How is RSD diagnosed?

In the early stages of RSD the limb is swollen and tender, and the diagnosis may not be straightforward, as it can mimic many other diseases, such as inflammatory arthritis, cellulitis, osteomyelitis, deep venous thrombosis, lymphatic obstruction and malignancy. In the late intractable disease, when the limb becomes cold, chronic arterial insufficiency needs to be considered.

There is no diagnostic test for RSD, and tests are only required to rule out the other causes of a painful swollen limb as listed above. Routine investigations, such as a full blood count and erythrocyte sedimentation rate should be normal, and if not an explanation should be sought. In terms of positive features supporting RSD

Table 20.2 Diagnostic criteria for RSD

1. The presence of an initiating noxious event, or a cause of immobilization
2. Continuing pain, allodynia or hyperalgesia, in which the pain is disproportionate to any inciting event
3. Evidence at some time of oedema, changes in skin blood flow, or abnormal sudomotor activity in the region of the pain
4. This diagnosis is excluded by the existence of conditions that would otherwise account for the degree of pain and dysfunction

Note: criteria 2–4 must be satisfied

Table 20.3 Treatment modalities for RSD (modified and simplified from Stanton-Hicks, 2002)

Medical	Rehabilitation	Psychological
Medications	Motivation	Counselling
NSAIDs	Desensitization	Behaviour modification
Opioids	Isometric exercises	Coping skills
Tricyclics	Mobilization	Relaxation therapy
Adrenoceptor	Flexibility	Hypnosis
antagonists	Strength exercises	
Corticosteroids		
Calcitonin		
Neurologic blocks		
Sympathetic		
Regional		
Epidural		
Neurostimulation		
Peripheral		
Epidural		

NSAIDs = non-steroidal anti-inflammatory drugs

(Table 20.2), X-rays may show patchy osteoporosis, especially in the juxta-articular region. Joint space is usually preserved, but may be lost in late disease with ankylosis. On bone scanning there is increased uptake in early disease, and reduced uptake in late disease. Patients with markedly increased uptake may have a better prognosis, possibly reflecting the fact that they have not yet progressed to late-stage disease. Thermography detects asymmetry in limb surface temperature, but is not widely available. Bone densitometry and magnetic resonance imaging (MRI) may show nonspecific changes, such as reduced bone density, soft-tissue swelling and bone-marrow oedema, but nothing specific to positively diagnose RSD. The greatest value of MRI is to rule out other causes of a painful swollen limb.

How is RSD treated?

Owing to our limited understanding of the aetiology and pathogenesis of RSD, much of the therapeutics is empirical, and what helps one patient may not help others. Because established RSD can be very challenging to treat, emphasis has been placed on prevention where possible and, failing that, early intervention. The main aims are to reduce pain and restore function. Early mobilization following predisposing conditions is important, and graded physiotherapy may be very helpful. A trial in 1999 showed that vitamin C, a powerful antioxidant, may prevent RSD, supporting the growing evidence for the role of oxygen-free radicals in RSD. This needs to be researched further.

Patients who are particularly vulnerable are patients with a previous history of RSD, particularly if they require surgery on the previously affected part. A controlled study found that the risk of RSD could be reduced by a stellate ganglion block after the operation. An uncontrolled study suggested pre-operative calcitonin may prevent recurrence.

Although many experts and committees have recommended physiotherapy, occupational therapy, vocational rehabilitation and behavioural therapy, the evidence base for these is weak or lacking. One study compared physiotherapy and occupational therapy with social work intervention as the control, and showed no differences in the three groups for pain at 12 months, with only small improvements in temperature and global impairment for the intervention arms of the trial. An algorithm of treatment has been proposed by Stanton-Hicks (2002) with a cautious start (heat, massage and gentle movement to restore normal sensory processing), then isometric exercises for strengthening, treatment of secondary myofascial pain syndrome, aerobic conditioning, through to complete functional rehabilitation. Because pain can be the main rate-limiting factor in rehabilitation, medical and psychological therapies often have to run side by side (Table 20.3).

The mainstay of drug interventions is analgesics and non-steroidal anti-inflammatories. Low-dose antidepressants and anticonvulsants are commonly used, but the evidence base is sparse. A systematic review of therapies concluded that the only trial data that consistently demonstrated analgesia was with oral corticosteroids. However, many clinicians have understandable concerns about using steroids for disease that has the potential to become chronic, and where the evidence base for ongoing inflammation driving the disease is limited. A plethora of other drugs have been tried in RSD, which is testimony to the difficulties in treating the condition. Intranasal calcitonin has shown conflicting results. Drugs that do show promise are the bisphosphonates, justified initially on osteoporosis being a significant feature of RSD. A controlled trial of alendronate showed improved bone mineral content of the affected limb, but only small benefits to pain management. By contrast, a trial of intravenous clodronate showed substantial improvements in pain management at 6 months, with highly significant pain reduction compared with placebo.

The role of sympathetic blockade is controversial. For paravertebral blockade, the stellate ganglion for upper limb RSD is blocked with a series of local anaesthetics, depending on response, and the lumbar sympathetic chain for lower limb RSD. Another technique is intravenous blockade, usually with guanethidine. However, a systematic review found this treatment to be ineffective, so its use may decline in future. Continuous blockade of the brachial or lumbar plexus has been advocated with drugs such as morphine, so that whenever the catheter is in place, the patient can take advantage of the pain relief to maximize their rehabilitation.

Intrathecal baclofen proved to be effective for the upper limb dystonias in six out of seven patients, but did not improve pain. Spinal-cord stimulation has been shown to be effective in relieving pain in controlled trials. The procedure is, however, not without risk, as it involves placing an electrode on the dorsal aspect of the spinal cord, and an electric current produces paraesthesias that block the pain in the affected area. However, the average improvement in pain is sustained but not substantial, and functional and quality-of-life benefits have not been demonstrated. This leaves the dilemma of whether invasive and costly interventions that provide modest pain relief are justified. Clearly these concerns and the risks involved mean that patients have to be carefully selected.

Further reading

Amit S, Williams K, Raja SN. Advances in treatment of complex regional pain syndrome: recent insights on a perplexing disease. *Current Opinion in Anaesthesiology* 2006; **19**: 566–572.

Birklein F. Complex regional pain syndrome. *Journal of Neurology* 2005; **252**: 131–138.

Gispen JG. Painful shoulder and the reflex sympathetic dystrophy syndrome. In: Koopman WJ, ed. *Arthritis and Allied Conditions*, 14th edn. Lippincott Williams & Wilkins, Baltimore, 2001: 2126–2134.

Harden RN, Bruehl SP. Diagnosis of complex regional pain syndrome: signs, symptoms and new empirically derived diagnostic criteria. *Clinical Journal of Pain* 2006; **22**: 415–419.

Herrick A. Reflex sympathetic dystrophy (complex regional pain syndrome type 1). In: Hochberg MC, Silman AJ, Smolen JS, Weinblatt ME, Weisman MH, eds. *Rheumatology*. Mosby, Edinburgh, 2003.

Merritt WH. The challenge to manage reflex sympathetic dystrophy/complex regional pain syndrome. *Clinics in Plastic Surgery* 2005; **32**: 575–604.

Stanton-Hicks MD, Burton AW, Bruehl SP *et al.* An updated interdisciplinary clinical pathway for CRPS: report of an expert panel. *Pain Practice* 2002; **2**: 1–16.

CHAPTER 21

Is it a Connective Tissue Disease?

Peter J Maddison[1] and Mohammed Tikly[2]

[1]Bangor University, Bangor, UK
[2]University of the Witwatersrand, Johannesburg, South Africa

OVERVIEW

- Raynaud's phenomenon and sicca symptoms are common presenting features of connective tissue diseases.
- The indirect immunofluorescence test is sufficient as a screening test for antinuclear antibodies, which are the serological hallmark of connective tissue diseases.
- Patients frequently present initially with non-specific features of a connective tissue disease but do not fulfil criteria for any specific disorder.
- Less than one-third of patients with undifferentiated connective tissue evolve clinically to fulfil classification criteria of a defined connective tissue disease.
- Not only is it important to recognize and treat potentially aggressive disease, but also to avoid over-treatment where the diagnosis is unclear or the disease has a potentially benign course.

Diagnosis of connective tissue diseases is often challenging because of the protean clinical features and the fact that no single symptom or sign is pathognomic of a specific connective tissue disease. Classification criteria for the major connective tissue diseases (see Chapters 18 and 19) were developed primarily as a means of standardizing patient populations for clinical research rather than for diagnosis. In practice, they are extremely limited for early diagnosis of connective tissue diseases. In many patients attending connective disease clinics, it is not possible to make definitive diagnosis, especially early in the course of a systemic rheumatic illness. Many, but not all, of these patients eventually fulfil classification criteria for one or more of the major connective tissue disease entities, a process that may take 10–20 years.

A substantial proportion of these patients have non-specific symptoms or signs—most commonly either isolated Raynaud's phenomenon, or an early inflammatory polyarthritis, or constitutional symptoms of fever, malaise and fatigue. Serological tests often show abnormalities that are suggestive of a connective tissue disease but not sufficiently specific to classify the patient as having one of the major connective tissue diseases. This has prompted the

introduction of additional terms such as "overlap syndrome" and "undifferentiated connective tissue disease."

From a management perspective, it is important not only to recognize and treat potentially aggressive disease, but also to avoid over-treatment in patients where either the diagnosis is unclear or the disease has a potentially benign course.

Autoantibody profile in diagnosis

Antinuclear antibodies are a hallmark of connective tissue diseases. Serology is of particular value in situations in which clinical expression of the disease is incomplete, when the presence of a particular antinuclear antibody profile can be diagnostic. These antibodies can be found in a variety of clinical settings, however, and their occurrence does not necessarily indicate the presence of any specific disease. It is therefore imperative that requests for antinuclear antibody tests and the interpretation of results thereof be done in the light of the clinical findings.

The indirect immunofluorescence test, using the HEp-2 cell substrate, is the gold standard for detecting antinuclear antibodies. In both systemic lupus erythematosus and scleroderma, antinuclear antibodies can be detected in 95% or more of untreated patients with active disease by this method (Table 21.1). In cases suspected of having either of these diseases, the indirect immunofluorescence test is enough as a screening test for antinuclear antibodies, and it is not cost effective to test automatically for anti-nDNA or other antibody specificities. The individual antinuclear antibody fluorescent patterns are of limited diagnostic utility but may provide guidance to more specific immunological tests. In some instances, a false negative result may occur if either the antigen is outside the nucleus (for example, anti-Jo-1 and anti-ribosomal P-protein antibodies, both often categorized under the umbrella term "antinuclear antibodies") or if it is present in a form not recognised by a particular autoantibody (for example, when anti-Ro is directed exclusively to determinants on the native Ro molecule not expressed in cultured HEp-2 cells). In such cases, the clinical picture dictates that specific autoantibody assays should be undertaken.

Once antinuclear antibodies have been detected with a screening test, it is important to determine their specificity. This is now part of the standard operating procedure of serology laboratories, but the process is greatly facilitated by the doctor giving sufficient clinical information when antinuclear antibody testing is requested.

Table 21.1 Antinuclear antibodies in various diseases detected by indirect immunofluorescence

Condition	Frequency of antinuclear antibodies (%)
Autoimmune rheumatic disease	
• Drug-induced lupus	100
• Systemic lupus erythematosus	98
• Systemic sclerosis (scleroderma)	95
• Sjögren's syndrome	80
• Pauciarticular juvenile idiopathic arthritis	70
• Polymyositis or dermatomyositis	60
• Rheumatoid arthritis	50
Organ-specific autoimmunity	
• Primary autoimmune cholangitis	100
• Autoimmune hepatitis	70
• Myasthenia gravis	50
• Autoimmune thyroid disease	45
• Idiopathic pulmonary hypertension	40
Other conditions	
• Waldenström's macroglobulinaemia	20
• Subacute bacterial endocarditis	20
• Infectious mononucleosis	15
• Leprosy	15
• HIV	10
Normal population	
• Children	8
• Adults	15

Box 21.1 **Characteristics of undifferentiated connective tissue disease**

- Common manifestations
  - Raynaud's phenomenon
  - Arthralgia or myalgia
  - Rash
  - Sicca symptoms
  - Constitutional symptoms (fever, malaise, fatigue)
- One-third evolve into a defined connective tissue disease, usually within 5 years

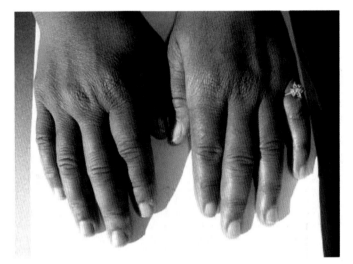

Figure 21.1 Swollen "puffy" fingers of patient with undifferentiated connective tissue disease

Specific antinuclear antibody tests are often helpful in stratifying patients into clinical subsets, which may be useful in the further management of specific clinical manifestations and prognostication (Table 21.2). These autoantibodies are usually present from the beginning of the clinical presentation and are detectable throughout the course of the disease. In some instances, such as the anti-nDNA test, autoantibody titres may fluctuate with disease activity. Many serology laboratories these days use commercial kits to detect specific autoantibodies. Although these tests are less labour intensive, they vary in sensitivity, and sometimes produce false-positive results. This is especially the case with the anti-nDNA and anti-Sm assays.

Undifferentiated connective tissue disease

The term "undifferentiated connective tissue disease" was first coined in 1980 by LeRoy and colleagues (LeRoy *et al.*, 1980). This was to counter the concept of mixed connective tissue disease being a distinct disease entity and to point out that many patients designated as having mixed connective tissue disease presented with an early phase of disease that later evolved into one of the "classic" connective tissue diseases, particularly scleroderma. Subsequently, undifferentiated connective tissue disease has been embraced by others and, rather than replacing mixed connective tissue disease, it has been used to describe patients with clinical and laboratory features of connective tissue disease (Box 21.1) who

do not fulfil criteria for any one disorder (Figure 21.1). Although no universally agreed definition of "undifferentiated connective tissue disease" exists, this term should be distinguished from other commonly used terms such as "overlap syndrome," in which patients meet the criteria for two or more connective tissue diseases or specific criteria for mixed connective tissue disease (Table 21.3) (see also Chapters 18 and 19). Other terms used in the literature that are synonymous with undifferentiated connective tissue disease include "lupus-like", "pre-lupus," "latent lupus" and "incomplete lupus."

Long-term, prospective follow-up studies of outcome show that these patients represent a large proportion (25–50%) of patients presenting to connective tissue disease clinics. Only a minority of patients, about 30%, evolve clinically to fulfil classification criteria of a defined connective tissue disease, usually in the first few years of follow-up. Spontaneous remission occurs in 5–10% of patients, but in the majority the undifferentiated connective tissue disease state persists. Major organ involvement is rare in these patients. Serositis, alopecia, photosensitivity, discoid rash (Figure 21.2) and the presence of either anti-nDNA antibodies or anti-Sm antibodies are predictors of evolution to SLE.

Table 21.2 Specificity of antinuclear antibodies in diagnosis and disease expression

Disease	Antibody	Frequency (%)	Clinical association
Systemic lupus erythematous	Anti-nDNA‡	70	• Lupus nephritis
	Anti-nucleosome	70	• Early disease, lupus nephritis, drug-induced lupus
	Anti-Sm	10–25*	• Vasculitis, central nervous system lupus
	Anti-U1RNP	30–50*	• Raynaud's phenomenon, swollen fingers, arthritis, myositis, mixed connective tissue disease
	Anti-Ro	40	• Photosensitive rash, subacute cutaneous lupus erythematosus, neonatal lupus, congenital heart block, Sjögren's syndrome
	Anti-La	15	• As for anti-Ro
	Anti-ribosomal P-protein	15	• Central nervous system lupus (psychosis or depression)
Sjögren's syndrome	Anti-Ro	60–90#	• Extraglandular disease, vasculitis, lymphoma
	Anti-La	35–85#	• As for anti-Ro
Systemic sclerosis	Anti-centromere	5–30†	• Limited cutaneous disease, microvascular or macrovascular disease, telangiectasia
	Anti-ThRNP	4	• Limited cutaneous disease
	Anti-topo-1	25	• Diffuse cutaneous disease, interstitial lung disease
	Anti-RNA polymerases	20	• Rapidly progressive diffuse cutaneous disease, scleroderma renal crisis
	Anti-U3RNP	5–20*	• Diffuse cutaneous disease, pulmonary hypertension
	Anti-PM-Scl	5	• Scleroderma–polymyositis overlap
	Anti-Ku	2	• Scleroderma–polymyositis overlap
Dermatomyositis and polymyositis	Anti Jo-1	30	• Anti-synthetase syndrome: mechanic's hands, interstitial lung disease
	(antibodies to other tRNA synthetases)	(3)	(anti-synthetase syndrome)
	Anti-SRP	4	• Severe myositis
	Anti-Mi2	10	• Dermatomyositis

‡Anti-double-stranded DNA antibody
*Higher frequency in people of African or Indian origin
With sensitive enzyme-linked immunosorbent assays
†Low frequency in people of African origin

Table 21.3 Terminology

Undifferentiated connective tissue disease	Patient has features seen in connective tissue disease but does not meet criteria for a defined connective tissue disease
Overlap syndrome	Patients meet criteria for two or more connective tissue diseases
Mixed connective tissue disease	Overlap of rheumatoid arthritis-like arthritis, systemic lupus erythematosus, scleroderma, and myositis with antibodies to U1RNP

Box 21.2 Raynaud's phenomenon—features suggestive of an underlying connective tissue disease

- Onset in early childhood or later adult life
- Asymmetrical involvement of fingers
- Evidence of digital ischaemic damage
- Abnormal morphology of nailfold capillaries (including dilated, distorted capillaries and areas of capillary dropout)
- Presence of autoantibodies associated with connective tissue disease

Raynaud's phenomenon

Raynaud's phenomenon is often the presenting manifestation of connective tissue diseases, especially scleroderma (Box 21.2). It is common, however, in otherwise healthy people.

Which connective tissue disease?

Although clinical presentation in the early stage can be similar between connective tissue diseases, the evolution of typical clinical features over weeks or months is usually enough to distinguish the

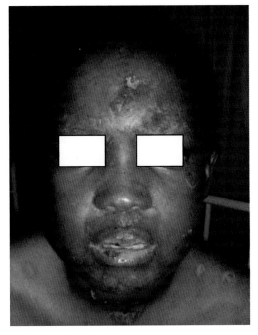

Figure 21.2 Active discoid lupus erythematosus

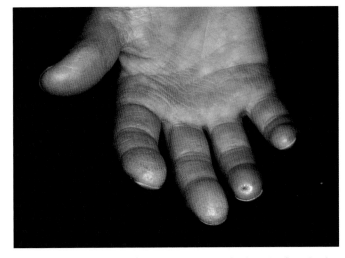

Figure 21.4 Finger pulp scars from previous digital ischaemic ulceration in a patient with systemic sclerosis

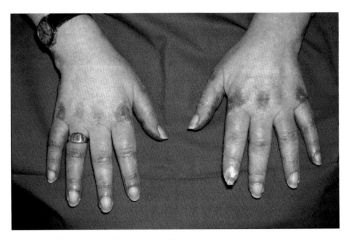

Figure 21.3 Hands in dermatomyositis

characteristic patterns associated with the different diseases. Early diagnosis is aided by recognition of distinctive serological profiles that are generally present with the earliest clinical manifestations. Diagnosis can also be facilitated by typical laboratory abnormalities and histological changes in the tissues involved. For example, microscopic polyangiitis, which presents with weight loss, fever, polyarthritis and active urinary sediment, can be distinguished from lupus by an autoimmune response characterized by pANCA antibodies directed against myeloperoxidase and the typical histological picture of pauci-immune focal necrotizing glomerulonephritis. Similarly, dermatomyositis sine myositis, which presents with photosensitive eruptions on the face, arms, and hands and is

associated with myalgia, can be distinguished from lupus by the distribution of the eruption, a raised serum creatine kinase, and typical changes on muscle biopsy, despite the absence of frank weakness (Figure 21.3).

Diagnosis is often complicated if lupus is part of an overlap syndrome and the patient fulfils classification criteria of more than one connective tissue disease (as opposed to undifferentiated connective tissue disease). The most common overlaps with systemic lupus erythematosus are patients who also have features of systemic sclerosis (Figure 21.4), polymyositis, or both, and patients with rheumatoid arthritis. Sometimes patients present with an overlap syndrome; at other times, the picture evolves sequentially. Development of Sjögren's syndrome during the course of systemic lupus erythematosus is well established, but occasionally patients with primary Sjögren's syndrome develop typical features of lupus, especially photosensitive eruptions typical of subacute cutaneous lupus erythematosus, after many years of disease.

Patients with an overlap of systemic lupus erythematosus and scleroderma or polymyositis, or both, often have a distinctive serological profile that includes high levels of antibodies to U1RNP. These patients have been suggested to have a distinctive connective tissue disease "mixed connective tissue disease." This concept is very controversial, however, with critics and protagonists.

A number of series report patients who fulfil criteria for both systemic lupus erythematosus and rheumatoid arthritis. For these patients, the term "rhupus" has been coined. These patients are usually easier to recognize when the rheumatoid arthritis develops first, but they are characterized ultimately by typical rheumatoid features such as erosive arthritis, subcutaneous nodules and rheumatoid factor. These features are accompanied by cutaneous, renal, haematological and other clinical manifestations characteristic of systemic lupus erythematosus, but unusual for rheumatoid arthritis, with the presence of anti-nDNA antibodies.

Differential diagnosis of connective tissue diseases

A common clinical conundrum is the distinction of systemic lupus erythematosus from other connective tissue diseases (Table 21.4). All frequently present with a mixture of systemic symptoms, including fever and weight loss, and musculoskeletal and/or mucocutaneous involvement. The combination of a careful history and physical examination, urine analysis, chest X-ray, laboratory tests for an acute-phase response, blood count, serum biochemistry, complement levels, creatine kinase and serological profile, however, results in the correct diagnosis in a high proportion of cases.

Drug-induced lupus

A carefully elicited drug history is essential to exclude drug-induced lupus. The management of this is very straightforward, involving discontinuation of the offending agent and short-term anti-inflammatory treatment. Procainamide and hydralazine carry the highest risk of inducing a lupus-like syndrome but are now seldom prescribed in clinical practice. In more recent years, several cases of drug-induced lupus have been reported in association with minocycline, a drug is prescribed often for acne, and sulfasalazine, a disease-modifying antirheumatic drug in rheumatoid arthritis, although individual risk of drug-induced lupus is low with these agents. In the context of rheumatoid arthritis, the diagnosis is sometimes difficult to make, particularly as antinuclear antibodies are present in up to 50% of patients with the condition. Drug-induced lupus is rare in people of African origin. The clinical presentation is similar to that of idiopathic systemic lupus erythematosus, with systemic features including fever and weight loss, arthralgia or frank arthritis, and serositis (particularly common with procainamide). Major organ involvement, such as nephritis and central nervous system manifestations, is less common, although renal disease can rarely occur in sulfasalazine-induced lupus. A high level of antinuclear antibodies usually shows a homogeneous pattern from the earliest presentation, and the typical preponder-

Table 21.4 Distinguishing features of connective tissue diseases

Condition	Distinguishing features
Systemic rheumatic diseases	
Rheumatoid arthritis	Prominent signs of synovitis; multisystem involvement uncommon at presentation; no autoantibodies associated with connective tissue disease
Systemic sclerosis	Pronounced Raynaud's phenomenon; scleroderma; characteristic serological profile
Dermatomyositis	Distinctive pattern of eruption; prominent muscle involvement; serological profile
Primary vasculitis	Distinctive renal involvement; neutrophilia (sometimes eosinophilia); serological profile
Behçet's syndrome	Lack of typical serological features
Adult Still's disease	Typical fever pattern; lack of typical serological features
Hereditary periodic fever syndromes (familial Mediterranean fever, TNF-associated periodic syndrome, hyperimmunoglobulin D, etc)	Intermittent manifestations; no autoantibodies associated with connective tissue disease
Other systemic disorders	
Autoimmune hepatitis	Typical liver involvement; absence of typical lupus features
Sarcoidosis	Typical histology; no autoantibodies associated with connective tissue disease
Histiocytic necrotizing lymphadenitis (Kikuchi–Fujimoto's disease)	Typical histology; lymphadenopathy, fever, neutropaenia and occasional antinuclear antibodies
Angioimmunoblastic lymphadenopathy	Typical histology; no autoantibodies associated with connective tissue disease
Other causes of photosensitivity and red face	
Polymorphous light eruption	Lack of systemic features; different histology; absent autoantibodies
Rosacea	Papulopustular eruption; non-systemic; absent autoantibodies
Seborrhoeic dermatitis	Different morphology and histology; non-systemic, absent autoantibodies
Contact dermatitis	History of allergen contact; pseudovesicle; no autoantibodies
Jessner's benign lymphocytic infiltration	Typical histology; negative serology
Erythrohepatic protoporphyria	Vesicobullous lesions; urinary and plasma porphyrin profile; no antibodies associated with systemic lupus erythematosus
Syphilis	Typical histology; diagnostic serology
Lupus vulgaris	Painful nodular cutaneous form of tuberculosis
Other causes of fatigue and musculoskeletal pain	
Fibromyalgia	No objective inflammation; no autoantibodies associated with connective tissue disease
Hypothyroidism	Little objective inflammation. May have Raynaud's phenomenon and carpal tunnel syndrome

ance of anti-histone antibodies can be shown with specific assays. Antibodies to native DNA and "extractable nuclear antigens" commonly associated with idiopathic systemic lupus erythematosus are invariably negative, except in the case of minocycline-induced lupus. The gold standard for diagnosis of drug-induced lupus, however, is that it resolves after the drug is stopped; the symptoms improve within days to weeks, although the antinuclear antibodies may take a year or two to disappear.

The anti-TNF agents, mainly used in the treatment of rheumatoid arthritis, but also for Crohn's disease and ankylosing spondylitis, also induce antinuclear antibody and, specifically, anti-nDNA antibody production. This phenomenon has been observed with all of the anti-TNF agents currently on the market, although more often with infliximab than adalimumab or etanercept. Only a very small proportion of patients develop a lupus-like illness, manifesting mainly with skin rashes, worsening polyarthritis and serositis. In all cases the illness has been reported to be mild and has resolved on discontinuation of the anti-TNF agent. As in the case of sulfasalazine-induced lupus, diagnosis can be challenging in patients with rheumatoid arthritis who have pre-existing antinuclear antibodies.

Other disorders of the skin

One of the most common conundrums in the connective tissue disease clinic is the patient referred with a history of photosensitivity or red face in association with musculoskeletal symptoms and, perhaps, systemic features such as fatigue. Photosensitive eruptions are common in the normal female population or may be induced by, for example, non-steroidal anti-inflammatory drugs. About 10% of women develop polymorphous light eruption—a pruritic papular eruption that occurs within hours of sun exposure, typically on normally covered sites, that spares the face and hands, and that resolves within days without epidermal change (Figure 21.5). In contrast, photosensitivity in systemic lupus erythematosus also affects the face and hands. The latent period after sun exposure is usually longer, the skin is less pruritic, and the eruption persists longer.

Similarly, the facial erythematous rash that is seen typically in patients with systemic lupus erythematosus must be distinguished from other causes. Typical rosacea consists of papulopustular lesions on a background of telangiectasia (Figure 21.6). Sometimes, light exposure aggravates this condition and a biopsy is sometimes needed to distinguish atypical forms from lupus. Benign lymphocytic infiltration, such as Jessner's (Figure 21.7), may produce papular or annular lesions that are indistinguishable clinically from subacute cutaneous lupus erythematosus (Figure 21.8) and tumid (papular) lupus erythematosus. The typical histological appearance includes a dense dermal lymphocytic infiltrate without the characteristic epidermal changes of lupus. Seborrhoeic dermatitis may affect the cheeks and paranasal folds and is usually pruritic and associated with desquamation. Contact dermatitis, which may be caused by cosmetics, produces superficial erythema, pseudovesicles and sometimes eyelid swelling. Lupus vulgaris, a painful nodular cutaneous form of tuberculosis, often affects skin over the nose and ears.

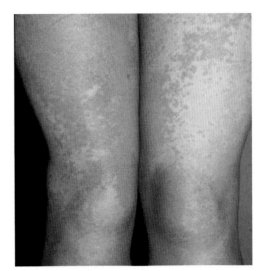

Figure 21.5 Polymorphous light eruption

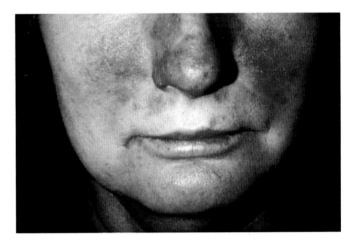

Figure 21.6 Rosacea papules and pustules

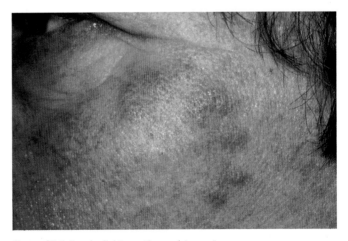

Figure 21.7 Papular light eruption and Jessner's

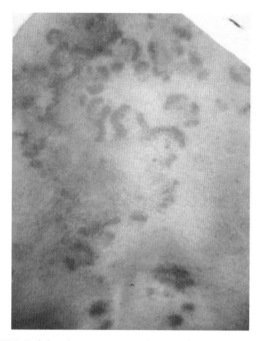

Figure 21.8 Rash in subacute cutaneous lupus erythematosus

Fibromyalgia

Fibromyalgia syndrome (see Chapter 8) is often mistaken for lupus, especially if the test for antinuclear antibodies is also positive, and sometimes is treated inappropriately (e.g. with corticosteroids). In addition, a significant proportion of people with fibromyalgia have other features that could be interpreted as manifestations of a connective tissue disease such as Raynaud's phenomenon, sicca symptoms and cognitive dysfunction. In those mistakenly treated with corticosteroids, although no evidence shows therapeutic efficacy in fibromyalgia, steroid withdrawal can make the symptoms worse. No evidence exists of an increased prevalence of positive antinuclear antibodies or the occurrence of connective tissue disease in patients with fibromyalgia. It has become increasingly apparent, however, that patients with connective tissue disease—especially those with systemic lupus erythematosus and Sjögren's syndrome—have a high prevalence of fibromyalgia that makes a considerable contribution to morbidity but is unrelated to the activity of the disease.

Endocrine disorders

Hypothyroidism can mimic a connective tissue disease because of non-specific symptoms of malaise, arthralgia and myalgia, which may be further confounded by Raynaud's phenomenon and carpal tunnel syndrome. The diagnosis should be considered in the peri- and postmenopausal patient in whom acute-phase reactants are normal and rheumatoid factor and antinuclear antibody tests are negative.

Diabetic cheiropathy is seen especially in patients with long-standing, severe type 1 diabetes. It causes painless generalized puffiness and induration of the fingers, resembling scleroderma. An inability to fully extend the fingers produces the so-called "prayer sign". Optimal glycaemic control and exercises may prevent worsening. Scleredema, another mimic of scleroderma in poorly controlled diabetes, presents as a thickened, indurated infiltrative skin disease. Unlike scleroderma, it occurs mostly on the upper back and is not associated with either Raynaud's phenomenon or antinuclear antibodies. It often clears spontaneously with good glycaemic control.

Is it infection?

Some infections can mimic connective tissue disease, especially systemic lupus erythematosus; these include HIV, syphilis, tuberculosis and persistent Epstein–Barr virus and cytomegalovirus infections. They can present with mucocutaneous manifestations, fever, malaise, polyarthralgia, lymphadenopathy and serological abnormalities, such as positive tests for antinuclear antibodies and rheumatoid factor. Distinguishing systemic lupus erythematosus from HIV infection can be especially challenging because of the additional overlapping clinical features of neuropsychiatric complications, nephropathy and haematological abnormalities such as leucopaenia and thrombocytopaenia.

A common clinical conundrum is how to distinguish an acute infection from a disease flare in a patient with systemic lupus erythematosus. To complicate matters further acute infections not infrequently trigger a lupus flare. Both bacterial infections and tuberculosis occur more commonly in lupus patients than in matched controls. Even patients in remission have an increased risk of infection, and this risk is enhanced by corticosteroids and other immunosuppressive agents such as cyclophosphamide. Bacterial infections involve the commonly occurring pyogenic organisms such as *Staphylococcus* species and *Escherichia coli*. Opportunistic infections also occur, especially in patients who take high-dose corticosteroids and immunosuppressive agents.

Measurement of C-reactive protein (CRP) has been suggested as a way of distinguishing between infection and a lupus flare. CRP levels are higher in patients with infection compared with those with active lupus; levels of CRP >60 mg/l strongly indicate infection, whereas levels <30 mg/l make infection highly unlikely. Occasionally, high levels of CRP can be seen with lupus flares of arthritis or serositis in the absence of infection. Prospective longitudinal studies have, however, shown CRP to be an unreliable predictor of infection.

In the absence of useful surrogate markers of infection in systemic lupus erythematosus, exhaustive microbiological investigations and early and often repeated cultures, sometimes from affected tissues, are needed to make a definitive diagnosis.

Reference

LeRoy EC, Maricq HR, Kahaleh MB. Undifferentiated connective tissue syndromes. *Arthritis and Rheumatism* 1980; **23**: 341–343.

Further reading

Atzeni F, Turiel M, Capsoni F, Doria A, Meroni P, Sarzi-Puttini P. Autoimmunity and anti-TNF-alpha agents. *Annals of the New York Academy of Sciences* 2005; **1051**: 559–569.

Fessler BJ. Infectious diseases in systemic lupus erythematosus: risk factors, management and prophylaxis. *Baillière's Best Practice & Research. Clinical Rheumatology* 2002; **16**: 281–291.

Gould T, Tikly M. Systemic lupus erythematosus in a patient with human immunodeficiency virus infection—challenges in diagnosis and management. *Clinical Rheumatology* 2004; **23**: 166–169.

Lawson TM, Amos N, Bulgen D, Williams BD. Minocycline-induced lupus: clinical features and response to rechallenge. *Rheumatology* 2001; **40**: 329–335.

Maddison PJ. MCTD: overlap syndromes. *Baillière's Best Practice & Research. Clinical Rheumatology* 2000; **14**: 111–124.

Mosca M, Tani C, Bombardieri S. Undifferentiated connective tissue diseases (UCTD): a new frontier for rheumatology. *Baillière's Best Practice & Research. Clinical Rheumatology* 2007; **21**: 1011–1023.

Solomon DH, Kavanaugh AJ, Schur PH. American College of Rheumatology Ad Hoc Committee on Immunologic Testing Guidelines. Evidence-based guidelines for the use of immunologic tests: antinuclear antibody testing. *Arthritis and Rheumatism* 2002; **47**: 434–444.

Swaak AJG, van de Brink H, Smeenk RJT *et al*. Incomplete lupus erythematosus: results of a multicentre study under the supervision of the EULAR Standing Committee on International Clinical Studies Including Therapeutic Trials (ESCISIT). *Rheumatology* 2001; **40**: 89–94.

CHAPTER 22

Sports and Exercise Medicine

Cathy Speed

Cambridge University Hospital, Cambridge, UK

OVERVIEW

- Sports and exercise medicine addresses the prevention and management of activity-related medical complaints, and the use of exercise for health-related benefit.

- Exercise and increased activity have proven benefits, both in the prevention and treatment of a wide range of conditions.

- Assessment of any sports injury requires an understanding of the potential intrinsic and extrinsic aetiological factors.

- Absolute rest is rarely if ever a component of a structured rehabilitation programme, which should aim to maintain physical fitness while restoring normal function.

- Increased activity can be beneficial to all, and be achieved by all, and it is incumbent on all health-care professionals to promote increases in physical activity.

Introduction

Sports and Exercise Medicine addresses the prevention and management of sports- and activity-related medical complaints, and the use of exercise for health-related benefit. Rheumatologists are often faced with sports injuries and have many patients who will benefit from an exercise prescription.

Sports injuries

Introduction

The key to managing sports-related injury is having an understanding of the patient and their sport. As with any patient, it is important to consider the patient's ideas, expectations and concerns. Those with an "athletic psyche" may have high anxiety levels about their injury and its implications, unrealistic expectations for recovery goals and time frames and a tendency to "overcomply" with rehabilitation programmes. An insight into the mechanics, training and techniques of the sport involved is also important, as this allows the underlying cause of the injury to be addressed (Figure 22.1).

ABC of Rheumatology, 4th edn. Edited by Ade Adebajo.
©2010 Blackwell Publishing Ltd. 9781405170680.

Assessment

When assessing sports injuries, it is helpful to consider intrinsic and extrinsic factors (Table 22.1).

Intrinsic factors encompass physical, physiological and psychological aspects of an individual that may contribute to injury. Importantly, what may be considered "abnormal"—for example, asymmetry of muscle development or joint range of motion—may be normal in relation to a trained athlete. Similarly, what is normal in the general population may be abnormal for an athlete—for example, average flexibility in a gymnast is likely to be abnormal.

Extrinsic factors play a significant role in the development of injury. Doing "too much, too soon, too often" is a common error in athletes of all levels. Other factors, such as inappropriate or recent change in equipment, environmental conditions and competing surfaces, also may play a role.

A central concept in the assessment of an athlete, in particular when considering injury, relates to the delicate balance that exists between optimal mobility of a joint or a series of joints, and optimal stability. Frequently this balance is disrupted in the development of injury and must be considered in diagnosis and treatment of any athletic complaint.

History—The history addresses the injury, training and competing habits, the potential role of other extrinsic factors, previous injury history and other medical issues. The mechanism of injury is important in elucidating the diagnosis, as it will implicate the structures involved and the severity of the injury.

Pain is most frequently the cardinal symptom and a usual pain history is taken: its site(s), radiation, timing of onset and subsequent temporal pattern, aggravating and relieving features and associated symptoms. The degree of swelling and its rapidity of onset after injury frequently correlate with the severity of injury. Instability or a feeling of "pre-instability" are highly relevant in sport and may indicate a true structural deficit or a lack of neuromuscular control. Clicking and clunking of a joint is relevant, particularly if new or painful. Neurological symptoms may be present and may indicate a true neurological deficit or, more frequently, neural irritation in association with a chronic soft-tissue injury.

A history of treatments used to date, a medication history (including vitamins and supplements) and a general medical background are all important. For example, underlying medical com-

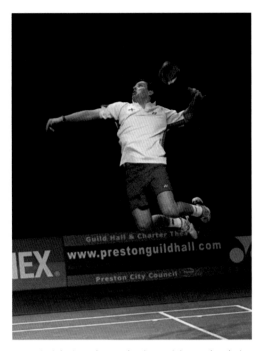

Figure 22.1 An insight into the mechanics, training and techniques of the sport is important in understanding sports injuries. This figure demonstrates the demands of a sport such as badminton, and the fine balance that exists between mobility and stability is a central concept in the consideration of sports injuries. Figure courtesy of Badminton England

Table 22.1 Common extrinsic and intrinsic factors in sports injuries

Intrinsic	Extrinsic
Hypermobility	Training: too much, too soon, too often
Muscle weakness/imbalance	Technique
Poor flexibility (local, general)	Equipment
Femoral anteversion	Surface
Tibia varum/valgum	Environment
Pes planus/cavus	Drugs (e.g. anabolic steroids/corticosteroids)
Presence of another injury	Poor nutrition
Chronic diseases (e.g. rheumatoid arthritis)	

plaints such as seronegative arthropathies will not infrequently masquerade as sports injuries, and other serious disorders including tumours should always be considered in an individual with regional musculoskeletal pain. In all athletes, underlying issues relating to bone health should always be considered. The age of the patient is also very important: children have fragile skeletons with vulnerable growth plates and an increased risk of avulsion injuries. The senior population have an increased susceptibility to soft-tissue injuries and the influence of co-morbidity requires consideration in diagnosis and management.

Examination—Examination commences with a general examination, in particular looking for stigmata of other disease, hypermo-

bility and assessment of the spine, as dysfunction here can contribute to injury. Assessment of asymmetry of muscle groups, flexibility and joint range of motion, is important but must be interpreted carefully. Core stability and control—the ability to control the body adequately during movement—should be assessed, as it is so often lacking in the injured athlete. Regional assessment of the injury follows the usual strategy of "look, feel, move and special tests". Identification of the site(s) of tenderness, swelling, instability and neurovascular status follows.

Although assessment commences with examination of the patient at relative rest, it is very important to proceed to dynamic assessment where there is any doubt about the nature and cause of the injury (Figure 22.2). It may be necessary to evaluate the individual during or after a rigorous set of exercises in order to reproduce symptoms. Video analysis may be very informative in illustrating the underlying factors contributing to injury; input from a coach or technical expert is also often helpful.

Investigations—Investigations (imaging in particular) are frequently required in the assessment of the injury, but should be requested only after a clinical diagnosis is made and interpreted carefully. No imaging is foolproof, and it is vital to request the correct test for the suspected injury.

Imaging includes plain X-rays, diagnostic ultrasound, magnetic resonance imaging (MRI), computed tomography (CT) and isotope bone scans. Plain X-rays assess for fractures, myositis ossificans, loose bodies and underlying joint damage but are not sensitive to early stress injuries. Stress views may be necessary to assess for instability. Diagnostic ultrasound demonstrates soft-tissue anatomy and impingements and allows dynamic assessment of the joint in question. MRI provides further information of the surrounding anatomy, bone oedema and some soft-tissue injuries (Figure 22.3), but MR arthrography is necessary to evaluate the labra of shoulder and hip most accurately. CT scanning for loose bodies, and scintigraphy for stress injuries in particular, may be indicated. Laboratory investigations for underlying medical complaints may be necessary.

Compartment studies, involving measurement of muscle compartment pressures before, during and after exercise are important in the evaluation of individuals with possible chronic exertional compartment syndromes.

Other investigations, such as dual X-ray absorptiometry scanning for those with recurrent stress fractures may be warranted. The sites of low bone density in athletes may differ from the general population in view of the different patterns of skeletal loading; scanning of sites such as the forearm is often necessary.

Management

The management of sports related injuries commences with an accurate diagnosis and identification of all the contributing factors. Education and counselling in relation to the injury, and discussion and agreement on an appropriate management strategy are vital. Appropriate levels of compliance will be enhanced by ensuring the athlete has a clear understanding of the injury, its implications and treatment. Clear goals need to be set, and reviewed regularly. Pain

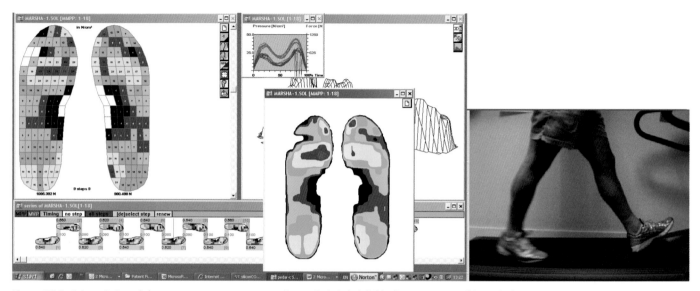

Figure 22.2 Gait analysis and shoe pressure measurement can be particularly helpful in the assessment of lower limb injuries

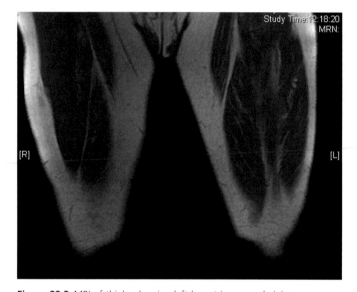

Figure 22.3 MRI of thighs showing left hamstrings muscle injury

Box 22.1 **Principles of management of sports injuries**

- Early diagnosis, identify and correct the mechanism
- In the acute phase: PRICES
- Control pain in order to allow rehabilitation to proceed
- Rehabilitation addresses flexibility, strengthening, proprioception, sports-specific work such as agility, speed, power, technique
- Graduated return to sport

Pain control may be necessary in order to allow rehabilitation to proceed. This may be in the form of ice/heat modalities, simple analgesics or non-steroidal anti-inflammatory drugs. Injections may be useful. For example, local anaesthetic may be used to identify the source of pain, and corticosteroid for chronic injuries in which inflammation is ongoing. Injudicious loading under the influence of analgesia, and in particular corticosteroid, must be avoided.

Surgery may be required—either early, or if other management approaches fail. The decision to intervene operatively will depend upon the nature of the injury and the circumstances of the athlete. For example, elite athletes may choose to have surgical intervention in the hope it will speed recovery to promote a swift return to sport. Surgery is never an isolated treatment; rehabilitation remains an essential part of management. Examples of indications for early surgical intervention include fractures, acute traumatic tendon ruptures, significant loose bodies and labral injuries, and exertional compartment syndromes.

Even when surgery is likely to be indicated, many injuries may be managed in the initial phases with rehabilitation (Figure 22.4). This may be termed "pre-habilitation": where strength and proprioception can be partly restored, enhancing the pace of postoperative recovery.

management is important, principally to allow rehabilitation to proceed. In the acute injury, the classical PRICES regime (protect, rest, ice, compression (if necessary), elevation, support) is followed. Rest is relative; the unaffected areas can and should continue to be exercised; for example, swimming or aquajogging after a tibial stress fracture. Supports and braces—such as a splint in ankle sprain, or boot in stress fractures of the foot—enable the individual to mobilize without overstressing the site of injury.

The most important aspect of management is rehabilitation, which, after the PRICE regime if necessary, addresses joint range of motion, proprioception, flexibility and strength issues initially. Underlying asymmetries in strength and flexibility are focused on, core stability is addressed and the patient then moves towards sports specific rehabilitation to include power, agility and control during appropriate activities (Box 22.1).

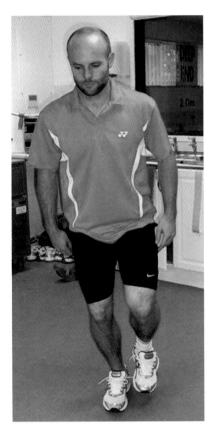

Figure 22.4 Rehabilitation involves progression from basic flexibility and strength exercises to sports-specific activities. Here, the athlete performs a single leg squat, a simple core stability exercise. Figure courtesy of Badminton England

Common sports injuries—the acute injury

Sports injuries can be broadly divided into acute injury and chronic overuse injury. The most common acute injuries involve ligaments (sprain) or muscles (strain) and vary enormously in severity in terms of the extent of injury (from a simple sprain/strain to a complete rupture), the muscle or ligament affected (e.g. a straight-forward long head of biceps tear to the problematic hamstring) and the location within the muscle/tendon complex (a midsubstance tear compared with a tear at the musculotendinous junction). The impact of any injury is of course further complicated by the functional aspirations of the individual and their age, which will affect the site of injury and the potential for healing. The most common acute sports injury is undoubtedly the ankle sprain.

Ankle sprain—Inversion injuries to the lateral ligament complex of the ankle are one of the most common causes of long-term disability after injury. Injuries initially occur in plantar flexion and slight inversion, such as at push off (Figure 22.5). Recurrent injuries can occur with minimal trauma, e.g. slipping on a kerb, indicating instability: functional (muscle weakness, loss of proprioception) or mechanical (significant ligament disruption).

After the acute injury, the degree of soft-tissue damage can be estimated by the extent of the swelling, and the likelihood of bone injury by clinical features (Box 22.2). Ankle sprain can result in additional damage that may cause either ongoing instability or chronic pain (Box 22.3). Popping, clicking, locking and neuralgia may all be significant.

Clinical assessment includes assessment of balance and proprioception, mechanical stability, sites and degree of tenderness, and neurovascular status. Management of the acute injury should focus on early mobilization, range of motion and strengthening exercises (particularly the peroneals) and proprioceptive work. Use of an ankle brace may help in an earlier return to sport.

Box 22.2 Ottawa Ankle Rules: when to X-ray for bony injury after ankle sprain

- Inability to bear weight and/or
- Bone tenderness at the posterior edge of the tibia or fibula or tip of either malleolus

---

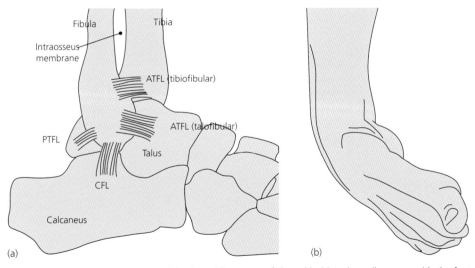

Figure 22.5 An ankle sprain involves a tear to one or more of the lateral ligaments of the ankle (a) and usually occurs with the foot in plantar flexion in slight inversion (b).

Box 22.3 Causes of pain and instability after ankle sprain

Articular injury
- Chondral/osteochondral fracture
- Meniscoid lesion

Bony injury
- Fibula

Nerve injury
- Superficial peroneal/posterior tibial/sural

Tendon injury
- Tibialis posterior (tear, tendinosis)
- Peroneal (subluxation/dislocation/tear/tendinosis)

Ligament injury
- Mechanical instability due to lateral ligament damage
- Syndesmosis/subtalar joint

Impingement
- Anterior osteophyte/anteroinferior tibiofibular ligament

Miscellaneous
- Failure to regain normal motion (tight Achilles tendon)
- Proprioceptive deficit with repetitive sprains (functional instability)

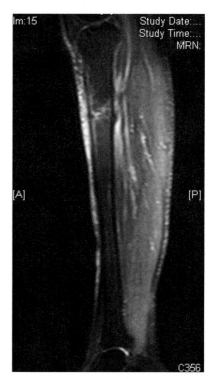

Figure 22.6 MRI showing a severe stress fracture of the proximal tibia

Box 22.4 Components of an exercise prescription

- Aerobic
  - Activities selection
    - Duration
    - Frequency
    - Intensity
- Resistance training
- Flexibility training

Address issues such as adverse biomechanics from osteoarthritis before commencing; counselling, supervision and progression of programme

Common sports injuries—the chronic/overuse injury

Whereas acute injuries are more common while working in a competitive sporting environment, the injury that presents most commonly to a sports medicine clinic is the overuse injury. Overuse injuries are defined by the inability of a normal structure to cope with an excessive load, as opposed to an insufficiency injury, in which a pathologically weak structure is unable to cope with a normal load. Overuse injury can affect the tendon (e.g. tendinopathy of which Achilles, patella and common elbow extensor and flexor are common), muscle (examples of which are chronic exertional compartment syndrome and medial tibial stress syndrome) and bone. The classical overuse bone injury is the stress fracture, the most common sites being the tibia, metatarsals and lumbar spine (spondylolysis), but they can occur in any loaded bone (e.g. ribs in rowers).

Stress fractures—Stress injuries to bone are a common reaction to repetitive loading of the skeleton without adequate time for remodelling. Although most stress injuries are fatigue-related, the possibility of insufficiency fractures, particularly in lightweight athletes, must always be considered. Most stress fractures will respond to relative rest, support and correction of the underlying cause (training, biomechanics, equipment errors). However, certain stress fractures are associated with an increased risk of poor healing/completion, including the superior surface of the femoral neck, anterior tibial cortex and navicular. These are areas that are under tension (rather than compression) and/or have poor vascular supply. They are managed either by non-weight-bearing and close monitoring or early surgical intervention (Figure 22.6).

Exercise prescription

The benefits of exercise in the prevention and management of disease are well established. Many patients with rheumatological diseases should be given an exercise prescription, as many are at increased risk of medical complications such as osteoporosis and cardiovascular events. Current recommendations are that adults aged 18 to 65 years need moderate-intensity aerobic physical activity for a minimum of 30 minutes on 5 days each week or vigorous-intensity aerobic physical activity for a minimum of 20 minutes on 3 days each week and strengthening exercise two to three times weekly. This may need to be modified for those with diseases such as rheumatoid arthritis, but provides a target.

The exercise prescription has a number of components (Box 22.4), which are adjusted according to the individual's needs, characteristics (e.g. age) and preferences. Patients in moderate- to severe-cardiac-risk groups should be assessed with an exercise test before commencing a programme. Supervision of patients may be necessary. Compliance is enhanced by education and counselling, careful prescription in choice of activities, written information about the programme, goal setting and frequent follow up, which may be done by telephone.

Summary

The evidence supporting the benefits of exercise/an active lifestyle both in preserving and restoring health is irrefutable. An active lifestyle will inevitably result in occasional musculoskeletal "injury", and while sports and exercise medicine has now been recognized as a medical specialty and thus should have increased NHS provision, the rheumatologist will still have a valuable role in contributing to the wider impact of activity-related musculoskeletal injury. It is therefore important that rheumatologists are confident in the assessment and rehabilitation of the exercising individual.

Further reading

Brukner P, Kahn K. *Clinical Sports Medicine*, 3rd edn. McGraw-Hill, Australia, 2007.

MacAuley D. *Oxford Handbook of Sport and Exercise Medicine*, 1st edn. Oxford University Press, Oxford, 2007.

MacAuley D, Best T. *Evidenced-based Sports Medicine*, 1st edn. BMJ Publishing Group, London, 2002.

CHAPTER 23

Vasculitis and Related Rashes

Richard A Watts[1,2] and David G I Scott[3]

[1]University of East Anglia, Norwich, UK
[2]Ipswich Hospital NHS Trust, Ipswich, UK
[3]Norfolk and Norwich University Hospital NHS Trust, Norwich, UK

OVERVIEW

- Systemic vasculitis should be considered in the differential diagnosis of all patients presenting with multi-system illness.
- Cytoplasmic anti-neutrophil cytoplasmic antibodies (cANCA) with proteinase 3 antibodies are associated with Wegener's granulomatosis, and perinuclear ANCA (pANCA) with myeloperoxidase antibodies are associated with microscopic polyangiitis.
- Urinalysis is a key investigation, as renal involvement is a major determinant of outcome.
- Treatment depends on the type of vasculitis, following guidelines from the British Society for Rheumatology and the European League against Rheumatism.
- Cyclophosphamide therapy should be used only for induction of remission; maintenance therapy should be with azathioprine or methotrexate in combination with glucocorticoids.

The vasculitides are a heterogeneous group of uncommon diseases characterized by inflammatory cell infiltration and necrosis of blood-vessel walls. Systemic necrotizing vasculitis can be rapidly life-threatening, so early accurate diagnosis and treatment is vital. Vasculitis may be primary (Wegener's granulomatosis, Churg–Strauss syndrome, microscopic polyangiitis and polyarteritis nodosa) or secondary to established connective tissue disease (such as rheumatoid arthritis), infection or malignancy. The severity of vasculitis is related to the size and site of the vessels affected. Classification is based on vessel size and determines the treatment approach (Table 23.1; Box 23.1).

Large-vessel vasculitis

Large-vessel vasculitis includes giant cell arteritis and Takayasu's arteritis. Giant cell arteritis is described elsewhere (Chapter 17). Takayasu's arteritis is uncommon and affects young adults, who initially present with a non-specific illness and later with loss of pulse, claudication (especially of the upper limbs) and stroke.

Medium-vessel vasculitis

Classical polyarteritis nodosa

A multi-system vasculitis characterized by formation of microaneurysms in medium-sized arteries. Patients present with a consti-

---

Box 23.1 **Symptoms suggestive of vasculitis**

Systemic
- Malaise
- Fever
- Weight loss
- Myalgia
- Arthralgia

Skin
- Purpura (palpable)
- Ulceration
- Infarction

Gastrointestinal
- Mouth ulcers
- Abdominal pain
- Diarrhoea

Respiratory
- Cough
- Wheeze
- Haemoptysis
- Dyspnoea

Ear, nose and throat
- Epistaxis
- Crusting
- Sinusitis
- Deafness

Cardiac
- Chest pain

Neurological
- Sensory or motor impairment

ABC of Rheumatology, 4th edn. Edited by Ade Adebajo.
©2010 Blackwell Publishing Ltd. 9781405170680.

Table 23.1 Classification of vasculitis

Vessels predominantly affected	Primary	Secondary
Large arteries	Giant cell arteritis Takayasu's arteritis	Aortitis associated with rheumatoid arthritis Infection (syphilis) Infection (hepatitis B)
Medium arteries	Classic polyarteritis nodosa Kawasaki disease	
Medium arteries and small vessels	Wegener's granulomatosis Churg–Strauss syndrome Microscopic polyangiitis	Rheumatoid arthritis, systemic lupus erythematosus Sjögren's syndrome Drugs Infection (HIV)
Small vessels (leucocytoclastic)	Henoch–Schönlein purpura Cryoglobulinaemia Leucocytoclastic vasculitis	Drugs Infection (hepatitis C)

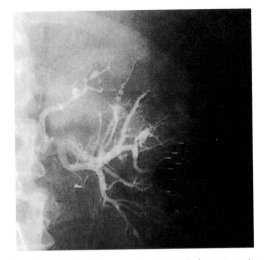

Figure 23.1 Coeliac axis arteriogram showing typical aneurysm in polyarteritis nodosa

tutional illness, which is often associated with rash, mononeuritis multiplex, vascular hypertension and organ infarction. Polyarteritis nodosa may be confined to the skin. Angiography shows typical microaneurysms (Figure 23.1). Polyarteritis nodosa is associated with hepatitis B infection.

Kawasaki disease (mucocutaneous lymph node syndrome)

An acute vasculitis that primarily affects infants and young children. It presents with fever, rash, lymphadenopathy and palmoplantar erythema. Coronary arteries become affected in up to one-quarter of untreated patients; this can lead to myocardial ischaemia and infarction.

Medium- and small-vessel vasculitis

This group includes the major necrotizing vasculitides: microscopic polyangiitis, Wegener's granulomatosis and Churg–Strauss syndrome, with involvement of both medium and small arteries. These may occur at any age, with the peak incidence at 60–70 years and are slightly more common in men. The annual incidence is about 20 cases per million people. The symptoms depend on the size and site of the vessel affected and on the individual diagnosis. They are associated with the presence of anti-neutrophil cytoplasmic antibodies (ANCA).

Wegener's granulomatosis

This is characterized by a granulomatous vasculitis of the upper and lower respiratory tracts and glomerulonephritis, but almost any organ system can be affected (Figure 23.2). The lungs are affected in 45% of patients at diagnosis. Symptoms in the ear, nose and throat (such as epistaxis, crusting and deafness) are particularly associated with this condition, and they should be sought in all patients with suspected vasculitis. Patients with limited Wegener's

granulomatosis—disease without renal involvement—may have a better prognosis. Biopsy of affected organs shows a necrotizing arteritis, often with formation of granulomas (Figure 23.3).

Microscopic polyangiitis

This is characterized by a vasculitis that commonly affects the kidneys. Lung involvement usually presents with haemoptysis caused by pulmonary capillaritis and haemorrhage (pulmonary-renal syndrome).

Biopsy of the kidney shows a focal segmental necrotizing glomerulonephritis with few immune deposits (sometimes called pauci-immune vasculitis).

Churg–Strauss syndrome

This syndrome is characterized by atopy (especially late-onset asthma), pulmonary involvement (75% of patients have radiographic evidence of infiltration) and eosinophilia in the tissues and peripheral blood ($>1 \times 10^9$/l). Such features can develop several years before the onset of systemic vasculitis. Cardiac involvement is a particular feature of Churg–Strauss syndrome and determines prognosis. Neuropathy is common.

Small-vessel vasculitis

Small-vessel vasculitis (leucocytoclastic or hypersensitivity) is usually confined to the skin, but it may be part of a systemic illness. The rash is purpuric, sometimes palpable, and occurs in dependent areas. The lesions may become bullous and ulcerate. Nailfold infarcts occur. Biopsy shows a cellular infiltrate of small vessels often with leucocytoclasis (fragmented polymorphonuclear cells and nuclear dust). Small-vessel vasculitis has a number of causes, of which drugs and infection are the most common.

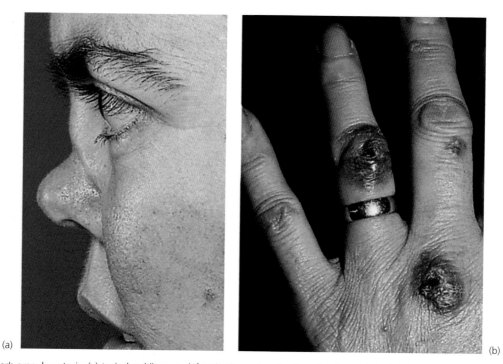

Figure 23.2 Wegener's granulomatosis; (a) typical saddle nose deformity (reproduced with patient's permission); (b) vasculitic rash

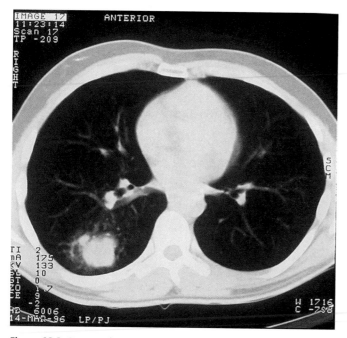

Figure 23.3 Computed tomography scan of thorax, showing a granuloma in Wegener's granulomatosis

Henoch–Schönlein purpura

This is a form of small-vessel vasculitis that occurs mainly in children and young adults. Patients present with rash, arthritis, abdominal pain and, sometimes, renal involvement (Figure 23.4). Deposits of immunoglobulin A can be detected histologically in the skin and renal mesangium.

Cryoglobulinaemia

Cryoglobulins are plasma proteins that precipitate in the cold. The condition presents with rash (including purpura digital ischaemia and ulcers) (Figure 23.5), arthralgia and neuropathy. A strong link exists between infection with hepatitis C virus and essential mixed cryoglobulinaemia: 80–90% of such patients are positive for anti-hepatitis C virus antibodies.

Behçet's syndrome

Behçet's syndrome is a systemic vasculitis of unknown aetiology, characterized by oro-genital ulceration. It is most common in Turkey and Japan. Ocular involvement occurs early in the disease course and affects 50% of patients. The pathergy phenomenon is characteristic and is a non-specific hyperreactivity in response to minor trauma.

Investigation

Investigation aims to establish and confirm the diagnosis, the extent and severity of organ involvement, and disease activity (Box 23.2).

Urine analysis

This is the most important investigation, because the severity of renal involvement is one of the key determinants of prognosis. Detection of proteinuria or haematuria in a patient with systemic illness needs immediate further investigation, and the patient is a medical emergency.

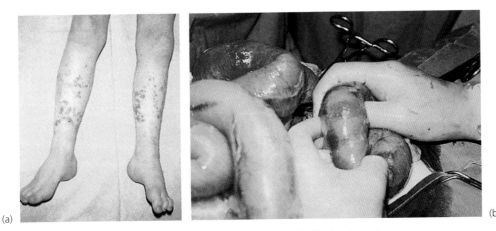

(a)   (b)

Figure 23.4 Small-vessel vasculitis in Henoch–Schönlein purpura; (a) affecting the skin; (b) affecting the gut

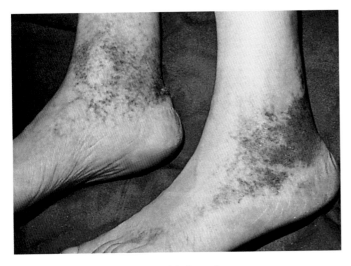

Figure 23.5 Vasculitic rash in cryoglobulinaemia

Blood tests

Leucocytosis suggests a primary vasculitis or infection. Leucopaenia is associated with vasculitis secondary to a connective tissue disease (typically systemic lupus erythematosus). Eosinophilia suggests Churg–Strauss syndrome or a drug reaction.

Liver function tests

Abnormal results suggest viral infection (hepatitis A, B or C) or may be non-specific.

Immunology

ANCA are associated with the primary systemic necrotizing vasculitides. ANCA in association with proteinase 3 antibodies are highly specific (>90%) for Wegener's granulomatosis. Perinuclear ANCA (pANCA) associated with myeloperoxidase antibodies occur in microscopic polyangiitis and Churg–Strauss syndrome. Rheumatoid factors and antinuclear antibodies may indicate vasculitis associated with connective tissue disease. Complement levels are low in infection, lupus and cryoglobulinaemia.

> **Box 23.2 Investigation of vasculitis**
>
> **Assessing inflammation**
> - Blood count and differential (total white cell count, eosinophils)
> - Acute-phase response (erythrocyte sedimentation rate, C-reactive protein)
> - Liver function
>
> **Assessment of organ involvement**
> - Urine analysis (proteinuria, haematuria, protein excretion)
> - Renal function (creatinine clearance, 24-hour protein excretion, urine protein/creatinine ratio biopsy)
> - Chest radiograph
> - Liver function
> - Nervous system (nerve-conduction studies, biopsy)
> - Cardiac function (electrocardiography, echocardiography)
> - Gut (angiography)
>
> **Immunological tests**
> - Antineutrophil cytoplasmic antibodies (including proteinase 3 and myeloperoxidase antibodies)
> - Other autoantibodies (rheumatoid factor, antinuclear antibodies, anticardiolipin antibodies)
> - Complement
> - Cryoglobulins
>
> **Differential diagnosis**
> - Blood cultures
> - Viral serology
> - Echocardiography

Biopsy

Tissue biopsy is important to confirm the diagnosis before treatment with potentially toxic immunosuppressive drugs. The choice of tissue to biopsy is crucial.

Other investigations

Angiography can show aneurysms. Blood cultures, viral serology and echocardiography are important to exclude infection and other conditions that may present as systemic multi-system disease and mimic vasculitis (Boxes 23.3 and 23.4).

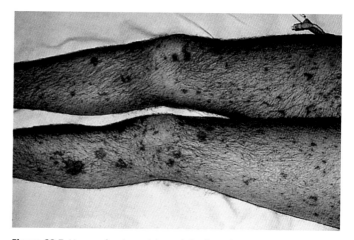

Figure 23.7 Haemorrhagic pustular rash in disseminated infection with *Neisseria meningitidis*

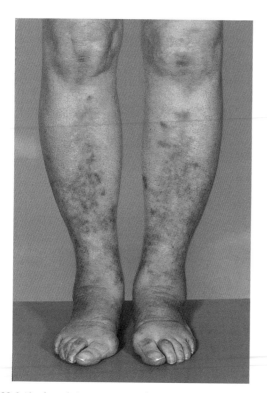

Figure 23.6 Livedo rash in cutaneous polyarteritis nodosa

Differential diagnosis

Livedo reticularis

Livedo reticularis is characterized by persistent patchy reddish-blue mottling of the legs (and occasionally arms) that is exacerbated by cold weather. It may lead to ulceration and is associated with vascular thrombosis (Sneddon's syndrome) and the presence of antiphospholipid antibodies. It is also a feature of polyarteritis nodosa (Figure 23.6) and cryoglobulinaemia.

Bacterial infections

Direct bacterial infection of small arteries and arterioles causes a necrotizing vasculitis or thrombosis. *Neisseria meningitidis* (Figure 23.7), *N. gonorrhoeae* (Figure 23.8) and *Streptobacillus moniliformis*, for example, may infect the vascular endothelium directly and cause maculopapular or purpuric skin lesions. Biopsies of early lesions show small-vessel vasculitis. The organisms can be cultured from an aspirate of the lesions.

Infective endocarditis

Several organisms—streptococci, staphylococci, Gram-negative bacilli and *Coxiella*—can cause endocarditis. Polyarthritis may be accompanied by splinter haemorrhages, Janeway's lesions (red macules over thenar and hypothenar eminences) (Figure 23.9), Osler's nodes (tender papules over extremities of fingers and toes) and clubbing. Diagnosis is by blood culture and echocardiography.

Cholesterol embolism

Cholesterol embolism (Figure 23.10) may occur spontaneously or after trauma to the aortic wall during vascular surgery or angiographic procedures. Typical cutaneous manifestations are ischaemia of the digits, particularly the toes, from abdominal atheroma, emboli and livedo reticularis. Digital ischaemia usually presents as sudden onset of a small, cool, cyanotic and painful area of the foot (usually the toe). The lesions are tender to touch and may progress to ulceration, digital infarction and gangrene; this mimics systemic vasculitis. Presentation may be with a systemic illness caused by tissue inflammation; features include eosinophilia and a positive test for ANCA.

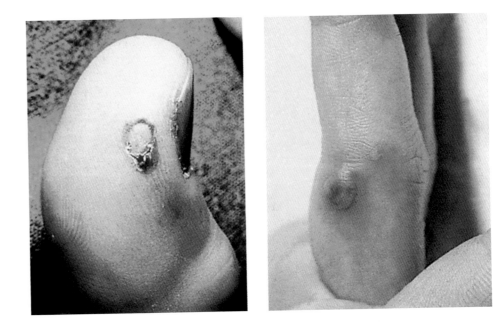

Figure 23.8 Gonococcal pustules in disseminated infection with *Neisseria gonorrhoeae*

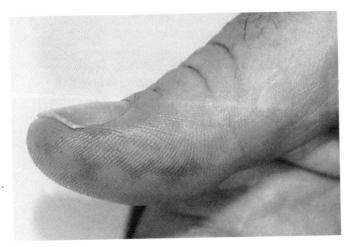

Figure 23.9 Janeway's lesions in infective endocarditis

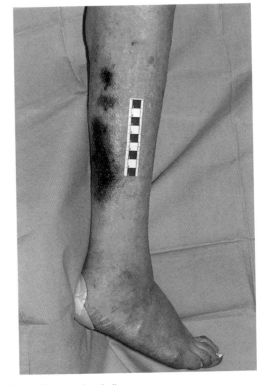

Figure 23.10 Cholesterol emboli

Atrial myxoma

Cardiac myxomata are rare benign tumours found most often in the left atrium (90% of cases). Constitutional symptoms and systemic embolization may lead to a wrong diagnosis of vasculitis. Systemic manifestations seen in 90% of cases include fever, weight loss, Raynaud's phenomenon, clubbing, elevated acute-phase proteins and hypergammaglobulinaemia. It is treated by surgical resection of the primary tumour and emboli.

Antiphospholipid antibody syndrome

Antiphospholipid antibody syndrome may present as catastrophic widespread thrombosis, and this can mimic systemic vasculitis. Livedo reticularis is the most typical cutaneous lesion, and it occurs in association with thrombosis and recurrent fetal loss.

Cocaine abuse

Cocaine abuse can cause destruction of the nasal mucosa and septum, mimicking systemic vasculitis.

Prognosis

The natural history of untreated primary systemic vasculitis is of a rapidly progressive, usually fatal disease. Before corticosteroids were introduced in Wegener's granulomatosis, the median survival was 5 months, with 82% of patients dying within 1 year and more than 90% within 2 years. The introduction of corticosteroids improved survival in polyarteritis nodosa to 50% at 5 years. The median survival in Wegener's granulomatosis was only 12.5 months using corticosteroids alone, with most patients dying of sepsis or uncontrolled disease. The introduction of oral low-dose cyclophosphamide combined with prednisolone resulted in a significant improvement in the mortality of Wegener's granulomatosis, with a survival rate at 5 years of 82%.

Small-vessel vasculitis confined to the skin without necrotizing features has an excellent prognosis. Takayasu's arteritis has a good prognosis (3% mortality) but typically relapses.

Treatment

Treatment depends on the size of vessel involved (Box 23.5). Small vessel vasculitis can often be treated conservatively. Takayasu's arteritis requires high-dose corticosteroids (oral prednisolone 40–60 mg/day), and additional immunosuppression with methotrexate or azathioprine. The dose of corticosteroid should be reduced rapidly according to clinical and laboratory parameters.

Box 23.5 **Aims of management of vasculitis**

- Induction of remission
- Maintenance of remission
- Recognition and early treatment of relapse
- Avoidance of drug toxicity

Table 23.2 Treatment regimens for cyclophosphamide

Drug	Dose
Continuous low oral dose	
Cyclophosphamide	2 mg/kg/day
Prednisolone	1 mg/kg/day
Intravenous pulse*	
Cyclophosphamide	10–15 mg/kg†
Prednisolone	1 g

Cyclophosphamide dose should be adjusted according to white cell count, renal function and clinical response
*Pulse frequency: fortnightly (×3), then three-weekly; adjusted according to clinical response and toxicity
†White cell count should be checked 7, 10 and 14 days after the first two pulses and immediately before subsequent pulses. For oral cylophosphamide the white cell count should be checked weekly for one month, fortnightly for two months and then every month.

The recently completed European randomized controlled trials in ANCA-associated vasculitis now guide the treatment approach. For patients with generalized disease, cyclophosphamide (Table 23.2) is used for remission induction and can be given either as continuous low-dose oral therapy or intermittent pulse therapy. Both routes are equally effective at inducing remission, but pulse therapy is probably associated with a slightly higher relapse rate. The major toxicities of cyclophosphamide are haemorrhagic cystitis, formation of bladder tumours, infertility and infection. Toxicity depends on the cumulative dose, so pulse therapy is less toxic. Mesna may reduce the frequency of bladder toxicity with intravenous cyclophosphamide. The risk of ovarian failure depends on age and cumulative dose of cyclophosphamide. Fertile males should be offered sperm storage before they are given cyclophosphamide. Prophylaxis with co-trimoxazole should be considered to prevent infection with *Pneumocystis jiroveci*. Immunosuppressed patients should receive vaccination with influenza and polyvalent pneumococcal vaccination.

Corticosteroids are started at a dose of 1 mg/kg, and the dose is reduced quite rapidly so that the drug can be discontinued at around 12 months. Alternate-day dosing may reduce the risk of infection. Intravenous methylprednisolone is often given with the first two pulses.

Once remission has been achieved with cyclophosphamide (usually after 3–6 months), azathioprine (or weekly oral methotrexate) is substituted for maintenance therapy. Cyclophosphamide should not be continued for more than 1 year because of the risks of toxicity. Survival has improved and remission can be obtained in most patients (85%) with cyclophosphamide, but many need prolonged immunosuppressive therapy (5–10 years), and the rate of relapse is still substantial (50% at 5 years).

Methotrexate may be considered in patients with localized disease, as an alternative to cyclophosphamide.

Patients with life-threatening disease (pulmonary haemorrhage) or a creatinine >500 μmol/l should receive plasma exchange in addition to intravenous methylprednisolone.

Regular assessment of disease activity is required, and treatment is tailored accordingly. Minor relapses may require an increase in maintenance therapy. Major relapses will require a further course of cyclophosphamide.

Intravenous immunoglobulin is effective in the treatment of Kawasaki disease, but its role in other vasculitides, where it induces temporary improvement, remains controversial at present. Etanercept does not improve relapse rate when used as adjunctive therapy to conventional therapy for remission maintenance. The role of tumour-necrosis-factor-α-blocking drugs in induction is uncertain. B-cell depletion with rituximab is a promising approach that is being investigated.

Further reading

Ball GV, Bridges L, eds. *Vasculitis*, 2nd edn. Oxford: Oxford University Press, Oxford, 2007.
Birck R, Scmitt W, Kaelsch IA, van Der Woude FJ. Serial ANCA determinations for monitoring disease activity in patients with ANCA-associated vasculitis: systematic review. *American Journal of Kidney Diseases* 2006; **47**: 15–23.

De Groot K, Rasmussen N, Bacon P *et al*. Randomised trial of cyclophosphamide versus methotrexate for induction of remission in early systemic antineutrophil cytoplasmic antibody associated vasculitis. *Arthritis and Rheumatism* 2005; **52**: 2462–2468.

Jayne D, Rasmussen N, Andrassy K *et al*. A randomised trial of maintenance therapy for vasculitis associated with antineutrophil cytoplasmic auto antibodies. *New England Journal of Medicine* 2003; **349**: 36–44.

Jayne D, Gaskin G, Rasmussen N *et al*. Randomised trial of plasma exchange or high dose methylprednisolone as adjunctive therapy for severe renal vasculitis. *Journal of the American Society of Nephrology* 2007; **18**: 2180–2188.

Lapraik C, Watts RA, Scott DG. BSR & BHPR guidelines for the management of adults with ANCA associated vasculitis. *Rheumatology* 2007; **46**: 1615–1616.

Maksimowicz-McKinnon K, Clark TM, Hoffman GC. Limitations of therapy and a guarded prognosis in an American cohort of Takayasu arteritis patients. *Arthritis and Rheumatism* 2007; **56**: 1000–1009.

Mukhtyar C, Guillevin L, Dasgupta B *et al*. EULAR recommendations for the management of primary small and medium vessel vasculitis. *Annals of the Rheumatic Diseases* 2009; **68**: 310–317.

Mukhtyar C, Guillevin L, Cid M *et al*. EULAR recommendations for the management of large vessel vasculitis. *Annals of the Rheumatic Diseases* 2009; **68**: 318–323.

Reinhold-Keller E, Beuge N, Latza U *et al*. An interdisciplinary approach to the care of patients with Wegener's granulomatosis. *Arthritis and Rheumatism* 2000; **43**: 1021–1032.

CHAPTER 24

Laboratory Tests

Cynthia Aranow[1], Margaret J Larché[2] and David A Isenberg[3]

[1]Feinstein Institute for Medical Research, Manhasset, USA
[2]McMaster University, Hamilton, Ontario, Canada
[3]University College Hospital, London, UK

OVERVIEW

- Abnormal laboratory tests occur frequently in patients with rheumatologic disorders.
- Laboratory abnormalities suggesting non-specific inflammation are common and accompany many rheumatologic disorders.
- Routine blood tests (haematology and chemistry) are useful to monitor known rheumatologic diseases and may be helpful in diagnosis. Abnormalities may reflect adverse effects of medications or may indicate organ involvement from an underlying rheumatologic disease.
- Immunological testing is primarily for diagnostic purposes and may help subsetting patients (e.g. patients with systemic lupus erythematosus who are anti-Ro positive are more likely to be photosensitive); however, the antinuclear antibody test is not a diagnostic test.
- Genetic testing (such as HLA-B27) is expensive and not a diagnostic tool.

This chapter describes investigations that may be performed in a patient with suspected and known rheumatologic disorders. Abnormal haematology tests, particularly anaemias and platelet abnormalities, are found commonly. Biochemical abnormalities include raised protein and globulin levels and reflect a non-specific inflammatory response. Haematological and biochemical investigations are useful for both diagnostic and monitoring purposes, while most immunological investigations are mainly used to facilitate diagnosis.

Haematology investigations

A full blood count and erythrocyte sedimentation rate (ESR) are used to monitor disease activity, to assess the effects of drug treatment, to exclude factors such as dietary deficiency or haemolysis that may be contributing to the morbidity of a rheumatological

disease, and (rarely) to exclude a primary haematologic malignancy that can mimic various forms of arthritis (Table 24.1).

Platelet abnormalities

Platelet abnormalities are often seen in rheumatic disorders; the most common abnormality is a mild to moderate thrombocytosis, which correlates with disease activity. Thrombocytopenia may occur as a side effect of interventional treatments such as methotrexate, cyclophosphamide or mycophenolate mofetil. Thrombocytopenia may also be observed in patients receiving treatment with gold or penicillamine; however, these medications are now rarely used. An autoimmune thrombocytopenia (usually chronic but occasionally acute) occurs in up to 20% of patients with lupus and in patients with primary antiphospholipid antibody syndrome. In some of these patients it has been possible to demonstrate the presence of antiplatelet antibodies. Approximately 15% of patients with "idiopathic" thrombocytopenia later develop lupus. Thrombocytopenia may also be seen in the subset of rheumatoid arthritis with Felty's syndrome (see below). Infections associated with arthralgia such as cytomegalovirus, hepatitis C and HIV can additionally be associated with thrombocytopenia.

White blood cell abnormalities

Felty's syndrome, the association of rheumatoid arthritis with leucopenia (predominantly neutropenia) and splenomegaly (and often leg ulcers), is rare. Leucopenia, particularly lymphopenia, is common in lupus. Bone-marrow suppression is a well-recognized complication of immunosuppressive drugs such as azathioprine, methotrexate, leflunomide, sulfasalazine, cyclophosphamide and mycophenolate mofetil, which are used to treat rheumatoid arthritis, psoriatic arthritis and lupus. Patients taking these drugs require regular haematological assessments to allow early detection of bone-marrow suppression. Leucocytosis is occasionally found in flares of lupus, but is more often a reflection of corticosteroid-induced demargination of neutrophils. Infective causes of a leucocytosis (particularly neutrophilia) must be excluded. Less common abnormalities, such as monocytopenia and eosinophilia in rheumatoid arthritis and basopenia in lupus, are well described. A range of blood test abnormalities in rheumatological disease are shown in Table 24.2.

ABC of Rheumatology, 4th edn. Edited by Ade Adebajo.
©2010 Blackwell Publishing Ltd. 9781405170680.

Coagulation abnormalities

Lupus anticoagulant is discussed in the section on antiphospholipid antibodies.

Acute-phase response

This response defines a coordinated set of systemic and local events associated with the inflammation that is the consequence of tissue damage. The term is misleading, as changes may occur in both acute and chronic inflammation. About 30 acute-phase proteins are

known. Elevated serum concentrations of these proteins often last for several days after the initiating event, and their synthesis in the liver is triggered by cytokines—particularly interleukin-1 (IL-1), IL-6 and tumour necrosis factor-α (TNF-α). These cytokines derive from activated macrophages that have been demonstrated at the site of the injury. Other types of cells such as fibroblasts and endothelial cells are also sources of cytokines. There is some specificity in the cytokine–acute-phase reactant interactions: for example, the synthesis of C-reactive protein (CRP) is dependent on IL-6, while haptoglobin production is influenced by the three cytokines mentioned above.

Measurement of the acute-phase response is helpful to ascertain inflammatory disease, as well as for the assessment of disease activity, monitoring of therapy and the detection of intercurrent infection.

It is impractical and unnecessary to measure all aspects of the acute-phase response; the most widely used measurements are the ESR and CRP (Table 24.3). Less common measurements include plasma viscosity, serum amyloid A (SAA) protein, haptoglobin and fibrinogen.

Plasma levels of cytokines such as IL-6, IL-1 and TNF-α are not commercially available and are currently used solely as research tools. Other tests of potential use in the future are SAA protein and matrix metalloproteinase-3 (MMP-3); both may predict bone damage in early rheumatoid arthritis.

Biochemical investigations

The majority of biochemical tests are useful in monitoring organ-specific complications of disease or in assessment of side effects of therapy.

Hepatic function

Abnormalities in hepatic function may reflect disease activity in some rheumatic diseases (for example, elevated alkaline

Table 24.1 Anaemia and rheumatologic disease

Type	Indices	Causes

Iron-deficient	↓Serum Fe
	↑Serum TIBC
	Microcytosis, hypochromasia
		NSAIDs ⎱ Peptic
		Corticosteroids ⎰ ulcer disease
		Disease *per se*:
		  e.g. oesophagitis in
		  scleroderma

Megaloblastic	Macrocytosis ↓Folate ↓B$_{12}$ ↓TFTs	Azathioprine Methotrexate (↓folate) Pernicious anaemia
Haemolytic	Reticulocytes Haptoglobins Positive direct Coombs' test	SLE Drugs e.g. dapsone

Chronic disease	Normochromic,
	  normocytic
	↓serum iron, ↓TIBC,
	  ↑ferritin
		Multifactorial, ↓EPO, abnormal
		  erythrocyte development,
		  ↑cytokines e.g. IL-1, TNF-α

EPO = erythropoietin; IL-1 = interleukin-1; NSAIDs = non-steroidal anti-inflammatory drugs; TFT = thyroid function test; TIBC = total iron-binding capacity; TNF-α = tumour necrosis factor alpha

Table 24.2 Blood test abnormalities in some rheumatological diseases

		RA	SLE	PMR	Crystals	myositis	SSc	Osteoporosis	Osteo malacia
Anaemia	Chronic disease	++	++	+	−	−	++	−	−
	Microcytic/hypochromic	++	+	++	−	−	++	−	−
	Megaloblastic	++	−	−	−	−	−	−	−
Acute-phase response	ESR	++	++	+++	+/−	+	+	−	−
	CRP	+	−	+	+/−	−	−	−	−
Abnormal renal function		+	++	+/−	+	+/−	+	−	−
Abnormal liver function		+	+	−	−	−	−	−	−
Uric acid		−	−	−	+	−	−	−	−
Bone biochemistry	Alk phos	−	−	+	−	−	−	−	+/−
	Ca^{2+}	−	−	−	−	−	−	−	↓/−
	PO^{4-}	−	−	−	−	−	−	−	↓/−

Alk phos = alkaline phosphatase; CRP = C-reactive protein; ESR = erythrocyte sedimentation rate; PMR = polymyalgia rheumatica; RA = rheumatoid arthritis; SLE = systemic lupus erythematosus; SSc = systemic sclerosis

Table 24.3 Acute-phase reactants

Parameter	Measurement	Pathophysiology	Affected by
ESR	Distance in mm that RBC column falls in 1 hour	Dependant upon rouleaux formation (aggregation of red cells) and PCV Indirect reflection of acute-phase proteins and immunoglobulins	Plasma proteins (i.e. fibrinogen, β2 microglobulin and immunoglobulins) Anaemia, ↓ in sickle cell anaemia
CRP	Immunoassay (mg/l)	Pentameric protein released from liver under influence of IL-6 within 4 hours of tissue injury	↑↑ in infection, often normal in SLE

CRP = C-reactive protein; ESR = erythrocyte sedimentation rate; IL-6 = interleukin-6; PCV = packed cell volume; RBC = red blood cell; SLE = systemic lupus erythematosus

phosphatase activity has been reported in rheumatoid arthritis and polymyalgia rheumatica). Raised enzyme activities may be more frequent because of toxicity from drugs used to treat rheumatic diseases, notably methotrexate, azathioprine, cyclophosphamide, sulphasalazine and leflunomide. The recommended frequency of hepatic monitoring is dependent upon the particular pharmacologic intervention being used; however, a baseline assessment is generally recommended before initiating any of the drugs mentioned above.

Many of the "hepatic" enzymes and proteins originate in tissues other than the liver. Thus a common cause of an isolated rise in alkaline phosphatase activity is in Paget's disease, in which the patient's bone is the site of origin. Similarly, liver transaminases may be elevated in myositis due to muscle damage.

Renal function

Abnormal renal function may be a component of a rheumatic disease or a consequence of treatment. Non-steroidal anti-inflammatory drugs and methotrexate are often implicated in renal dysfunction and may necessitate a dose reduction or discontinuation of therapy. Measurement of plasma creatinine concentration is widely used as a test of renal function. However, it is not sensitive and requires a substantial loss of glomerular function before beginning to rise. The blood urea concentration is also an insensitive marker of renal function and is influenced by factors that include the rate of protein metabolism, adsorption of blood from the enteric tract and fluid balance. The chromium 51-labelled EDTA test, is an available and accurate measure of glomerular function. It is infrequently performed, as it is cumbersome to obtain and impractical for serial use.

Urinalysis is a simple method to detect renal involvement in patients with rheumatological disease. Patients with glomerulonephritis (accompanying vasculitis, lupus or other connective tissue diseases) will have an active urinary sediment with protein and/or blood on dipstick testing and red cells and granular or cellular casts on light microscopy.

Twenty-four-hour urine collection is the gold standard for quantification of proteinuria and to assess creatinine clearance. A spot urine protein : creatinine ratio is increasingly used, given its reliability and its ease of determination. Serial estimations of urinary

protein excretion are helpful to monitor treatment in rheumatologic patients with renal involvement.

Bone biochemistry

The main diseases of bone presented to rheumatologists are osteoporosis, osteomalacia and Paget's disease. The most commonly measured markers are serum alkaline phosphatase activity and serum calcium and phosphate concentrations. All three tend to be normal in osteoporosis, while a raised alkaline phosphatase activity of bone origin is the key biochemical feature of Paget's disease. Severe cases of osteomalacia are associated with hypocalcaemia, hypophosphataemia and increased alkaline phosphatase activity. Parathyroid hormone levels may be high, while vitamin D levels are usually low with this condition.

Biochemical markers of bone and cartilage turnover, such as the cross-linked collagen derivatives, pyridinoline, deoxypyridinoline and N-telopeptides, may be used to assess bone turnover in osteopenia and osteoporosis. During periods of high bone turnover, such as after menopause, Paget's disease and hyperparathyroidism, increased levels of these compounds are found in urine.

Other biochemical tests

Recent epidemiological studies suggest that patients with chronic inflammatory diseases such as rheumatoid arthritis and systemic lupus erythematosus (SLE) are predisposed to atherosclerosis independently of other risk factors. These patients should be screened for modifiable conditions such as diabetes and hyperlipidemia, which may confer increased atherosclerotic risk. Assessment of fasting glucose, lipids and perhaps homocysteine should be made in all patients with chronic inflammatory diseases.

Plasma urate is discussed in Chapter 10.

Muscle disease is associated with a rise in creatine kinase (CK) activity. This enzyme occurs as three isoenzymes: CK MM originates from skeletal muscle, CK BB from brain and thyroid, and CK MB from myocardium and regenerating skeletal muscle. Serial measurements of CK activity often reflect disease activity in myositis, but interpretation of markedly elevated values should include consideration of the effects of vigorous exercise and intramuscular injections, which can dramatically but temporarily raise enzyme activity. Levels of cardiac troponin I are typically absent in noncardiac muscle disease and a negative troponin I will help to exclude a potential cardiac origin for an elevated CK.

Immunological investigations

Autoantibodies

Autoantibodies are immunoglobulins that bind to self-antigens (molecules present in the patient's own tissues). Low concentrations of autoantibodies are present in the plasma of normal individuals and have a higher prevalence in the normal elderly population. These antibodies are overexpressed in autoimmune conditions, owing to a variety of factors, including genetic predisposition and environmental triggers such as infection. Autoantibodies may be divided into those directed against organ-specific antigens (such as the acetylcholine receptor in myasthenia gravis or intrinsic factor in pernicious anaemia) and those that bind to more ubiquitous antigens such as DNA or the phospholipid component of cell membranes (such as cardiolipin). Relatives of patients with rheumatic diseases may make autoantibodies reflecting a genetic tendency to autoimmunity; these antibodies are usually not organ-specific.

Detection of autoantibodies in rheumatic disorders (Table 24.4) is generally more useful for diagnosis than for monitoring disease activity.

Rheumatoid factors

These antibodies are immunoglobulins (Ig) that bind the Fc (constant region) of IgG. Several assays are available, including the classic Rose-Waaler test, which relies on the ability of rheumatoid factors to agglutinate sheep erythrocytes coated with anti-sheep immunoglobulin, and the latex agglutination test, in which latex particles coated with human IgG aggregate in the presence of IgM rheumatoid factor. These tests identify only the IgM isotype. Detection of IgG and IgA rheumatoid factors by enzyme-linked immunosorbent assay (ELISA) is now widely available. Oligoarticular rheumatoid arthritis may be associated with a negative test for IgM rheumatoid factor but a positive test for IgG rheumatoid factor. The clinical specificity of IgA rheumatoid factor is not clear, but has been found early in the course of rheumatoid arthritis. Reference ranges vary between laboratories.

An elevated rheumatoid factor has a definite but limited value as a diagnostic test for rheumatoid arthritis. The test is positive in 70–80% of patients with rheumatoid arthritis and in some patients with other disorders, including other arthritic conditions (such as lupus and Sjögren's syndrome). Rheumatoid factor positivity is additionally seen in infections such as tuberculosis, hepatitis B, hepatitis C and syphilis.

Antinuclear antibodies

Antinuclear antibodies (ANAs) are immunoglobulins that bind to antigens in the cell nucleus. ANAs are classically detected by immunofluorescence using murine liver or kidney cells, or a human epithelial cell line (HEp-2) (Figure 24.1). A titre of greater than 1:80 is usually considered positive, although autoimmune disease is generally associated with higher titres (ε1:320). Newer assays using ELISA or fluorescent microspheres (bead) technology) are increasingly utilized by commercial laboratories. A positive test for ANA is not diagnostic of SLE, as an ANA may occur in several

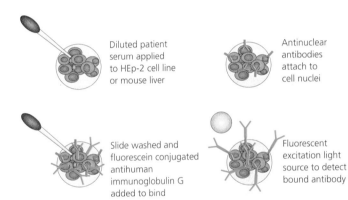

Figure 24.1 Indirect immunofluorescence for antinuclear antibodies. Serum from patients is diluted in serial doubling dilutions. A titre of 1:80 means that the patient's serum has been diluted by a factor of 80. The HEp-2 cell line is derived from human epithelial cells, which are cultured as a monolayer

Table 24.4 Autoantibodies associated with some rheumatological diseases

	RF	ANA	dsDNA	Ro	La	Sm	RNP	ANCA	Jo-1	Topoisomerase	Cardiolipin
RA	+++	+	–	+/–	+/–	–	–	–	–	–	–
SLE	+	+++	+++	++	++	++	++	–	–	–	++
Sjögrens	+	++	–	+++	+++	–	–	–	–	–	–
Myositis	–	++	–	–	–	–	–	–	+	–	–
SSc	–	++	–	–	–	–	–	–	+	+	–
Antiphospholipid syndrome	–	–	–	–	–	–	–	–	–	–	+++
Vasculitides	+	–	–	–	–	–	–	++	–	–	–

ANA = antinuclear antibody; ANCA = antineutrophil cytoplasmic antibody; DsDNA = double-stranded DNA; RA = rheumatoid arthritis; RF = rheumatoid factor; RNP = ribonuclear protein; SLE = systemic lupus erythematosus; SSc = systemic sclerosis conditions, including hepatic, pulmonary and haematological diseases and malignancy. In infectious diseases the test tends to be positive only transiently, but in the right clinical context a positive test is strongly suggestive of an autoimmune rheumatic disease.

The pattern of immunofluorescence varies according to which nuclear or cytoplasmic antigens are recognized (Table 24.5).

Antibodies to DNA

Anti-DNA antibodies are typically detected by an ELISA or immunofluorescence test with the haemoflagellated organism *Crithidia luciliae* (Figure 24.2).

Crithidia contains pure double-stranded DNA (dsDNA) in a very large mitochondrion, and a positive assay is virtually specific to patients with lupus. Antibodies to dsDNA are often found in high titres in lupus and are especially likely to be found in patients with renal disease. These antibodies are monitored in lupus patients, as they may reflect disease activity, and a rising titre may be predictive of a flare. There are reports of the development of anti-dsDNA antibodies following treatment with TNF-α antagonists. These

Table 24.5 Antinuclear antibody staining patterns: associations with immunological disease

ANA staining patterns	Antigen	Disease associations
Homogeneous	DNA or histone proteins	SLE
Speckled	RNA, Sm, Ro and La proteins	Sjögrens syndrome, overlap syndromes
Nucleolar	Nucleolar proteins	Scleroderma
Centromere	Proteins in centromere	Limited scleroderma

ANA = antinuclear antibody; SLE = systemic lupus erythematosus

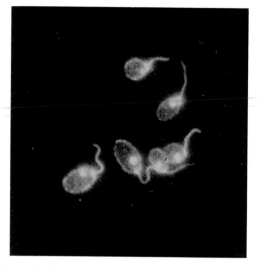

Figure 24.2 *Crithidia* staining

antibodies are predominantly of the IgM subtype and are rarely associated with a lupus-like syndrome.

Antibodies to extractable nuclear antigens

Antibodies to extractable nuclear antigens (ENAs) are directed against antigens such as Ro, La, Sm, ribonuclear protein (RNP), centromere and topoisomerase. They were initially detected by counter-immunoelectrophoresis, a technique in which serum is tested against a saline extract of mammalian nuclei and compared with reference sera to determine a line of precipitation. More specific tests for each antigen (which consist of varying combinations of RNA and protein) are now available in many laboratories and are performed using immunoblot or ELISA.

The identification of antibodies to one or more antigens in a patient's serum can be helpful in the diagnosis of an autoimmune disease (Table 24.4). For instance, antibodies to Sm are specific for lupus. Similarly, antibodies to Ro and La (also known as SS-A and SS-B) are often found in Sjögren's syndrome. Some antibodies relate to specific subtypes of disease—anti-topoisomerase-1 is found in 25% of patients with systemic sclerosis with pulmonary and cardiac involvement, while anti-Jo-1 antibodies are specific to patients with myositis (polymyositis or dermatomyositis) and pulmonary fibrosis. However, as seen in Table 24.4, there is considerable overlap between expression of clinical disease and expression of particular antibodies.

Longitudinal measurement of antibodies to ENAs is usually unnecessary, as there is no consistent association between titres and disease activity. However, the presence of high titres of ENAs in an asymptomatic subject may pre-date the onset of clinical disease.

Antibodies to cyclic citrullinated peptides

Antibodies to proteins involved in epithelial cell differentiation, known as filaggrins, are found in patients with rheumatoid arthritis. Antibodies to cyclic citrullinated peptides (CCPs), which cross-react with anti-filaggrin antibodies are 90% specific for rheumatoid arthritis. These antibodies are measured by ELISA and are available in many immunology labs.

Antiphospholipid antibodies

In the rheumatological context, antiphospholipid antibodies bind chiefly to negatively charged phospholipids such as cardiolipin. There are four tests available. The lupus anticoagulant test measures the ability of antiphospholipid antibodies to prolong clotting times (e.g. partial thromboplastin time, Russell's viper venom time) (Figure 24.3). The simplest and cheapest antiphospholipid test is the ELISA for anticardiolipin antibodies. It allows detection and quantitation of IgG, IgM or IgA antibodies against the phospholipid cardiolipin. The Venereal Disease Research Laboratory test is used in the diagnosis of syphilis and utilizes a variety of phospholipids. Antibodies in test plasma may bind to these, creating a false-positive test for syphilis. This test is of limited diagnostic value for the detection of antiphospholipid antibodies. A fourth overlapping population of antiphospholipid antibodies comprises antibodies to a co-factor-binding protein, β2 glycoprotein-I. Similar to antibodies that directly bind phospholipid, anti-β2 glycoprotein-I antibodies are useful as markers of future thrombotic

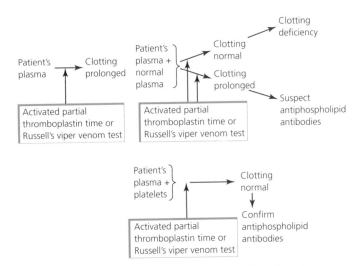

Table 24.6 Changes in C3, C4 and/or CH50 in diseases

Change in C3, C4 or CH50	Characteristic conditions	Cause
↑↑ ↑	Bacterial infections Inflammatory diseases, including RA and seronegative arthritides	Part of acute-phase response
↓	SLE, especially lupus nephritis, other vasculitides	Consumption by immune complexes
↓	Hereditary hypocomplementemic syndromes	Hereditary

RA = rheumatoid arthritis; SLE = systemic lupus erythematosus

Figure 24.3 Detection of the lupus anticoagulant. Although the lupus anticoagulant is associated with thrombotic episodes *in vivo*, paradoxically the *in vitro* test relies on prolongation of the activated partial thromboplastin time (or Russell's viper venom test, or the kaolin-cephalin clotting time). This is thought to be due to the interaction with the phospholipid portion of the prothrombin activator complex of the clotting cascade. When normal plasma is added to patient plasma, clotting factors are replenished and a clotting-factor-deficiency-related clotting prolongation will be corrected; however, if antiphospholipid antibodies are the cause of an abnormal test result, the clotting time will not correct. An excess of phospholipids may be added in the form of platelets, which should then correct the clotting prolongation

or neurological events in patients with SLE and/or anti-phospholipid antibody syndrome (APLS).

Persistently raised concentrations of antiphospholipid antibodies (notably of the IgG isotype) associate with APLS. This syndrome consists of several clinical features including thrombosis (both arterial and venous), recurrent fetal loss, thrombocytopenia and various neurological disorders. APLS may occur in isolation or in the context of a connective tissue disease such as lupus.

Antineutrophil cytoplasmic antibodies

These are antibodies that bind to antigens in the cytoplasm of neutrophils and are often found in patients with vasculitides. The standard test is immunofluorescence demonstrated on normal neutrophils. Usually, one of two patterns is seen: a diffuse "cytoplasmic" staining (cANCA) or a "peripheral or perinuclear" staining pattern around the edge of the nucleus (pANCA). Different proteins are bound by cANCA and pANCA; cANCA binds almost exclusively to serine proteinase 3, while pANCA binds to myeloperoxidase (MPO) as well as other proteins. Antibodies to serine proteinase 3 and MPO may be directly measured by ELISA.

Antibodies to serine proteinase 3 are found in about 80% of patients with Wegener's granulomatosis. Those against MPO are seen in patients with vasculitides such as microscopic polyangiitis and Churg–Strauss syndrome. Antibodies to other antigens, including lactoferrin, elastase, cathepsin G, catalase and lysozyme, stain as a pANCA and have been identified in patients with lupus, rheumatoid arthritis and inflammatory bowel diseases.

Immunoglobulins

A polyclonal rise in immunoglobulins is common in inflammation. In Sjögren's syndrome total IgG concentrations may be substantially raised, often up to 30 g/l or more. Quantification of immunoglobulins and determination of their subtype by protein electrophoresis should be performed in patients with Sjögren's syndrome, as these patients have approximately a 40 times increased risk of developing lymphoma.

Complement

Proteins of the complement cascade play a central role in cell lysis, opsonization of bacteria and clearance of immune complexes. C3 and C4 components are most commonly measured (and in some laboratories CH50, which is a measure of overall integrity of the complement pathway) and are useful in screening for complement deficiencies (Table 24.6).

Complement degradation products, particularly C3d and C4d, are currently available as research tools as markers of SLE disease activity.

Genetic associations

Most rheumatic disorders are polygenic, and analysis of genetic markers is of limited value. Close human leucocyte antigen (HLA) associations are found with diseases such as ankylosing spondylitis and rheumatoid arthritis. In the former, 95% of patients possess an HLA-B27 allele. The frequency of B27 in the general population is around 10%. However, HLA typing is expensive and usually unnecessary, as it is never diagnostic. A thorough clinical assessment with appropriate haematological, biochemical, immunological and radiological investigations should lead to a definitive diagnosis. HLA haplotype determinations are not tests for specific diseases, because HLA haplotypes do not associate with individual rheumatological diseases; furthermore, family members of patients with rheumatic diseases (e.g. ankylosing spondylitis) may have a rheumatic-disease-associated HLA and no clinical disease.

Microbiology

The differential diagnosis in any acute monoarthropathy must include septic arthritis. This is easily excluded by joint aspiration, with culture of synovial fluid and blood. It is necessary to inform the laboratory if tuberculosis or gonococcal infections are suspected, as specific culture media and techniques are required. Polyarthropathies may be associated with several viral and bacterial infections. Chronic hepatitis B or C or HIV infection may cause polyarthralgia. Acute rheumatic fever, which is still a major killer on a worldwide scale but rare in the Western world, is associated with streptococcal infection (i.e. positive anti-streptolysin O titre or *Streptococcus* species in blood or throat cultures). The seronegative spondyloarthropathies may be related temporally to a diarrhoeal illness or to urethritis. Organisms often implicated in these diseases include *Salmonella*, *Yersinia*, *Campylobacter* and *Chlamydia*. Parvovirus B19 has been associated with a self-limiting polyarthritis similar to rheumatoid arthritis. Other viruses such as rubella and human T-lymphotropic virus may present with an arthralgia. Lyme disease is associated with a rash and polyarthropathy and the diagnosis depends on demonstration of antibodies to the spirochaete *Borrelia burgdorferi*.

Conclusions

Blood tests are useful in terms of assessment, diagnosis and monitoring in rheumatological diseases. There is a trend for laboratories (particularly in the USA) to use "rheumatology screens" with an array of markers often including rheumatoid factor, antinuclear antibody and ESR and CRP. This is not to be recommended, as it leads to many false-positive results. Blood tests should be used judiciously where there is an indication.

Further reading

Hakim G, Clunie A. Haq I. *Oxford Handbook of Rheumatology*, 2nd edn. Oxford University Press, Oxford, 2002.

Hochberg MC, Silman AJ, Smolen JS, Weinblatt ME, Weisman MH, *Rheumatology*, 4th edn. Mosby, St Louis, 2008.

Playfair JHL, Chain B. *Immunology at a Glance*, 9th edn. Wiley, Chichester, 2009.

Shipley M, Black CM, Compston J, O'Grabaigh D. Rheumatology. In: Kumar R, Clark M, eds. *Clinical Medicine*, 5th edn. WB Saunders, Philadelphia, PA, 2002.

CHAPTER 25

The Team Approach

Janet Cushnaghan[1], Elaine M Hay[2] and Louise Warburton[3]

[1]Southampton General Hospital, Southampton, UK
[2]Staffordshire Rheumatology Centre, Stoke-on-Trent, UK
[3]Shawbirch Medical Practice, Telford, UK

OVERVIEW

- Understand the meaning of a multidisciplinary team (MDT).
- Know which professionals make up the MDT.
- Understand the role of each professional and how this contributes to the holistic care of the patient.
- Understand how to refer to each professional and what conditions are managed by each.
- Understand the role of the general practitioner as gate-keeper to the service.

Background

Traditionally, the patient journey involved an initial consultation with a general practitioner (GP), sometimes followed by onward referral to a consultant rheumatologist in secondary care. The consultant, or one of their medical team, would assess the patient and formulate a treatment plan. Whether or not the patient saw anyone else in the team, such as a physiotherapist, depended very much on the local facilities. It would not have been unusual for a patient with a musculoskeletal problem only ever to see their GP and/or a consultant rheumatologist in the course of their treatment.

However, times have changed, and with this comes an increasing recognition of the potential benefits that patients may gain from a multidisciplinary approach to their management. Implicit within this is the changing role of patients themselves: the crucial function of the multidisciplinary team (MDT) is to use different approaches to empower patients to take an active role in their management. A multidisciplinary approach to management is subtly different to "shared care", where therapists and doctors from primary and secondary care manage patients and share records. Shared care is not a new concept; it has been used for years in diabetic and antenatal care, but is often led by the needs of the doctors and therapists, rather than the needs of the patient.

The changing world of musculoskeletal service provision

Integrated-care pathways (ICPs) have been introduced as a core concept in the UK Department of Health document Musculoskeletal Services (MSK) Framework (Department of Health, 2006). The Framework proposes a redesign for musculoskeletal services, based on the patient's entire journey. The development of multidisciplinary clinical assessment and treatment services (CATS) is the keystone of the service. CATS bring together skilled professionals from primary and secondary care, including allied health professionals (AHPS), extended-scope physiotherapists (ESPs), GPs with special interest (GPwSI), chiropractors, osteopaths and nurse practitioners, as well as hospital consultants and other specialists.

One of the main targets of the MSK framework is to reduce the waiting time for patients from first presentation to definitive treatment. However, the spin-off from this is an integrated team approach to the patient, according to which patients will be seen and assessed by the most appropriate specialist (doctor or AHP). Consequently there is enhanced opportunity for patient education and promotion of self-management by improving patients' skills to cope with their pain.

This service redesign is in keeping with Standards of Care (see http://www.arma.uk.net/care.html) produced by the UK Arthritis and Musculoskeletal Alliance (ARMA), an umbrella organization that brings together a variety of national societies concerned with rheumatic and musculoskeletal diseases. These Standards highlight the importance of a multidisciplinary approach to the management of musculoskeletal conditions; for example, Standard 10 of this document states that "People with inflammatory arthritis should have ongoing access to the local multidisciplinary team, whether this is based in secondary care, or in the community".

The multidisciplinary team

A few essential ingredients are needed to ensure the success of the MDT (Figure 25.1; Box 25.1). The first, and most important of these, is effective communication. It is vital that members of the team have the opportunity to talk to each other, that they have a shared agenda and that they speak the same language. Second, clinical-care pathways should be developed that, wherever possible, are underpinned by a robust evidence base. The evidence base

ABC of Rheumatology, 4th edn. Edited by Ade Adebajo.
©2010 Blackwell Publishing Ltd. 9781405170680.

Key components of the multidisciplinary team

Multidisciplinary team

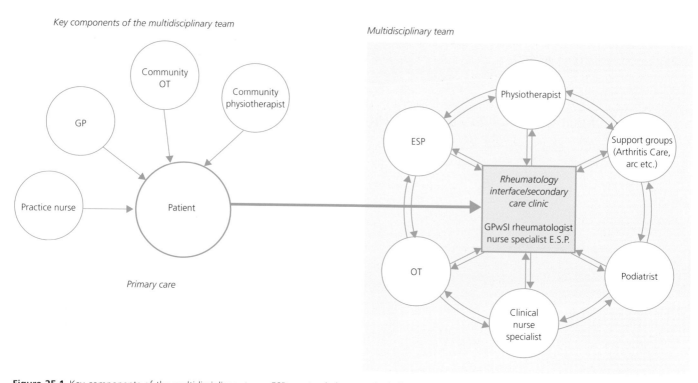

Figure 25.1 Key components of the multidisciplinary team. ESP = extended-scope physiotherapist; GP = general practitioner; OT = occupational therapist

Box 25.1 **Members of the multidisciplinary team**

- General practitioners
- GPs with a special interest
- Physiotherapists
- Extended-scope physiotherapists
- Occupational therapists
- Nurse specialists
- Podiatrists and chiropodists
- Consultant rheumatologists
- Support agencies

Box 25.2 **Recommendations from NICE guidelines CG79 on the management of rheumatoid arthritis**

1 Refer for specialist opinion any person with suspected persistent synovitis of undetermined cause. Refer urgently if any of the following apply:
   - the small joints of the hands or feet are affected
   - more than one joint is affected
   - there has been a delay of 3 months or longer between onset of symptoms and seeking medical advice.
2 Do not avoid referring urgently any person with suspected persistent synovitis of undetermined cause whose blood tests show a normal acute-phase response or negative rheumatoid factor.

www.nice..org.uk

should be debated and discussed between members of the MDT to formulate care pathways that are acceptable to the whole team, and to the patient. For care pathways to be translated into effective patient care, all individuals involved must have ownership, be involved in team collaboration and participate actively in their development and subsequent implementation.

General practitioners

The GP is, traditionally, the gate-keeper to musculoskeletal services, although this is changing with initiatives such as Physio-Direct. Most musculoskeletal conditions will be managed solely by the GP with first-line treatment such as advice and prescription of analgesics. However, the GP also fulfils the crucial role of screening for "red-flags"—signs and symptoms of potentially serious disease, which need urgent referral to secondary care. In addition, it is vital

that GPs are able to recognize certain specific diagnoses, such as the early signs of inflammatory arthritis, to facilitate early referral to secondary care (Box 25.2). The British Society for Rheumatology (BSR) has recently published guidelines for the management of rheumatoid arthritis in the first 2 years (Luqmani *et al.*, 2006), which stress the importance of early referral. The Primary Care Rheumatology Society (http://www.pcrsociety.org.uk) and the Arthritis Research Campaign (http://www.arc.org.uk) take an active role in supporting and educating GPs in these important functions.

Onward referral options for the GP will increasingly include a multidisciplinary clinic such as the CATS described above. However, the precise options available will depend upon the local service provision.

GPwSIs

GPwSIs are GPs who have developed an area of expertise above and beyond that demanded of normal general practice, and they may have obtained a diploma or further postgraduate qualification in a relevant area. Many GPwSIs will work in interface clinics (e.g. CATS) or in secondary care in the context of an integrated musculoskeletal service. A competency framework for musculoskeletal/rheumatology GPwSIs has been published (Hay *et al.*, 2007).

Physiotherapists

Physiotherapists are trained in the assessment and management of locomotor and muscular problems. A pivotal part of their role is educating patients about biomechanical dysfunction and actively promoting self-management through appropriate exercise regimes. Some physiotherapists may undertake more specialist roles within rheumatology, including management of flares of inflammatory arthritis, manual therapy or hydrotherapy.

Extended-scope physiotherapists

ESPs have extra expertise in diagnosing, as well as treating, patients with musculoskeletal problems and may assess new referrals in a similar way to GpwSIs. They will diagnose and formulate a treatment plan as part of the MDT and may have additional skills, such as joint and soft-tissue injections, or limited prescribing.

Occupational therapists

Occupational therapists (OTs) (Table 25.1) work with other members of the MDT to maintain the function of the patient in the context of a working or home environment. OTs are particularly skilled in assessing and treating hand problems, through advice, exercises, prescription of orthotics (appliances) and provision of labour- and pain-saving devices—for example specially adapted knives and forks with padded handles, which are easier to grip. Community-based OTs will perform domiciliary visits to assess the need for home aids such as stairlifts. As well as providing practical advice, OTs are skilled in helping patients deal with the psychological consequences of their disease using cognitive behavioural approaches and relaxation techniques.

Nurse specialists

In secondary care, nurse specialists play an important role in assessing and managing patients with a range of rheumatological complaints (Table 25.2). One particular area of expertise lies in counselling and follow-up of rheumatology patients receiving disease-modifying anti-rheumatic drugs and anti-tumour necrosis factor (anti-TNF) drugs. Nurses often take a lead role in monitoring patients with inflammatory arthritis for side effects and effectiveness, including blood and urine testing, performing disease activity scores and liaising with consultants and GPs as appropriate.

In accordance with agreed protocols, nurse specialists may administer drugs (e.g. intramuscular steroids or intra-articular injections) and teach patients to self-administer certain drugs, such as subcutaneous methotrexate or anti-TNF.

Nurse specialists often act as a crucial link between primary and secondary care, and between the patient and specialist services, through providing telephone helplines or drop-in clinics where patients can receive advice about acute problems such as flare-ups. Nurse specialists are key in the delivery of patient education.

Chiropodists and podiatrists

Chiropodists and podiatrists are specifically trained to assess, diagnose and manage foot- and gait-related pathology. This includes the direct treatment of painful lesions (i.e. corns and callouses) as well as more serious complications such as infection and ulceration. They will assess foot and lower limb function, footwear and gait to determine if this is contributing to soft-tissue and joint pathology. Treatment may involve patient education, prescription footwear, orthoses (custom shoe inserts) or injection therapy (i.e.

Table 25.1 Functions of an occupational therapist

Activity	Methods employed to improve patient care
Assess patient hand function; measure grip strength and assess dysfuntion	Prescription of hand orthotics such as wrist splints
	Prescription of exercises
	Injection of specific problems such as trigger finger
Assess activities of daily living	Prescription of devices such as stairlifts, bath rails, walking aids
Assess how the patient manages in their own home	
Assess patient's psychological well-being and coping strategies	Use cognitive-behaviour techniques and counselling to improve coping mechanisms

Table 25.2 Functions of a rheumatology nurse specialist

Function of nurse specialist	Activities undertaken and benefits to patient
Seeing patients at diagnosis	Helping patients to come to terms with the diagnosis and understand the implications of the disease
Discussing drug therapies	Discussing possible side effects of drug therapies; discussing how to take medications
Drug monitoring	Coordinating blood and urine testing and interpreting results
Performing regular patient reviews	Assessing disease activity with disease activity scores
	Exploring patient's perceptions and needs
Adminstering drug treatments	Administering subcutaneous and intramuscular injections
	Administering joint injections
Providing a patient telephone helpline	Offering support and advice to patients when required
	Coordinating further care
Liaising with other members of the team to act upon information received from telephone helpline or face-to-face interaction	Formulating a care plan and modifying in response to changing circumstances

Table 25.3 Support agencies available

Name of support agency	Contact details
Arthritis Research Campaign	http://www.arc.org.uk 0870 850 5000
Arthritis Care	http://www.arthritiscare.org.uk 0845 600 6868
National Rheumatoid Arthritis Society	http://www.rheumatoid.org.uk 0800 298 7650

Table 25.4 Wider aspects of team working that contribute to the care of patients with rheumatoid arthritis

Members of the wider team	Function of the group
Patients, stakeholders, doctors and allied health professionals, nurses	Development of guidelines for the management of rheumatoid arthritis such as by the National Institute for Health and Clinical Excellence (NICE) and the British Society for Rheumatology (BSR)
Doctors, allied health professionals, nurses	Development of patient advice leaflets in consultation with experts in the team; this contributes to patient education

steroid injections) for soft-tissue and joint conditions. Some podiatrists (podiatric surgeons) are trained to perform foot surgery.

Consultant rheumatologists

Consultant rheumatologists are trained to assess and manage patients with a range of musculoskeletal complaints, ranging from non-specific back and neck pain to complex multi-system conditions such as rheumatoid arthritis. Traditionally, they were the first point of contact for a GP referral into the musculoskeletal service, although, as we have seen, this pattern is changing with the developments in service provision outlined above. Consultants often take on the role of coordinating the MDT and have overall responsibility for ensuring holistic care for the patient. They may be responsible for ensuring clinical governance for the MDT through continuing professional development, appraisal and training of the staff.

Support agencies

Agencies such as the Arthritis Research Campaign (arc) and Arthritis Care (Table 25.3) offer educational resources and direct advice to patients with arthritis. They provide an invaluable service, both to patients and to professionals, who can use their resources as part of their treatment plan.

Wider aspects of team working

These professionals not only work together directly in the care of patients with rheumatoid arthritis, they also collaborate in the drawing up of guidelines for the management of the disease and the production of patient literature (Table 25.4).

Although the multidisciplinary team described in this chapter is based on the new UK model, the role and activities of the multidisciplinary team are generally the same worldwide. It has not been possible to focus on every single professional that may be involved in the complex care of patients with a rheumatological condition. Instead we have highlighted the philosophy of care that can be adapted to suit all conditions and embrace all members of the multidisciplinary team.

References

Department of Health. The Musculoskeletal Framework: A joint responsibility: doing it differently. Department of Health, London, 2006.

Hay EM, Campbell A, Linney S, Wise E, Musculoskeletal GpwSI Working Group. Development of a competency framework for general practitioners with a special interest in musculoskeletal/rheumatology practice. *Rheumatology (Oxford)* 2007; **46**: 360–362.

Luqmani R, Hennell S, Estrach C *et al*. British Society for Rheumatology and British Health Professionals in Rheumatology guideline for the management of rheumatoid arthritis (the first 2 years). *Rheumatology (Oxford)* 2006; **45**: 1167–1169. Available online at: http://www.rheumatology.org.uk

CHAPTER 26

Epidemiology of the Rheumatic Diseases

Alan Silman and Jacqueline Oliver

Arthritis Research Campaign, Chesterfield, UK

OVERVIEW

- Rheumatoid arthritis affects 0.8% of the population and has definite genetic and lifestyle risk factors.
- Osteoarthritis is the commonest arthritic complaint; although age is the key risk factor, both genetic and lifestyle risks are implicated.
- Musculoskeletal pain syndromes are almost universal in the population, but accurately documenting their occurrence is difficult.
- Mechanical factors are important for most musculoskeletal pain syndromes.
- Other autoimmune rheumatic diseases are much less common but affect younger age groups.

Musculoskeletal diseases account for around 10% of general practitioner (GP) consultations in the UK each year. The most common diseases are osteoarthritis (OA) and low back pain (LBP) (Figure 26.1). These diseases generally are more common in women than men and increase with age. It is estimated that the proportion of over 65s in the population will increase 3-fold in the next 30 years, increasing the burden on health-care systems from musculoskeletal disorders.

Rheumatoid arthritis

Rheumatoid arthritis (RA) is estimated to have a prevalence of around 0.8% of the adult population. It is three times more likely to occur in women than men (Figure 26.2). However, estimates are considerably higher in some populations and a prevalence of 6.8% has been recorded in some Native American populations. The disease most commonly presents in the sixth and seventh decades.

A number of genetic and environmental factors have been linked with the risk of developing RA (Box 26.1). Some factors increase the risk, whereas others are thought to offer a protective role in

disease development. Data from national twin studies have shown that the heritability of RA is around 60%. This source of the genetic component has been extensively investigated, and links to genes encoding HLA-DRB1 alleles are well established. Other genes, albeit with weaker effects, have also been identified, and with the increasing use of whole genome screens it is likely that more candidate genes will be discovered in future.

Several studies have implicated hormonal factors in RA, although the results have been conflicting. The higher incidence in women may suggest a hormonal influence on disease onset. A consistent finding is that current or ever use of the oral contraceptive pill has a protective role. RA onset is also reduced by 70% during pregnancy, but there is a 5-fold increased risk in the post-partum period.

Socio-economic factors have not been consistently associated with RA, but several lifestyle factors have been associated with the disease. Cigarette smoking has been the subject of many studies, and one study reported that the risk of RA was increased 3-fold for males who smoke. Heavy smoking (increased risk of over 13-fold) and passive smoking have also been linked with RA, while the cessation of smoking has been shown to reduce the risk of RA. Dietary factors are an increasing area of interest for epidemiological studies. Low fruit and vitamin C intake and high red meat intake have both been linked with a 2-fold increased risk of RA. High intakes of antioxidants (β-cryptoxanthin and zeaxanthin) found in some fruits and vegetables may reduce the risk. The benefits of following a Mediterranean diet (high proportion of oily fish and vegetables) may confer a protective role. The role of caffeine intake on RA is not yet clear, and studies so far have produced mixed results. Infectious agents have been implicated as a risk factor for RA. Both pet ownership and prior blood transfusion have been shown to

---

Box 26.1 **Risk factors for rheumatoid arthritis**

- Age
- Gender (more common in women)
- Genetic factors
- Infectious agents
- Hormonal factors
- Lifestyle factors

ABC of Rheumatology, 4th edn. Edited by Ade Adebajo.
©2010 Blackwell Publishing Ltd. 9781405170680.

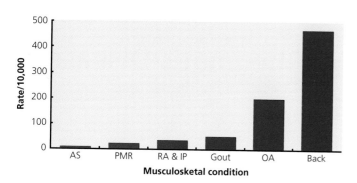

Figure 26.1 GP consultation for major musculoskeletal conditions in 2006. AS = ankylosing spondylitis; IP = inflammatory polyarthritis; OA = osteoarthritis; PMR = polymyalgia rheumatica; RA = rheumatoid arthritis

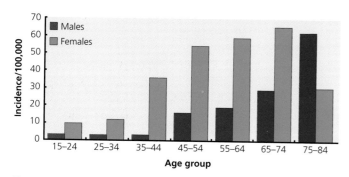

Figure 26.2 Incidence of rheumatoid arthritis by age and gender in Norfolk, UK

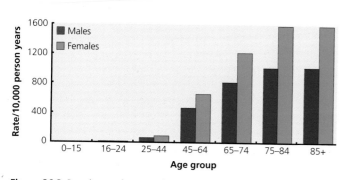

Figure 26.3 Prevalence of osteoarthritis by age and gender

increase the risk of RA 5-fold. There is an association between Epstein–Barr virus and RA—an observation that has been recognized for over 25 years, although its role in the causation is not clear.

Osteoarthritis

OA is the most common form of arthritis and a leading cause of disability. The prevalence is around 10–20% in people aged over 65 years (Figure 26.3). OA is more common in women than men and is age-dependent, being uncommon in those under 40 years. Each

Box 26.2 **Risk factors for osteoarthritis**

• Genetic factors/family history
• Obesity
• Gender (more common in women)
• Age
• Joint injury
• Occupation

year it is estimated that over 2 million people in the UK visit their GP with OA symptoms. The site most frequently affected is the knee, although the hip and hand are also commonly affected. Hip OA is less common but is more disabling than knee OA.

A number of risk factors are associated with OA, of which the strongest is age (Box 26.2). Genetic factors are important, and OA in some families displays classical Mendelian inheritance. The heritability of cartilage volume, as a marker of degeneration, has been estimated at over 70%. Congenital joint deformities may increase the stress on the cartilage and contribute to OA development. The increase of obesity in the population is one of the major factors associated with both the development of knee OA and with the progression of the disease. Having a high body mass index has been associated with an up to 9-fold increased risk of knee OA. Joint injury can also increase the risk of OA. This may be due to direct cartilage damage or a result of increased stress on the cartilage due to the injury. Certain occupations are at an increased risk, e.g. jobs that have excessive knee-bending and farming. Factors that affect the progression of OA are also increasingly being studied. Recent studies have shown that a low vitamin D intake can increase the risk of OA, and a high vitamin C intake may reduce the risk.

Musculoskeletal pain

Most patients presenting with musculoskeletal pain do not have a definite arthritis such as RA or OA. The most commonly reported causes of musculoskeletal pain are LBP, shoulder pain and fibromyalgia/chronic widespread pain (CWP). Estimates of the occurrence of musculoskeletal pain vary widely. It is difficult to gain robust estimates due to the episodic nature of most musculoskeletal pain syndromes; the onset of pain is not always clearly defined and is subject to recall bias.

Low back pain

LBP is common, and at least 50% of the general population will report an episode of LBP in their lifetime. A recent study estimated that the prevalence of LBP has tripled in men and doubled in women over the past 40 years. LBP is generally more common in women and the prevalence increases with age (Figure 26.4). A number of risk factors are implicated with LBP, including poor posture, occupation, poor job satisfaction, smoking, obesity, previous LBP episode and low social class (Box 26.3). In both men and women as the number of children increases so does their risk of LBP.

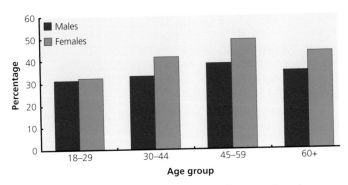

Figure 26.4 One month prevalence of back pain by age and gender

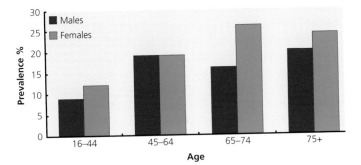

Figure 26.5 Prevalence of shoulder pain

Box 26.3 **Risk factors for low back pain**

- Age
- Number of children
- Previous episode of low back pain
- Obesity
- Smoking
- Fitness
- Occupation (heavy lifting, prolonged sitting)

Shoulder pain

Up to one-third of the population will report an episode of shoulder pain at some time. Reported rates are dependent on how shoulder pain is classified (i.e. what is the shoulder?) and how the data are collected. Population studies based on self-reported symptoms estimate shoulder pain prevalence is between 20 and 40%. A recent study estimated that the prevalence of shoulder pain has doubled in men and quadrupled in women over the past 40 years. The number of patients who consult their GPs with shoulder pain increases with age (Figure 26.5) and is generally higher in women than men.

Risk factors for shoulder pain include social class and mechanical and psychosocial factors. Workplace risk factors for men developing shoulder pain include carrying weights, damp and cold working environment, working with hands above shoulder level or stretching below knee level and using arms or wrists in a repetitive manner. Performing monotonous work has been associated with a 3-fold increased risk of shoulder pain in both sexes.

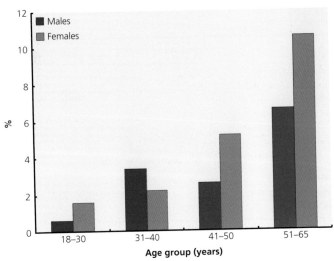

Figure 26.6 Prevalence of chronic widespread pain by age and gender

Fibromyalgia/chronic widespread pain

CWP, defined as both axial and limb pain affecting both upper and lower limbs on both sides of the body, is more common in women and is more likely to develop with increasing age (Figure 26.6). The prevalence estimates for CWP are consistent, between 11 and 14%. CWP has been reported more frequently in South Asian women. There is some evidence that patients with depressive symptoms are at an increased risk of developing CWP. Subjects with an increased tendency to visit their GP were found to be nine times more likely to develop CWP. The fibromyalgia syndrome (CWP plus widespread tender points) has a prevalence of between 1 and 11%, the variation being due to the method of ascertainment.

Other rheumatic diseases

The incidence of some of the other rheumatic diseases seen in rheumatological practice is summarized in Table 26.1.

Ankylosing spondylitis—Ankylosing spondylitis (AS) is three times more common in males than females, and peak onset is between 20 and 40 years of age. Prevalence is around 0.5–2.0/1000 in European populations. It is relatively rare in some African and Japanese populations but more frequent in Native Americans, with a prevalence of 6% reported in Haida and Bella Indians. The causes of the disease are still unknown, although a strong link with HLA-B27 has been established, with the frequency of the gene in white AS patients at around 90%. There is an increased risk of the disease in relatives of probands, and results of twin studies show concordance rates of 50–75% in monozygotic twins. Infection may play a part in the disease, but the data are conflicting despite several decades of study.

Psoriatic arthritis—Psoriatic arthritis (PsA) has a prevalence of around 0.1–0.2%, and there is little difference in the rate between genders or age bands. Risk factors for the disease include family history, and there is some evidence that the disease is linked to HLA alleles. There are also a number of environmental triggers associated with PsA. The disease is known to start after HIV

Table 26.1 Incidence by gender of the major rheumatic and autoimmune diseases

	Incidence/100,000		Sex ratio (M:F)
	Men	Women	
Rheumatoid arthritis	14	36	1:3
Psoriatic arthritis	3.5	3.4	1:1
Ankylosing spondylitis	11.7	2.9	3:1
Systemic lupus erythematosus	0.5	6.8	1:8
Scleroderma*	1.1	6.2	1:8
Polymyalgia rheumatica	40	62	1:2–3
Giant cell arteritis	8	27	1:2–3
Gout**	190	70	3:1

*/million
**Varies widely between different populations

infection, and prior trauma has also been associated with disease onset.

Systemic lupus erythematosus—Systemic lupus erythematosus (SLE) has a prevalence of between 10 and 250/100,000. It is more common in women than men, with on onset between 35 and 50 years of age. It is noticeably higher in African American, Asian and Afro-Caribbean populations than in white populations. There is strong evidence for a genetic cause for the disease, and first-degree relatives of patients are at an up to 9-fold increased risk of disease development. Twin studies also show a high concordance rate, supporting a genetic contribution for the disease. Associations with HLA have been reported, but these vary between populations. Despite the high female excess, so far no hormonal link to the disease has been found, and there is limited support for environmental risk factors, although infectious agents and chemical exposure have all been studied.

Scleroderma—Scleroderma is a rare disease; it usually presents between the ages of 35 and 55, with an up to 8-fold female excess. Population prevalence studies estimate the prevalence of scleroderma to be between 30 and 1130/million—the wide variation is due to the lack of population studies, as the disease is rare. There is some evidence suggesting that the disease has a higher incidence in black African populations. So far only a weak association between HLA and scleroderma has been found, although stronger links have been found with specific autoantibodies

(anti-topoisomerase and anti-centromere antibodies). A number of environmental triggers are thought to be risk factors for the disease. Exposure to silica dust (stone masons and gold miners) has been linked with the disease but there is no evidence that silicone implants increase the disease risk. Exposure to organic solvents has been linked to an increased risk of scleroderma, and there is some evidence from case reports that specific drugs may be linked with the disease.

Gout—Gout is more common in men (around 1–2%) than women (around 0.2–0.5%). The prevalence varies in different populations. Extremely high rates are found in Polynesians (up to 10% in New Zealand Maori males), whereas gout is rarely found in African populations. Two recent studies in the USA and New Zealand suggest that the incidence of gout has increased 2-fold over the past 30 years. The main susceptibility factor for gout is hyperuricaemia. Risk factors for hyperuricaemia include obesity, hypertension, alcohol consumption, diet and some genetic factors.

Polymyalgia rheumatica and giant cell arteritis—Polymyalgia rheumatica (PMR) and giant cell arteritis (GCA) are related disorders that usually present in the over 50s. Prevalence over the age of 50 is between 0.2 and 2.2/1000 for GCA and 5.5 and 10.9/1000 for PMR. Both diseases are more common (2- to 3-fold higher) in women than men. Both diseases increase with age, peaking at around 70 years with a decline after that. There is some evidence that there is a genetic link for HLA alleles and PMR/GCA, but results have not been consistent in different populations. Reports suggest that both diseases may be seasonal in incidence, but again the results have been inconsistent. There are a number of reports that suggest infectious agents as a risk factor for these diseases, and peak incidences have followed outbreaks of *Mycoplasma pneumoniae*, human parvovirus B19 and *Chlamydia pneumoniae*.

Further reading

McBeth J, Jones K. Epidemiology of chronic musculoskeletal pain. *Best Practice and Research. Clinical Rheumatology* 2007; **21**: 403–425.

Oliver JE, Silman AJ. Risk factors for the development of rheumatoid arthritis. *Scandinavian Journal of Rheumatology* 2006; **35**: 169–174.

Royal College of General Practitioners/Birmingham Research Unit. *Annual Prevalence Report 2006*. Available online at: http://www.rcgp.org.uk/pdf/Annual%20prevalence%20report%202006.pdf

Sharma L, Kapoor D, Issa S. Epidemiology of osteoarthritis: an update. *Current Opinion in Rheumatology* 2006; **18**: 147–156.

Silman AJ, Hochberg MC. *Epidemiology of the Rheumatic Diseases*, 2nd edn. Oxford University Press, Oxford, 2001.

Index